Stephen Z. Fadem • José A. Moura-Neto
Thomas A. Golper
Editors

Complications in Dialysis

A Clinical Guide

Springer

Editors
Stephen Z. Fadem
Section of Nephrology
Baylor College of Medicine
Houston, TX, USA

José A. Moura-Neto
Escola Bahiana de Medicina e
Saúde Pública
Salvador, Bahia, Brazil

Thomas A. Golper
Salisbury, VT, USA

ISBN 978-3-031-44559-0 ISBN 978-3-031-44557-6 (eBook)
https://doi.org/10.1007/978-3-031-44557-6

This Springer imprint is published by the registered company Springer Nature Switzerland AG
The registered company address is: Gewerbestrasse 11, 6330 Cham, Switzerland

Paper in this product is recyclable.

Complications in Dialysis

Foreword

It was nearly a hundred years ago that the first attempts were made to use dialysis to treat kidney failure, focused variously on both extracorporeal therapy and peritoneal dialysis. It took nearly 40 years of improvisation after these initial attempts, culminating with the introduction of the Scribner shunt, which made long-term treatment with hemodialysis a reality. As such, the first outpatient dialysis facility opened its doors in 1962 in Seattle. The path for peritoneal dialysis was longer, even with the introduction of the Tenckhoff indwelling catheter in the late 1960s. It took nearly a decade after that for the partnership of a nephrologist with a physicist that led to the introduction of continuous ambulatory peritoneal dialysis (CAPD) in 1978 for the long-term treatment of uremia.

Today, nearly 3.8 million people around the world are receiving maintenance dialysis care, of which over 400,000 are being treated with peritoneal dialysis and 24,000 patients with home hemodialysis. Indeed, given the limited availability of organs for transplantation, kidney failure is the only organ failure for which dialysis treatment is available—with long-term dialysis—upon demand in many parts of the world. While we celebrate the introduction of many new treatments to prevent kidney failure, particularly from diabetic kidney disease, we anticipate a growing need for dialysis as hundreds of millions of people continue to be lifted out of poverty worldwide and demand access to lifesaving treatments such as long-term dialysis.

Even though the fundamentals of dialysis treatment have remained unchanged from the time they were first envisioned, there continue to be substantial changes in dialysis care. As such, there has been a decrease in emphasis on small-solute clearances as a measure of dose of dialysis, lower hemoglobin targets, less use of erythropoietin, more use of parenteral iron and calcimimetics, wariness about aggressive ultrafiltration over short periods of treatment, longer treatment times, and a greater recognition of patient-reported outcomes. Hemodialysis treatments have become safer with technological innovations; in several parts of the world, there has been a rapid expansion in the use of home dialysis, particularly peritoneal dialysis, and there is an increasing use of automated peritoneal dialysis. There has been a substantial reduction in peritonitis with peritoneal dialysis and a lower risk of transfer of patients to hemodialysis. Up until just prior to the COVID pandemic, there has been a sustained decrease in the risk of death for patients treated with long-term dialysis.

With a growing population of patients worldwide and continued changes in dialysis care, it is important for nephrology practitioners to have up-to-date information available to guide clinical practice. This textbook, "Complications in Dialysis—A Clinical Guide," fills this gap by providing succinct information on the state-of-the art care of patients undergoing long-term dialysis. Edited by three leading internationally recognized experts in dialysis care (Drs. Fadem, Golper, and Moura-Neto), it covers the entire range of topics necessary to provide high-quality care to patients with kidney failure with in-center or home hemodialysis or peritoneal dialysis. Organized logically into 22 chapters, it offers readers the full range of information including details of hemodialysis procedure, complications of uremia and their management, and complications with and management of complications of each dialysis modality. This book is a must-have reference for busy nephrology providers worldwide.

Division of Nephrology, Department of Medicine
University of Washington,
Seattle, WA, USA

Rajnish Mehrotra

Introduction

Introduction

In 1861, Thomas Graham, a Glasgow chemist, discovered that the proteins (colloids) in blood could be separated from fluids and crystalloids. He gave the world the discovery of dialysis. Once revealed, researchers immediately began to unearth a suitable semipermeable membrane and an anticoagulant such that dialysis could be achieved to treat uremia or Bright's disease. Bright's disease was universally fatal. It was discovered 35 years earlier by Richard Bright, a physician at Guy's Hospital in London. Attempts to dialyze with animal membranes and hirudin, a substance derived from leeches, were not tenable. Collodion, a flammable cellulose material that was the result of mixing strong acids with cotton, was mechanically unstable. It took advancements in technology to give us regenerated cellulose or cellophane—a product initially described as a method to prevent wine from staining tablecloths but popular in the meatpacking industry for sausage casing. The anticoagulant heparin was discovered in 1916 and retained the name it was given when it was initially thought to be made in the liver, not the intestines and lungs, as was later determined. It was not adequately purified or standardized until 1934 and is the prevailing anticoagulant in use today for the management of hemodialysis [1].

The story of Willem "Pim" Kolff's tribulations in building a functional dialysis machine includes a rotating wooden drum powered by a sewing machine engine, wrapped with 30–40 m of cellophane tubing, and churning through a tub filled with a balanced "dialysate" solution. Kolff built his first dialysis machine in 1940 and used box after box of sausage casing.

Kolff made 16 unsuccessful attempts between 1943 and 1945 to dialyze acutely ill patients as a last resort before he was able to achieve clinical success, saving a Nazi sympathizer who developed uremia as the consequence of a complicated recovery from acute cholecystitis. What is incomprehensible is that this achievement was carried out during the Nazi invasion of the Netherlands. Hospital conditions were nearly unworkable, and research had to be done at odd hours. The Wehrmacht had commandeered all manufacturing plants to make wartime supplies, confiscating all aluminum and leaving him only wood. Gestapo raids on the hospital were frequent; the glassblower responsible for making dialysis cannulation equipment was shot dead by Germans. Meanwhile, Kolff harbored a young Jewish boy, the son of a colleague captured by Nazis.

These efforts of Kolff symbolize that therapeutic advances can arise from the ability to overcome challenges. This theme of overcoming odds and defeating inevitable failure has underpinned the field of dialysis ever since [2].

The major impediment to successful dialysis was the damage done to arteries and veins during the process of cannulating them with the necessary dialysis tubing. It would not be until 1960 that the first patient with chronic kidney failure would successfully dialyze. Clyde Shields, a machinist, was first dialyzed by Belding Scribner in Seattle through a plastic, implanted shunt surgically placed in an artery and vein in the arm. Shields survived 11 years and died of heart disease. The Scribner shunt was replaced by the Brescia-Cimino arteriovenous fistula still used today [3]. To be able to sustain life with an artificial kidney was and still is truly miraculous, but even the best designed machine and the most optimal management do not approach the fully functioning kidney. Thus, it is natural that obstacles and barriers abound. The journey to develop the dialysis machine was fraught with challenges, and we continue to meet challenges every day when caring for the 400,000 patients who undergo dialysis each year—this translates to at least a fifth of a million procedures being performed each year.

Complications of Dialysis or Complications in Dialysis

To name this book Complications of Dialysis would limit it to adverse events that are related to a procedure. The end result, however, would differ based on the underlying condition of the subject. Advanced kidney disease is characterized by maladaptation, and it is necessary to accommodate the loss of all vital body functions, not just kidneys. The consequent derangement in mineral metabolism, cardiac function, and blood vessels and the results of chronic inflammation make the dialysis patient highly vulnerable to the slightest nuances in care that an otherwise healthy individual with normal body reserves could handle with less effort. It is impossible to separate the person from the procedure. This book will explore not just complications that are related to the dialysis procedure but also the comorbidities of patients who require dialysis and who are at a higher risk of having an unfortunate event. The book will also discuss safety principles that will help us not only chart misfortune but also reset a path toward its correction.

The Dialysis Procedure

First is the process of dialysis itself. Dialysis must start with pure water, but the water feeding into the dialysis facility or home is loaded with unwanted minerals. The water supplied by municipalities is chlorinated, and the removal of chlorine and a host of additional minerals, as well as filtering bacteria and endotoxins, will be essential. The dialysis solution must be proportioned and composed to remove toxins but not disrupt the balance of other critical electrolytes and minerals. The modern dialysis machine has built-in alarms and features that alert users when the concentrate used to mix the dialysis bath is outside a targeted range. Such a simple miscalculation could result in a fatality. Air in a dialysis line can also cause a fatal embolus. Most causes of death in dialysis patients are not the result of machine failure or performance. This is because of the forced vigilance built around this discipline.

Major Complications

Factors contributing to death in dialysis patients can occur because of inaccurate medication delivery or inappropriate dosing, hyperkalemia, access incidents that were improperly treated, or exposure to pathogens. Inappropriate administration of medications, either because of a prescription error, a dose that is incorrect for the degree of kidney function, or patient error, can lead to somnolence, hypotension, hypoglycemia, or hyperkalemia (see Chap. 18). Hyperkalemia deaths occur across the spectrum of CKD [4]. Currently, hyperkalemia is addressed not only by changing the dialysis plan but also by prescribing potassium binders. The newer formulations are more palatable and better tolerated. It will be worthwhile to determine what impact this has on hyperkalemia as a contributing factor to dialysis mortality (see Chap. 1).

Dialysis is, by design, intended to remove excess volume. However, excess fluid removal can result in a drop in blood pressure. A majority of dialysis patients are diabetic and have autonomic insufficiency. These drops in blood pressure may not trigger the regulatory mechanisms to increase vascular tone. Dialysis timing is essential so that excess fluids are removed safely without causing hypotension. Many dialysis patients have hypertensive changes that result in cardiac hypertrophy and fibrosis. Hence, excess shifts in volume can be harmful. Hypotension may occur at the end of the dialysis treatment and is multifactorial. Closely monitoring blood pressure use in dialysis patients, attention to dry weight, and close monitoring for several minutes after completing dialysis may help avert a catastrophic event such as a fall (see Chap. 2).

Access rupture is rare but can be catastrophic. The arteriovenous fistula can form an aneurysm. If an area thins and becomes shiny and pale, there is a likelihood that it could rupture. Proper inspection and preemptive management of outflow stenosis may prevent or at least alert caregivers of the possibility of a future incident (see Chap. 5). AV graft infections and catheter infections are more likely to lead to sepsis. Patients with a tunneled catheter have a significantly higher risk of death from sepsis (adjusted odds ratio 6.9). Infections are always a risk because direct contact with blood is necessary for hemodialysis and with the peritoneal membrane for peritoneal dialysis (see Chaps. 4 and 11). Blood-borne infections are preventable with careful precautions and attentiveness to hygiene during the dialysis procedure. Major challenges of infection control involve the emergence of resistant organisms. Viral infections such as hepatitis B are easily spread within a dialysis center if strict hygiene precautions are not followed. Iatrogenic infections accounted for 9.6% of deaths in one study (see Chap. 4) [5].

The patient response to dialysis is highly variable because of the underlying diseases that initially precipitated the kidneys to fail, the complications inherent in kidney disease, and the comorbidities accompanying disease conditions such as hypertension, diabetes, and chronic inflammatory states. These patients face dilemmas that include fatigue, gait and balance disorders, falls, mineral imbalance, anemia, heart failure, neuropathy, bleeding disorders, deep vein thromboses, cognitive decline, and frailty, to mention but a few. They require various medications to help adjust to underlying diseases or to the dialysis procedure. Furthermore, when kidney function has been impaired, the excretion of commonly used medications decreases (see Chaps. 3, 6–8, and 18).

Home Dialysis

Dialysis is now a generic term that includes home peritoneal dialysis (PD), home hemodialysis (HHD), and hemodialysis in the center (ICHD). Peritoneal dialysis has its own set of rewards, benefits, and complications. Peritoneal dialysis and home hemodialysis share common patient disease processes, particularly metabolic disorders, but each has major differences. Peritoneal dialysis involves a complex membrane, and it is vital for it to remain intact, or PD will fail. Repeated episodes of inflammation can result in its failure. Peritoneal dialysis complications can be catheter or cycler related. Infectious complications of peritoneal dialysis include peritonitis, tunnel infections, and exit-site infections. Noninfectious complications include hemoperitoneum, hydrothorax, chyloperitoneum, icodextrin rash, pneumoperitoneum, membrane leaks, and hernias (see Chaps. 9 through 15).

HHD and PD share in common the psychological stresses associated with home dialysis. These stresses mount and take their toll on the patient and the caregiver. Improved support for the psychological challenges of resultant burnout could both improve acceptance of home dialysis and reduce the return to ICHD (see Chap. 16).

HHD is far safer because of the use of blood-leak detectors. The sharp learning curve for HHD is a detractor for most patients. The emergence of more patient-friendly home dialysis machines should simplify techniques for setting up the machines and make the procedure safer (see Chap. 17).

Frailty, Muscle Wasting, and Falls

The burdens dialysis patients encounter are heightened by the burdens and challenges inherent in age-related disorders that often culminate in the dwindling state of frailty. When cognitive function and patient independence decline, the chances for a dialysis-related complication increase. Muscle wasting is usually seen in aged dialysis patients but may be delayed through diet and exercise programs. Falls are especially common in the dialysis population. Understanding why patients fall and that there are remedial steps that can mitigate the risk of a serious injury with a fall may help reduce both the incidence and the consequences of falling (see Chaps. 3, 19, and 20).

Disaster Management

In the real world, we face natural disasters that can be the culmination of weather-related or other natural phenomena. These catastrophes remind us of how vulnerable the dialysis patient is. When disaster strikes, access to an intact facility with adequate electrical power and water is essential. Without this, a patient may be forced to miss dialysis for several days. Hurricanes, floods, wildfires, and earthquakes lead to both serious disruptions to the general population and havoc in the dialysis world (see Chap. 21).

Patient Safety

Patient safety indicators include anesthesia complications, postoperative hip fractures or hematomas, and metabolic, respiratory, or septic events. They also include deep vein thromboses or wound infections. A Veterans Administration review of these patient safety indicators demonstrated that among acute hospitalizations, CKD patients were at the highest risk of infection and death in diagnosis-related groups that were generally considered safe. The preadmission estimated glomerular filtration rate (eGFR) was an independent predictor of risk for patient safety indicators ($p = 0.001$) [6].

Despite its common use, dialysis is still a procedure that is evolving. Each day we learn new and better techniques and procedures that make care safer, more effective, and more efficient. The advancement of dialysis care is not possible without mechanisms in place to track deviations from safety and processes to ensure that improvements can be implemented and accessed (see Chap. 22).

Conclusion

Dialysis is a brilliant but highly unnatural event that is applied to fundamentally ill people. It evolved over several years as the consequence of persistence despite failure. As technology advances, scientists and investigators have used it to minimize complications and make the care that patients receive more gratifying and safer. Along the path, we encounter many complications, but through building a culture of safety, we learn from them and march forward.

Acknowledgments

Special gratitude to the many contributors who spent hours researching and developing chapters that readers will find both understandable and useful. We would like to also thank the people whom we invited to review our chapters and who returned highly valuable suggestions—Ruth Wintz, Jeff Giullian, Judy Geraci, Doc Berryhill, Sylvia Donato-Moore, and William Mitch.

References

1. Cameron JS. Practical haemodialysis began with cellophane and heparin: the crucial role of William Thalhimer (1884–1961). Nephrol Dial Transplant. 2000;15(7):1086–91. https://doi.org/10.1093/ndt/15.7.1086.
2. Boers H. Inventor for life. Kanoeb: B&Vmedia Publishers; 2007.
3. Fadem S. Issues in dialysis. 1st ed. New York: Nova Science Publishers; 2012.
4. Einhorn LM, Zhan M, Hsu VD, Walker LD, Moen MF, Seliger SL, et al. The frequency of hyperkalemia and its significance in chronic kidney disease. Arch Intern Med. 2009;169(12):1156–62. https://doi.org/10.1001/archinternmed.2009.132.
5. Bray BD, Boyd J, Daly C, Doyle A, Donaldson K, Fox JG, et al. How safe is renal replacement therapy? A national study of mortality and adverse events contributing to the death of renal replacement therapy recipients. Nephrol Dial Transplant. 2013;29(3):681–7. https://doi.org/10.1093/ndt/gft197.
6. Seliger SL, Zhan M, Hsu VD, Walker LD, Fink JC. Chronic kidney disease adversely influences patient safety. J Am Soc Nephrol. 2008;19(12):2414–9. https://doi.org/10.1681/asn.2008010022.

Section of Nephrology, Department of Medicine Stephen Z. Fadem
Baylor College of Medicine
Houston, TX, USA
Salisbury, VT, USA Thomas A. Golper
Bahiana School of Medicine and Public Health José A. Moura-Neto
Salvador, Bahia, Brazil

Contents

Contributors

Ibironke W. Apata Division of Healthcare Quality Promotion, Centers for Disease Control and Prevention, Atlanta, GA, USA

Division of Renal Medicine, Emory University School of Medicine, Atlanta, GA, USA

Matthew J. Arduino Division of Healthcare Quality Promotion, Centers for Disease Control and Prevention, Atlanta, GA, USA

George R. Aronoff DaVita Kidney Care, Denver, CO, USA

Tushar Bajaj Department of Medicine, University of Chicago Pritzker School of Medicine, Chicago, IL, USA

Shweta Bansal Division of Nephrology, Department of Medicine, University of Texas Health San Antonio, San Antonio, TX, USA

Brendan Bowman DaVita Kidney Care, Denver, CO, USA

Division of Nephrology, Department of Medicine, University of Virginia School of Medicine, Charlottesville, VA, USA

Viviane Calice-Silva Joinville Region University, Joinville, Santa Catarina, Brazil

Pro-Rim Foundation, Joinville, Santa Catarina, Brazil

Rafia Chaudhry University of California, San Francisco, San Francisco, CA, USA

Sylvia Donato-Moore DaVita Med Center at Home, Houston, TX, USA

Madeline Miller Drake Department of Vascular Surgery, Houston Methodist Hospital, Houston, TX, USA

Angelina R. Edwards Division of Kidney Diseases, Hypertension and Transplantation, Department of Medicine, Houston Methodist Hospital, Houston, TX, USA

Stephen Z. Fadem Section of Nephrology, Department of Medicine, Baylor College of Medicine, Houston, TX, USA

Rachel B. Fissell Division of Nephrology and Hypertension, Vanderbilt University Medical Center, Nashville, TN, USA

Nupur Gupta Indiana University School of Medicine, Indianapolis, IN, USA

Lucas G. da Luz Moinhos de Vento Hospital, Porto Alegre, Rio Grande do Sul, Brazil

Ana Flávia Moura Bahiana School of Medicine and Public Health, Salvador, Bahia, Brazil

José A. Moura-Neto Bahiana School of Medicine and Public Health, Salvador, Bahia, Brazil

Shannon Novosad Division of Healthcare Quality Promotion, Centers for Disease Control and Prevention, Atlanta, GA, USA

Joan Araujo Oliveira Moitinho Clinical and Academic Unit of Nephrology, Hospital Universitário Pedro Ernesto, Faculty of Medical Sciences, Rio de Janeiro State University, Rio de Janeiro, Brazil

Roberto Pecoits-Filho Pontifical Catholic University of Parana, Curitiba, Brazil

Arbor Research Collaborative for Health, Ann Arbor, MI, USA

Eric Kevin Peden Department of Vascular Surgery, Houston Methodist Hospital, Houston, TX, USA

Cibele Isaac Saad Rodrigues Pontifical Catholic University of São Paulo, São Paulo, Brazil

Santa Lucinda Hospital (FUNDASP), Sorocaba, São Paulo, Brazil

Megha Salani Vanderbilt University Medical Center, Nashville, TN, USA

Anjali Bhatt Saxena, MD Division of Nephrology, Stanford University, Stanford, CA, USA

Santa Clara Valley Medical Center, San Jose, CA, USA

Osama El Shamy Division of Nephrology and Hypertension, Vanderbilt University Medical Center, Nashville, TN, USA

Shashank Sharma Department of Vascular Surgery, Houston Methodist Hospital, Houston, TX, USA

Stuart M. Sprague Division of Nephrology and Hypertension, Department of Medicine, Northshore University Health System, University of Chicago Pritzker School of Medicine, Evanston, IL, USA

José H. R. Suassuna Clinical and Academic Unit of Nephrology, Hospital Universitário Pedro Ernesto, Faculty of Medical Sciences, Rio de Janeiro State University, Rio de Janeiro, Brazil

Karen Ugwu Value-Based Care, Panoramic Health, Tempe, AZ, USA

Jacob Basil Watson Department of Vascular Surgery, Houston Methodist Hospital, Houston, TX, USA

The Hemodialysis Procedure

1

Stephen Z. Fadem

Introduction

Over a period of several years, the dialysis community, a collaboration of dialysis manufacturers, healthcare professionals, and patients has established requirements for handling water and concentrates and has developed surveillance principles that reflect the highest possible levels of protection from chemical and microbial. These follow the International Organization for Standardization (ISO)'s publication ISO 23500-1-2019. The standards dictate that the dialysis facility medical director ensures that dialysis fluids meet all quality standards. Thus, medical directors and other dialysis personnel must be aware of the adverse events that can arise from mistakes and errors that breach the quality standard with respect to water treatment.

The implementation of these rigorous standards has been fruitful regarding the technical and medical device aspects of renal replacement therapy (RRT), leaving non-technical errors such as communicating and carrying out dialysis prescriptions as the major causes of dialysis-related death. In a review of 1357 RRT patients, deaths were mainly related to hyperkalemia, prescribing errors, out-of-hours care, infections, and vascular access [1].

Yet, the dialysis team must always keep its guard up. Biomedical mistakes can claim several lives at once. Within minutes seven dialysis patients in Dallas received blood heated above normal temperatures resulting in a fatal cardiac arrest in three of them [2]. In the dialysis filter (referred to as the dialyzer), only a 20–45 micron polyacrylic membrane separates blood and the dialysis fluid. Dialysis fluid journeys from being fed into the facility from a municipal water source. It then comes in contact with a multimedia filter (MMF) to reduce suspended solids, is then softened

S. Z. Fadem (✉)
Section of Nephrology, Department of Medicine, Baylor College of Medicine, Houston, TX, USA
e-mail: fadem@bcm.edu

S. Z. Fadem et al. (eds.), *Complications in Dialysis*,
https://doi.org/10.1007/978-3-031-44557-6_1

by sodium-embedded particles, and afterward dechlorinated with activated carbon. The water subsequently passes repeatedly through a reverse osmosis (RO) system until meeting standards for use. Afterward, the nearly pure water is combined with acid and bicarbonate either centrally or in the machine. What is delivered to the patient must be sterile and have the correct conductivity, temperature, pH, and mixture of sodium, potassium, calcium, and bicarbonate. Along the way, any disinfectants and contaminants such as chlorine, fluorine, or lead must be removed. Excess sodium from the softener or oxidant cleaning substances cannot be reintroduced. The Association for the Advancement of Medical Instrumentation (AAMI), in cooperation with the International Organization for Standards (ISO), has published standards establishing the maximum allowed concentration of potential contaminants and methodologies that minimize hazards and complications.

Most Common Contaminants

The information contained in this chapter glimpses the necessary basis for understanding the concepts and implementation procedures for water safety. The reader is referred to AAMI's extensive library of online publications, the CDC, CMS, and the manufacturer's specifications for a more thorough background.

Aluminum

When dialysis was first developed as a practical therapy, it was noticed that bone disorders and vascular calcification were complications not addressed. The practice of having patients ingest a substance to bind dietary phosphorus has been integral to therapy. Throughout the course of dialysis history, substances replaced some complications with others. Although effective as a phosphate binder, aluminum was associated with osteodystrophy as characterized by bone pain, osteomalacia, and fractures [3]. It was also associated with dementia [4].

Initially, tap water was used for dialysis, but as the therapy became more advanced, the use of sedimentation filters, water softeners, and carbon filters were used to remove sodium, potassium, magnesium, calcium, and chlorine. The discovery of aluminum toxicity in the 1970s lead to the use of RO-treated water for dialysis. Aluminum is now less associated with dialysis fluid than with the use of aluminum-based binders. The maximum allowed concentration in dialysis fluid is 0.01 mg/L. The practice of using aluminum to bind dietary phosphorus has shifted to either non-calcium-based binders such as sevelamer or calcium-based binders such as calcium acetate. In addition to bone disease and dementia, aluminum toxicity is associated with cardiomegaly [5].

Chlorine and Chloramine

Throughout the history of civilization, the availability of water has been essential to the establishment of a municipality. For a clearer perspective of this relationship, refer to *The Source* by James Michener, himself a dialysis patient (**http://nephron.com/nephsites/nic/michener.html**) [6]. Waterborne diseases were a major challenge to public health, and the ability to disinfect drinking water has been a major advancement. The chlorination of drinking water is the most common means of disinfecting surface water or water systems exposed to open air. The amount added varies and may also be a function of temperature. Chlorine (Cl_2) and chloramine (NH_2Cl) are routinely added to municipal water systems to reduce bacterial counts. Chlorine is a powerful bleach and an oxidant (meaning it takes electrons from other molecules) that has been added to drinking water. This practice has been ongoing since 1908. The disadvantages of chlorine are that it is volatile and produces disinfection by-products. Chloramine is a combination of chlorine and ammonia, is less volatile, and produces fewer environmental toxins. The amount of chlorine or chloramine added to potable water is unlikely to cause long-term health problems when consumed orally. If they come into contact with blood, these substances can cause hemolysis [7, 8]. If the contact is severe, it can be associated with methemoglobinemia and protein denaturing. The toxic patient may present with headache, nausea and vomiting, acute malaise, hypertension, shortness of breath, chest, back, and abdominal pain, cardiac arrhythmias, and hyperkalemia. Activated carbon, while an effective absorber of contaminants, is used inline with ion-exchange water softeners to reduce chlorine products to their nonoxidative state.

Copper, Brass, Galvanized Metal

The use of copper in plumbing dates to Egypt around 2500 BC. Copper piping was used to irrigate the Nile and as part of the drainage systems for the pyramids (**https://www.plumbingsupply.com/pmegypt.html**). Copper pipes are taken for granted as a common tool in modern plumbing. However, copper, brass, or galvanized metal are expressly prohibited at any point in the journal of water handling beyond water treatment. The maximum allowable concentration of copper in the water system is 0.1 mg/L. Currently, blood levels of copper are generally low [9]. Copper is a necessary element and serves as a cofactor in many enzymatic reactions. Cooking acidic foods in uncoated copper cookware or excessive amounts of copper in drinking water are the most likely causes of copper toxicity. Copper toxicity may be associated with gastrointestinal side effects, blue-green emesis and stool, altered mentation, and even coma. It can lead to rhabdomyolysis, hemolysis, multisystem failure, and death [10].

Fluoride

Since 1945, fluoride has been added to municipal water supplies and has been proven to prevent tooth decay (SOURCE: **https://www.cdc.gov/fluoridation/basics/timeline.html**). RO effectively removes fluoride from water used for dialysis treatment. On occasions where the reverse osmosis system is not working, standby deionization tanks must be placed inline as a substitute. Deionization (DI) is not recommended as a primary method for water purification because it does not remove aluminum, fluoride, or low-molecular weight bacterial toxins like microcystins. In addition to being used as a standby alternate method when RO fails, DI can be used for polishing treated reverse osmosis fluid. Faulty DI equipment has been associated with severe toxicity [11, 12]. Fluoride toxicity may cause ventricular fibrillation. The maximum allowable fluoride concentration in the treated water is 0.2 mg/L.

Lead

Lead is ubiquitous in our environment and has been extensively used in industry, especially in plumbing. Ancient Rome was oblivious to the damaging impact of its chronic use. Lead acetate was even used as a sweetener. Historians now suggest that this dark era was associated with infertility and incompetence, and the follies of the Roman emperors are often blamed on their excess consumption of lead [13]. Lead toxicity is still a major health challenge, especially for children (Source: World Health Organization). Lead toxicity can lead to hemolytic anemia, muscle weakness, and in high levels, encephalopathy and brain damage. The administration of recombinant erythropoietin may be associated with lowering lead levels in dialysis patients [14]. While lead toxicity can occur in hemodialysis patients, it is rare, with pH levels in the normal range. The maximum concentration of lead allowed in treated water is 0.005 mg/L. Lead toxicity has been associated with smoking cigarettes or cigars that have been produced with contaminated tobacco leaves [15].

Nitrates, Sulfates, Zinc, and Trace Elements

The maximum allowed concentration of nitrate in treated dialysis water is 2 mg/L. Dialysis has been shown to lower nitrate, nitrate, and cyclic guanosine monophosphate levels in patients [16].

Serum sulfate levels can be high in dialysis patients. The allowed concentration in treated water is 100 mg/L. The clinical effects are not well established, but it could possibly lead to osteodystrophy [17]. A small study looking at sulfur content in hemodialysis (HD) patients compared 94 patients on HD with 33 patients controls who were not on HD and had mean serum creatinine levels of 0.8 ± 0.37 mg/dL (0.56 ± 0.17 mM vs. 0.31 ± 0.13 mM, $p < 0.001$). The dialysate sulfur level was 0.4 μmol/L. There were no clinical differences. The reasons for the mild but significant elevation in sulfur were not explained [17].

The maximum allowable zinc concentration in treated dialysis water is 0.1 mg/L. In actuality, zinc deficiency is prevalent in the dialysis population [18].

Several other trace elements may be present in the potable water source. Their effect on kidney disease is not clear. They include antimony, arsenic, barium, beryllium, cadmium, chromium, mercury, nickel, manganese, selenium, silver, and thallium. In a systemic review of 128 studies, it was noted that cadmium, chromium, copper, lead, and vanadium tended to be higher in the dialysis population, while selenium, zinc, and manganese were lower. Zinc deficiency is associated with anorexia, dysgeusia, impaired cognitive function, delayed wound healing, and abnormal immune response. Selenium protects against the oxidant stress [18].

Standards by ANSI/AAMI/ISO 23500-1-5 dictate that all elements be kept below specific levels in water used for dialysis. Testing for these elements must be routinely performed [19]. Dialysis personnel should have a good working relationship and open lines of communication with those in charge of water fed into the dialysis system for their particular facilities.

Water Treatment Equipment

The water treatment system has built-in redundancy for safety reasons. In 1997, James Reason published *Managing the Risks of Organizational Accidents* [20]. He likened organizational accidents to the passage through the holes of multiple layers of Swiss cheese; all the holes lined up. Each hole represents a gap in a defense mechanism that has either been turned off or somehow defeated. In designing, implementing, maintaining, and using a water system, there are several steps. While a single mistake at any given time may not lead to catastrophe, a combination of mishaps can. Maintenance failures, the human factor, and machine wear and tear loom as potential antecedents of disaster.

The municipal water that feeds into the dialysis system must undergo treatment to remove microbes, chloramine, and chlorine, and other chemicals such as aluminum, nitrates, fluoride, and sulfates. The dialysis equipment must function to provide water that is safe for dialysis use, commonly referred to as dialysis quality water.

The availability of feed water for the well-functioning of treatment and distribution system is essential. A critical component of this system is the circulating pump. Each dialysis facility should develop contingency plans that deal with events that prevent or delay the dialysis procedure from being performed. These plans include not only natural disasters but also electrical outages, a water main break, or low water pressure. Plans to provide contingency operations when the concentrate preparation system fails should also be in place. The loss of available water at any point necessitates either the rescheduling or relocation of dialysis patients from their routine dialysis times to different ones. This threatens patient safety when rescheduling is not possible because of unavailable transportation. Patient satisfaction also declines if faulty and unpredicted water-related problems force disruptions.

Once installed, it must be demonstrated that the equipment performs according to standards. This includes records of testing, chemical, microbial, initial trend analysis, and meeting performance indicators.

Routine surveillance is required to ensure that water is neither contaminated with chemicals, microbes, or endotoxins nor can be produced in sufficient amounts and with ample pressure. The schedule varies depending on the chemical in question. However, for chlorine, surveillance is done daily.

Water storage tanks are sometimes necessary, particularly when the water supply from a municipal source is not predictable with respect to either quantity or pressure. Tanks must be routinely drained and disinfected. They should be fitted with inline pyrogenic filters to remove particles and molecules >1 kD.

Sediment Filter

Sediment filters are a popular way of removing particles from drinking water. They do not remove trace elements or contaminants, nor do they remove dissolved organic and inorganic substances. They are also referred to as multimedia filters and have progressively smaller particles. They tend to clog, and the increased resistance impedes the downflow water supply. This can be avoided by backwashing the filter on a timed schedule. Gauges can measure the change in pressure across the system and help determine the need for backwashing. Algae can contaminate these filters and they should be fitted with opaque housing since light is necessary for algae growth.

Cartridge Filters

Cartridge filters are cylindrical canisters housing a filter medium with a draining core in the center. The housing can be cleaned for algae when the cartridge is changed. Opaque housings prevent algae from growing. They can be fitted with gauges to determine the change in pressure that results from the accumulation of particulate material. Cartridge filters have the advantage over sediment filters of being able to filter particles of a smaller diameter.

Water Softeners

When water is fed into the dialysis system, it is said to have levels of hardness determined by the number of substances like calcium and magnesium that it contains. These are removed through ion exchange within the water softener, where calcium and magnesium ions are removed and replaced with sodium ions. Testing for hardness can be done using ethylenediaminetetraacetic acid (EDTA) testing strips. Online hardness monitors can also be used. Hardness checks should be performed at the end of the duty cycle to ensure that regeneration is adequate at the time of the

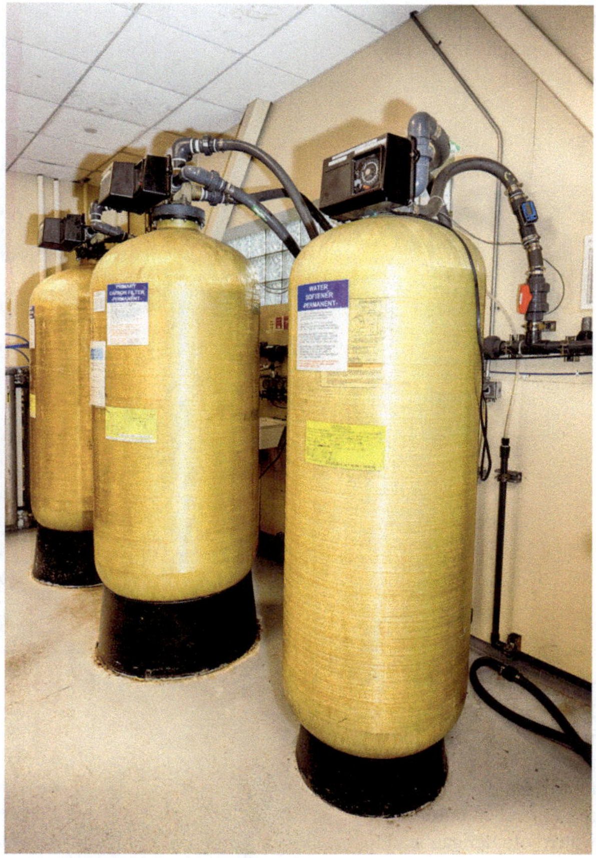

Fig. 1.1 The water softener tank is inline with the carbon filter tanks. In the background is the RO system. (Photograph by Stephen Z. Fadem)

worst-case condition. By design, the system should not enable the sodium chloride to enter the product water line during regeneration.

The softener is a tank that holds a resin with sodium ions attached—a sodium exchange resin. When the "hard" water-containing minerals come in contact with the sodium resin, the sodium is exchanged for the other positively charged molecules. After a period of time, there is little sodium remaining for the exchange reaction to take place, and the resin is said to be exhausted. It can be regenerated by exposure to a highly concentrated sodium chloride solution. Mechanisms that prevent water with a high sodium content from entering the product water line should be used. Water softening extends the life of the fragile reverse osmosis (RO) membranes by reducing the load of minerals that must be separated from the supplied water.

Figure 1.1 shows the water softener tank and then the two carbon tanks.

The brine tank (Fig. 1.2) contains the salt that is added to the water softener tank shown in Fig. 1.1. The brine test is checked daily to ensure that the salt level is above the red line (Fig. 1.3).

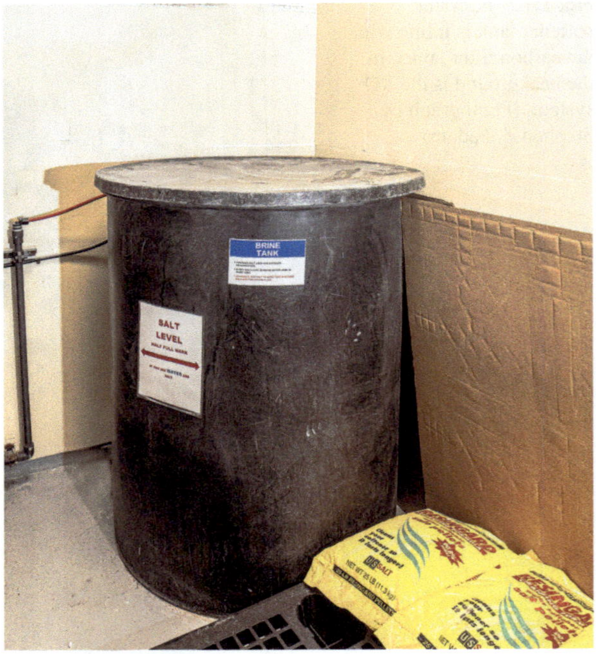
BRINE TANK
SALT LEVEL

Fig. 1.2 Salt brine tank. (Photography by Stephen Z. Fadem)

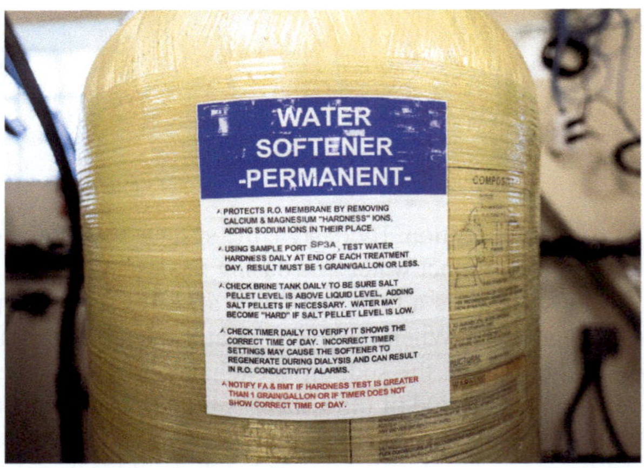
WATER SOFTENER -PERMANENT-
PROTECTS R.O. MEMBRANE BY REMOVING CALCIUM & MAGNESIUM "HARDNESS" IONS, ADDING SODIUM IONS IN THEIR PLACE.
USING SAMPLE PORT SP3A, TEST WATER HARDNESS DAILY AT END OF EACH TREATMENT DAY. RESULT MUST BE 1 GRAIN/GALLON OR LESS.
CHECK BRINE TANK DAILY TO BE SURE SALT PELLET LEVEL IS ABOVE LIQUID LEVEL, ADDING SALT PELLETS IF NECESSARY. WATER MAY BECOME "HARD" IF SALT PELLET LEVEL IS LOW.
CHECK TIMER DAILY TO VERIFY IT SHOWS THE CORRECT TIME OF DAY. INCORRECT TIMER SETTINGS MAY CAUSE THE SOFTENER TO REGENERATE DURING DIALYSIS AND CAN RESULT IN R.O. CONDUCTIVITY ALARMS.
NOTIFY FA & BMT IF HARDNESS TEST IS GREATER THAN 1 GRAIN/GALLON OR IF TIMER DOES NOT SHOW CORRECT TIME OF DAY.

Fig. 1.3 The hardness test is performed daily and must show a value of less than 1 grain/gallon. Failure to properly monitor the water softener can lead to excess minerals reaching the RO membrane and damaging it. (Photography by Stephen Z. Fadem)

Carbon Filters

Tanks embedded with carbon are used to remove total chlorine, and the maximum allowed chlorine in the treated water is 0.1 mg/L. Chlorine and chloramine are removed in tanks bedded with carbon, and the amount removed varies with both pH and temperature. The inability to predict the quantity of these substances removed mandates intense surveillance of the chlorine in the delivered water and the

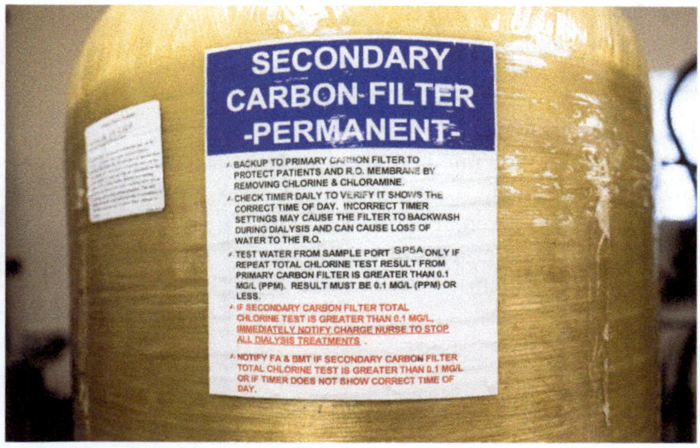

Fig. 1.4 Each carbon tank system must have a backup tank. If the total chlorine test from water processed through this tank is over 0.1 mg/L, then all dialysis procedures must be stopped

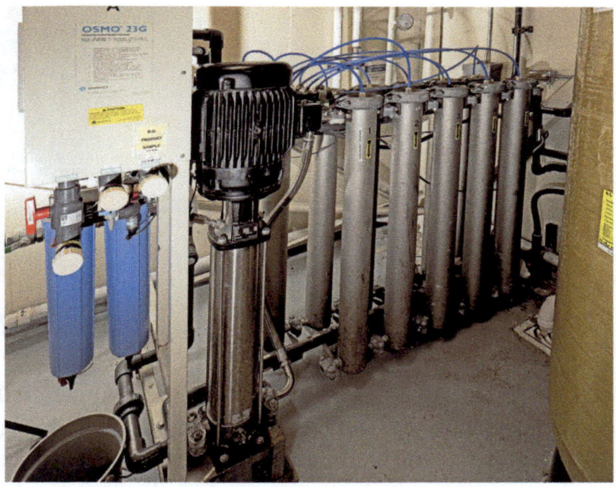

Fig. 1.5 An installed Mar Cor 23G-Series Reverse Osmosis System. (Photograph by Stephen Z. Fadem)

performance of the carbon bed. Two carbon tanks are placed in series such that when there is a breakthrough in one, the carbon is exhausted and embedded with virgin carbon. The new bed is always placed in the second position. The patient is protected by continuous online monitoring of total chlorine levels, and the system is shut down when the total chlorine level is greater than 0.1 mg/L. Chlorine test strips can be used to monitor total chlorine every 4 h as an alternative to continuous online monitoring (Figs. 1.1 and 1.4).

Reverse Osmosis (RO)

RO forces a solvent from a higher to a lower concentration across a semipermeable membrane. Since this is counter to the basic physics principles of osmosis, it requires energy to be put into the system and pressure generated. RO emerged out of the necessity to desalinate seawater for human consumption to alleviate the

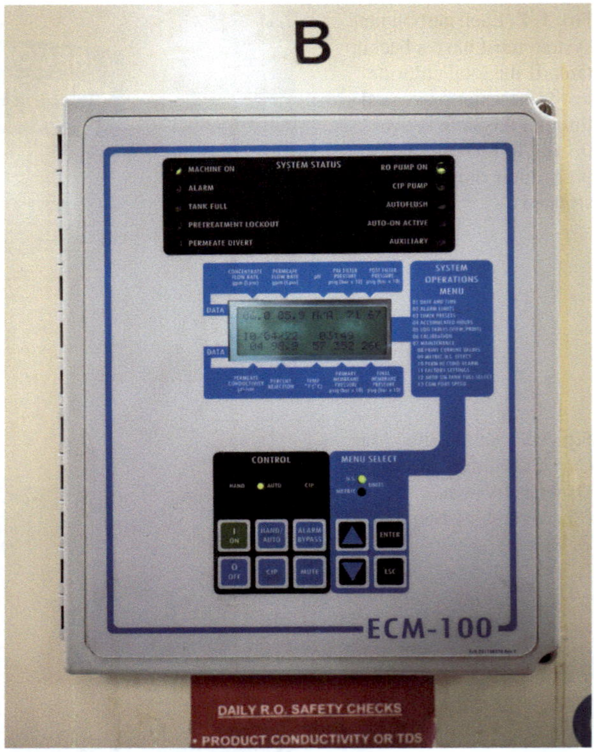

Fig. 1.6 The RO system is a series of fragile membranes packed into cylinders. The system must be monitored closely to ensure the rejection rate is over 90%. When the photograph was taken, it was 98.9%. (Photograph by Stephen Z. Fadem)

challenges of water shortage. It became commercially available when suitable membranes with low salt permeability were developed (Fig. 1.5).

The RO system in the dialysis facility is monitored continuously, measuring product water conductivity. This can be displayed as total dissolved solutes (S/m). A well-functioning RO machine will reject 98% of the solute in the feed water. This amount is normalized for pressure and temperature. If the rejection rate decrease is greater than 90%, then the system needs to be checked by chemical analysis. The operating log records daily water checks [21]. See Fig. 1.6.

Chemical contaminants also include organic compounds like pesticides and polyacrylic aromatic hydrocarbons. The exact impact they have on clinical outcomes is not well defined. RO should be effective in removing them, as should the activated carbon used in chlorine and chloramine removal.

Water that has been softened and dechlorinated (pretreated feedwater) passes through a 5-micron cartridge filter. This removes carbon fines that are released from the carbon tanks. Carbon fines can damage the RO and membranes. The water is then pumped through the membrane housing units. The pressure of the system is continuously monitored, and the system will alarm and shut down should it rise above a set point. A conductivity sensor is also attached inline. After traveling through the last membrane, the concentrate is recycled and mixed with feedwater at the inlet piping. This allows for a high machine recovery. In addition to pressure and conductivity, the machine monitors temperature. pH may be monitored as well.

RO machines specify a Langelier saturation index of −0.1. This is to minimize calcium scale formation on the membranes. Continuous chlorine must be less than 0.1 ppm and the slit density index less than 3. The hardness level should be less than 1 grain/gallon.

When the machine is operating, daily logs must be completed at the start of every day to verify that the water system is running within normal operating parameters. Manufacture's preventive maintenance recommendations are required to be followed to ensure the RO system runs as designed to avoid harm to patients. This may include maintenance of the pH buffer system and changing the pre-filter cartridges at least monthly or when pressures drop, flushing the machine, verifying product water quality, cleaning and calibrating the pH and conductivity probes, and cleaning and sanitizing the RO and dialysis water distribution system. All manufacture-required maintenance should only be performed by trained biomed personnel certified by the equipment manufacturer.

Initially, disinfection should be done monthly, but this may be extended to a maximum of 3 months. Cleaning and sanitizing the machine are vital to protect the membrane. Cleaning and sanitizing vary but may be required weekly or every 2 months. The manufactures' disinfection protocols should be followed and validated through culture and endotoxin sampling.

The AAMI water quality analysis should be done at least each year or as required by the manufacturer or regulatory agency.

Microbes and Endotoxins

Much of the water system maintenance ensures that microbes and endotoxins are reduced to safe dialysis quality levels. Endotoxins are lipopolysaccharides that are the breakdown remnants of bacteria. They can activate an innate pyrogenic cytokine response characterized by fever and chills. They can cause hypotension, multiorgan system failure, and even death. The horseshoe crab (*Limulus polyphemus*) blood cells are reactive to endotoxins, and the standard is to use the limulus amebocyte lysate (LAL) test to determine whether endotoxins are present. Action levels are warnings that the contaminant is at a high enough level to warrant action to interrupt the trend toward an unacceptable level.

With high flux dialysis membranes, endotoxin microbial remnants are able to pass bidirectionally because of back filtration, necessitating that water meets minimal standards for both cultured microbes and endotoxins. Ultraviolet light, ozone, and heat are alternatives to traditional disinfecting and allow for bacterial control. Culture schedules and techniques, disinfection schedules, and methods are outlined in AAMI and ISO standards, and further discussion can be found in the chapter on infection control. The maximum levels of bacteria and endotoxin allowed in dialysis water and the action levels are set forth in ISO 23500-3 through ISO 23500-5. Bacteria can produce a matrix component that adheres to surfaces and enables resident bacteria to become embedded within the film and protected. Strategies to prevent and eliminate biofilm generation involved disinfecting equipment on a timely basis.

Dialysis Fluids

All dialysis machines are designed to mix acid and bicarbonate concentrates with dialysis-quality water to produce an isotonic solution called dialysate, which is compatible with human blood. Proportioned and balanced dialysis fluids must contain the correct composition of acids and bicarbonate. The acid concentrate is a mixture of salts that are diluted with bicarbonate concentrate to yield the fluid used in dialysis. When treated, this water must meet ANSI/AAMI standard 13959 (the Standard) to be considered. These fluids have been cleared by the FDA and are available in a liquid form that is ready for use or a dry powder form. The dry powder should be reconstituted with water specified by the Standard. The process combines the first stream (acid concentrate), the second stream (bicarbonate concentrate), and water to constitute the final water used for dialysis. Errors can occur if there is an incorrect chemical formulation, contamination, or incorrect labeling. They can also occur if the system is contaminated with microbes or endotoxins. Metals that are known to be toxic to humans include copper, brass, galvanized metals, aluminum, zinc, and lead are specifically prohibited by the Standard.

The equipment used to mix the correct volume of purified water with the concentrates must mix the solution well enough to completely dissolve the ingredients before delivery to the central storage point or the point of dialysis service. The final step is proportioning with water.

To reduce the risk of microbial infection, all bicarbonate mixers, loops, and jugs should be drained and flushed at the end of the day. This is required by ANSI/AAMI 23500 and the Centers for Medicare and Medicaid Services (CMS). The standards also dictate that the manufacturer's instructions are critically followed to minimize the risk of a chemical mixing error or microbial contamination. Overmixing may result in the off-gassing of carbon dioxide. Failure modes can be related to incorrect assembly or calibration or failure to follow the operating instructions. The timing and proper temperature are critical. If the temperature is too cold, the ingredients will dissolve slowly. Additional time may be needed to allow ingredients to dissolve fully. The equipment must be mixed within the time outlined in the manufacturer's instructions. Failure can occur if the procedures and frequency standards with regard to maintenance or disinfection of equipment and the water system are not done properly. (See Figs. 1.7 and 1.8).

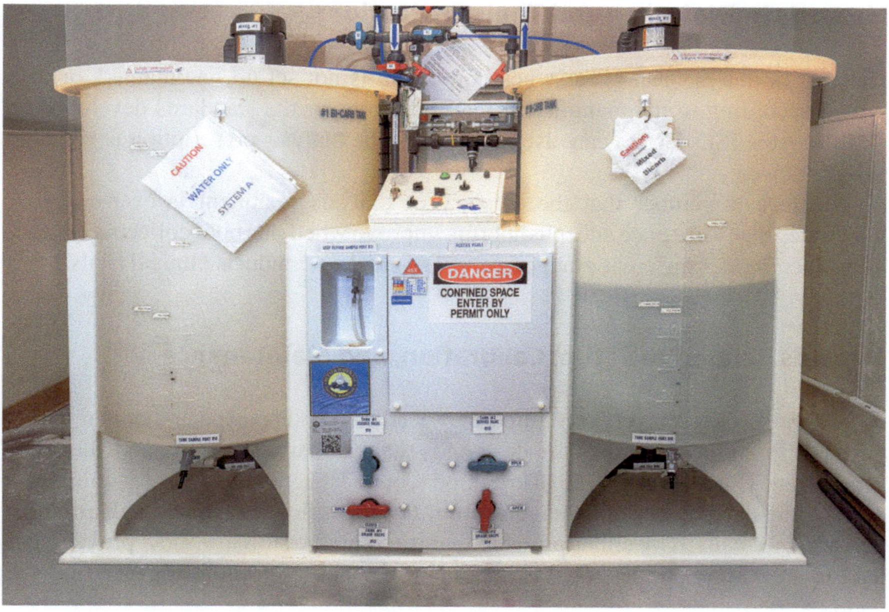

Fig. 1.7 Batch bicarbonate mixing. (Photograph by Stephen Z. Fadem)

Fig. 1.8 Batch acid mixing. (Photograph by Stephen Z. Fadem)

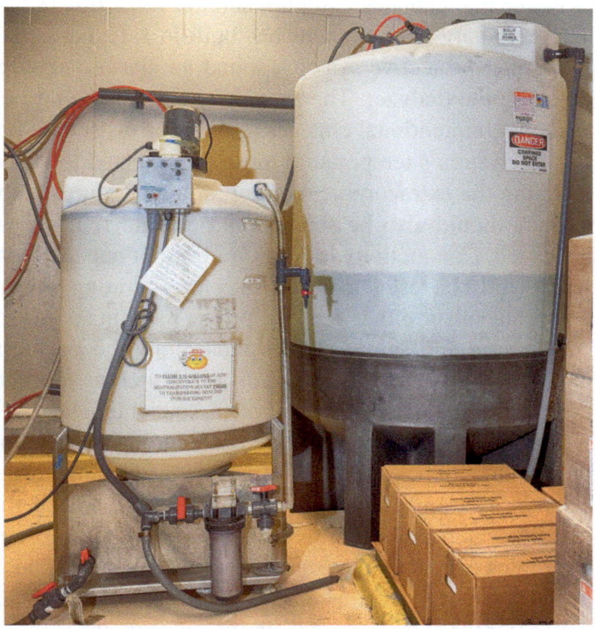

Hazards in Dialysis—and Their Protection

Hazards in dialysis can occur when equipment is not set up, maintained, or calibrated according to the manufacturer's instructions or the standards developed by ANSI/AAMI/ISO. Errors can also occur when the dialysis prescription is not carefully followed.

We must remember that the delivery of dialysis treatment is ever-evolving. Outcomes that were once accepted norms improve when our field collectively looks at data, compares different practice patterns, and then conducts clinical trials.

Hazards Related to Setup, Calibration, and Maintenance

Tube or pipe cuts not properly fitted may lead to pockets or gaps that can harbor bacteria. Piping terminations are dead ends that can harbor bacteria and should be minimized. The pressure in the distribution loop must be within the safe limits specified by the dialysis machine manufacturer. Improper flow can result in distribution performance caused by either pressure that is too high or too low. Low pressure can lead to stagnation and bacterial contamination resulting in biofilm generation and endotoxins.

The properly installed hemodialysis machine will be tested to ensure all vital parameters can meet the manufacturer's specifications. Routine scheduled dialysis machine maintenance is set up, and the validation process is implemented.

Hemodialysis equipment has built-in safeguards to protect against hazards. In particular, protective systems sound an alarm and stop unsafe dialysis fluid from reaching the dialyzer. The protective system should be independent of the control system. Unintentional changes to the controls should be prevented.

The system's temperature must be protected to keep the dialyzer and fluid from reaching the extracorporeal circuit at temperatures below 33° or above 42 °C. The system should also be set for the net fluid removal and alarm if this number is exceeded. Conductivity is monitored, and if outside preset limits, it must alarm. The alarms must be tested to ensure they are operating properly. System error and human error can both be either due to improper handling of the concentrate or the equipment.

Warning and safety notices must draw the operator's attention to precautions necessary to prevent cross-infection, as well as to the hazards associated with the connection and disconnection of the patients. Hazards may also be related to the incorrect choice of dialysis fluid concentrates. Alarm limits of the protective system are required to be posted. Warnings on the hazards related to transporting undesired substances from dialysis fluid to the blood side of the dialyzer are also posted. Hazards can occur if alarms are cleared without resolving the underlying problems. Examples of potential hazards are kinked cannula lines that are not detected by the protective system. Ultrasound gel may interfere with an ultrasonic air detector. Air may enter the extracorporeal circuit downstream of the air detector if the connection joints are not sufficiently tightened. Negative pressures can lead to the introduction of air when single-needle dialysis or central venous catheters is used.

Warnings are required regarding disinfection procedures—only those defined and validated by the manufacturer should be used. The required quality of incoming dialysis water and dialysis fluid concentrates should be posted. To avoid complications related to wear and tear, the intervals at which parts should be exchanged should also be available and adhered to.

There must be a warning that the blood flow rate will be reduced when pre-pump arterial pressure is extremely negative. The range and accuracy of the blood flow rate of the pumps, inlet, and outlet pressures should be accurately maintained.

Calibrating dialysis equipment should always be done according to the manufacturer's instructions. Failure to install, operate, or maintain dialysis machine equipment according to the instructions provided by the manufacturing company may cause injury or death to the patient or operator. Several warnings are present in the calibration manual for all dialysis equipment.

Maintenance should never be performed when the patient is connected to the machine. In fact, the machine should be removed from the treatment floor while it is being serviced. It should be appropriately labeled and not returned to be put back into use until it is fully tested. Conductivity and pH levels must be confirmed before returning to the floor for use in patient care.

Calibration involves making mechanical adjustments to hydraulics and electronics. It also involves storing data in the electronic memory of the machine. Calibration procedures should be performed only when needed following a repair or failed performance. It should not be performed routinely to verify normal operations. Instead of routine calibration, performance tests to be used are designated in the preventive maintenance procedures. Calibration procedures should either use primary standards or be traceable to the National Institute for Standards and Technology (NIST). Only original equipment manufacturer parts should be used to repair or upgrade hemodialysis machines, as they have been tested to meet ANSI/AAMI/ISO standards. The manufacturer also requires that if certain specified components are replaced, the calibrations must be conducted. The Fresenius 2008 T Hemodialysis System Calibration Procedures, available online, offer a good example of a manufacturer's calibration instruction manual (**https://fmcna.com/content/dam/fmcna/live/support/documents/techical-documentation/2008t-hemodialysis--systems/508032_Rev_H.pdf**).

Electric shocks can and do occur in dialysis and have been reported, but are exceedingly rare [22].

Conductivity

Materials are either able to conduct electricity or resist electrical flow. The two are reciprocal. Resistance is measured in ohms (Ω). Conductivity is measured in Siemens per meter (S/m). Liquids that carry atoms with an electrical charge or ions are known as electrolytes; pure water does not conduct electricity. Ions are either positively charged—cations, or negatively charged—anions. Sodium is the major cation in the body. The body's composition of electrolytes like sodium, potassium, chloride, and bicarbonate is held steady with functioning kidneys. The serum sodium levels range between 135 and 145 mEq/L, and it is hazardous for them to fall outside this range. The conductivity range in dialysis fluid is set to mirror the serum sodium and maintain it is a safe range.

Dialysis therapy helps control electrolyte composition as well as acid–base balance. To this end, dialysis fluids must be carefully balanced. Conductivity is an accurate, reliable, reproducible, and easy way to measure the salt content of dialysis solutions. However, it depends upon temperature. Part of the automated calibration process is to check conductivity to ensure it is in the target range using the appropriate temperature coefficient.

While physicians can control the composition of calcium, magnesium, bicarbonate, and potassium in the bath, they are limited by guidelines and standards to a specific range. They also have control over the sodium level, and the concept of sodium modeling was developed and demonstrated to be useful in alleviating cramping during dialysis. Online conductivity metering made this practical [23]. Sodium profiling is rarely done today because it leads to sodium loading, increased thirst, volume expansion, and hypertension. Ultrafiltration profiling may reduce intradialytic light-headedness [24]. Varying serum sodium levels with dialysis may be valuable to control symptoms, but management needs to be individualized. Randomized controlled trials are lacking [25].

Although the safety profile has been satisfactory, iatrogenic hypernatremia can occur during dialysis. It is associated with increased thirst, elevated blood pressure, and weight gain [26]. Erroneous conductivity measurements can account for dialysis against a high sodium bath. Meters such as the 90XLTechnician Meter and pHoenix meter must be accurately calibrated and rechecked. Incorrect bicarbonate or acid dialysate concentrate measures can interfere with measurements. Calcium carbonate precipitation can block monitoring sensor cells. Temperature errors can also affect the conductivity [26].

Air Embolism

If air is introduced into the lines and is able to enter the circulation, it can lead to fatal consequences. Dialysis machines are equipped with sophisticated air detection systems, but these must be tested each time the machine is set up for use. Staff training should emphasize that retrograde cerebral air emboli can occur if any of the steps in the manufacturer's instructions are bypassed or omitted. With proper setup, testing, and management, the incidence of air embolism is rare. Exposure of the blood circuit to air can result in its introduction into the brain, leading to hypoxic-ischemic encephalopathy. Emboli of air are also prothrombotic.

The likelihood of an air embolus is higher with a central venous catheter than with a fistula. When an air embolism is suspected, the patient must be immediately placed in the Trendelenburg position with the head lowered [27]. 100% oxygen should be started. Hyperbaric therapy may improve the outcome and reduce residual defects. Incidences of cerebral air emboli are now rare but do occur despite safeguards. Therefore, suspicion should be high with any sudden alteration in sudden difficulty in arousing, altered mental status, sudden onset blindness, or other focal defects.

Temperature

Dialysis fluid must be monitored for its temperature at the dialysis machine fluid outlet. Prolonged elevated temperatures will cause hypotension as the dialyzer is an efficient heat exchanger. The maximum dialysis fluid temperature is limited to ≤42 °C. Cold dialysate causes tachypnea, tachycardia, and shivering. Ventricular fibrillation can also occur with hypothermia.

Abnormally high dialysis bath temperatures may not be readily noticeable. Temperatures greater than 46 °C are associated with hemolysis and denaturation of blood components. The equipment should include a protective system that is independent of the temperature control system. This prevents dialysis fluid from reaching the dialyzer at a temperature below 33 °C or above 42 °C for the temperature that is measured at the hemodialysis equipment dialysis fluid outlet. Auditory and visual alarms should work to provide a safe condition. The dialysis flow should be stopped if the temperature is out of ranged. If heat is used for disinfection, the system must be monitored to ensure that the water is restored to a safe temperature before being used to prepare concentrate. Dialysis fluid temperature should be within the tolerances that have been specified in the manufacturer's instructions.

Temperature calibration is essential because the solution's conductivity is a function of temperature and increases if the temperature is elevated. To ensure an accurate conductivity reading, users must follow instructions provided by the manufacturer regarding the temperature coefficient for the particular model in use.

Fluid Protection

The equipment should include a protective system that is independent of the ultrafiltration control system to prevent a deviation in net fluid removal from the set value of the controlling parameters. Ultrafiltration controllers should also include an independent protective system to prevent unintentional changes in the control system that could lead to a hazard. The protective system should activate an auditory and visual alarm.

Disconnection

Although no system can perfectly prevent blood loss during the procedure, several protective measures can be taken. The measure of venous pressure during dialysis is closely monitored. The hemodialysis equipment should also include an alarm system to alert the operator to a rupture or separation of the extracorporeal circuit due to excess internal pressure. It should also include a system to protect against an accidentally disconnected line, rupture, or dislodged fistula needle. The drop in venous pressure that may indicate a dislodged needle or disconnected catheter connector may be small. Pressure pulse alarm systems may require at least a minute to detect the fault condition and turn the blood pump off. In this period, the patent may have already lost 500 cc of blood.

The optimal way to prevent the hazardous consequences of a bloodline disconnection is to always maintain the visibility of the access needle, keeping it in full view. The patient's head must remain uncovered at all times during dialysis to ensure an immediate detection and response to a needle dislodgement, disconnection, or disruption in the extracorporeal circuit. The facility should be adequately staffed, and the staff trained to be on the lookout for acute disconnections. The system should also contain a protective system to protect against blood leaks or blood loss due to coagulation.

Protective systems must be activated prior to the patient starting dialysis. The protective system is part of a redundancy that, in addition to the control system, lowers the likelihood of the system failing. The success of this redundancy has been corroborated by the low number of serious accidents resulting from hemodialysis malfunction in the USA.

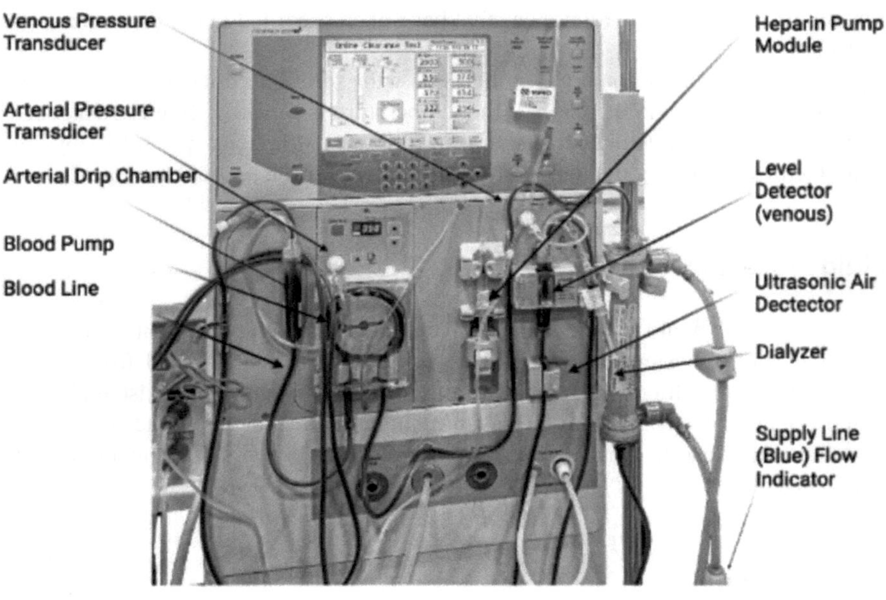

Fig. 1.9 Highlights some of the protections that are incorporated into the machine (Made with biorender.com). A dialysis machine commonly used on the dialysis floor. Note the monitoring protections incorporated into the machine. These must be tested and active for the machine to operate safely. (Photograph by Stephen Z. Fadem)

Batch and Proportioning Systems

Batch and proportioning systems differ in that acid and bicarbonate concentrate components are mixed in the final volume of water to create dialysis fluid when batched (see Figs. 1.7 and 1.9). In proportioning system, one of the concentrates is proportioned along with water while the other is added to that composition proportionate to what is required based on the machine dilution ratio. Opportunities for error can result from incorrect assembly, defective parts, or operator error, such as not following instructions when using the equipment. To avoid hazards, complete routine maintenance procedures are necessary. Calibration equipment must be accurate, especially with measuring pH and conductivity. The proportioning system must be calibrated properly and the proportioning ratio correct. Concentrates should be clearly labeled, for using the incorrect concentrate could also lead to hazards.

Prescription-Related

Acid–Base

Granuflo® is a concentrate of minerals that, when diluted with water, will create a bicarbonate and acetate solution. It was developed by Fresenius Medical Care in 2003, and its main advantage is that it is a powder, not a liquid. This eliminated the need for 55-gallon drums. It contained 8, rather than 4 mEq of acetate, a mineral metabolized to bicarbonate by the liver. On November 4, 2011, Fresenius issued an internal memo that they had performed a case-controlled study in 80,516 patients in 2010 and found an adjusted odds ratio of 4.7 for cardiac arrest associated with higher bicarbonate levels. They stated that the safety data confirmed alkalosis was a significant risk factor leading to cardiopulmonary arrest. They claimed in their memo that dialysis machines underestimated the total buffer patients received. The levels of acetate in their dialysate were leading to metabolic alkalosis and an increased risk of sudden death in dialysis patients. It was argued that dialysis machine settings would only account for bicarbonate and not the extra acetate. Other dialysis centers were not notified until March 2012, when the US FDA issued a Class I recall of Granuflo. The argument was that the extra alkalosis at the end of dialysis would cause hypotension, reduce respirations, bind free calcium, and lead to cardiac arrest. The alkalosis could also cause transient hypokalemia.

Despite cited observational literature [28] being questioned, several large jury awards were given to the families of patients who had died while being dialyzed using Granuflo. Although the DOPPS cohort study demonstrated a trend between higher dialysate concentrations and morbidity [29], the mortality relationship to serum bicarbonate was not duplicated in other studies. A large study of 76,462 dialysis patients failed to demonstrate an association between the dialysate buffer and SCD. The strongest association between SCD and dialysis was related to missed treatments, lower serum albumin, hemoglobin, potassium, body mass index, and a larger erythropoietin stimulating agent dose [30].

Sudden cardiac arrest (SCA) accounts for 29% of deaths in dialysis patients. The most likely causes are fluid and electrolyte fluxes, fluid removal, and a uremic milieu superimposed on underlying cardiovascular pathology. Whether dialysate bicarbonate–acetate concentrations result in a higher risk of cardiac death has been questioned by the academic renal community. An observational study looking at serum bicarbonate levels showed that a significant difference ($p < 0.001$) between measured bicarbonate levels in patients who had a higher incidence of death, but the values were 22.0 vs. 21.0 mEq/L for SCA patients vs. control [31]. In a large case-control study neither dialysate buffer or its bicarbonate component were associated with SCA during treatment [32].

Temperature

Physicians often elect to lower the dialysis bath temperature. In a systemic review of 26 trials studying 484 patients, reducing the bath temperature lowered the rate of intradialytic hypotension by 70% (95% CI 49–89%) and increased intradialytic mean arterial pressure. The odds of feeling cooler with a lowered bath temperature was 2.95 (95% CI 0.88–9.82). The standard bath temperatures varied between 36.0 and 38.5 °C. Bath temperatures were lowered into the 35 °C range, although in one case study, the temperature was lowered from 37 to 34 °C [33]. Studies of brain white matter microstructure with diffusion tensor imaging (DTI) suggested that using cooled dialysate would improve hemodynamic tolerability and that dialysis at 0.5 °C below core body temperature would protect patients from white matter changes [34]. As promising as this was, the same group has performed a multicenter trial in Ontario. They found that personalized cooler dialysate did not change cardiovascular outcomes when compared with standard temperature dialysate baths, questioning its benefits [35].

Fluid Removal

Rounding physicians establish a targeted weight to maintain adequate fluid balance. Historically, intradialytic weight gains above the "estimated dry weight" were removed by ultrafiltration, as excess gains put additional strain on the cardiovascular system. The Hemodialysis Study (HEMO Study) was a large trial of 1846 chronic hemodialysis patients who were followed for 7 years. They were dialyzed three times a week. The total amount ultrafiltered was expressed as mL/kg/h. Patients were divided into three categories, ≤10 mL/kg/h, between 10 and 13 mL/kg/h, and >13 mL/kg/h. Between 10 and 13 mL/kg/h, the hazard ratio was 1.59, and in the group having >13 mL/kg/h removed, the hazard ratio was 1.71. The all-cause cardiovascular mortality began to rise at ultrafiltration rates >10 mL/kg/h [36]. These findings suggest that large fluid gain removal achieved by either extending the dialysis time or by adding an additional weekly treatment.

Potassium Prescriptions

The serum potassium level ranges within a window that reflects the extremes of health. It is more abundant inside the cell, and the large differences across the cell wall create the electrical gradients that permit the transfer of substances essential for the cell to function. The normal kidney closely guards potassium homeostasis, and when kidney function is lost, hyperkalemia threatens to depolarize muscle cells resulting in their ability to contract. This can lead to paralysis in skeletal muscle and ventricular fibrillation in the heart. When the serum potassium falls too low, it generally reflects low total body potassium and can also lead to arrhythmias and muscle weakness. The patient who presents to dialysis with a serum potassium level >6 mEq/L (or mmol/L) is at risk for both all cause and cardiovascular mortality [37]. Acute changes in potassium during dialysis caused by a high serum-to-dialysate ratio are also associated with arrhythmia and ventricular events over the 12 h post-dialysis. A large drop in serum potassium during dialysis is most likely accompanied by metabolic alkalosis and hypotension-related ischemia. It may trigger arrhythmia and even death at the end of a dialysis session. Dialysate potassium baths less than 2.0 mEq/L have been associated with sudden death [31]. A DOPPS reviews the following year found that dialysate potassium baths less than 1.5 mEq/L were associated with sudden death (HR 1.28; 95% CI 1.12–1.74; $P = 0.004$). The same DOPPS study also found a higher HR 1.17 (95% CI 1.01–1.37, p 0.04) for dialysate K bath between 2 and 2.5) [38]. As low potassium rates are also associated with dialysis mortality, the dialysate prescription should be individualized.

Hospitalizations and death are more common on Mondays and Tuesdays following a 2-day interdialytic period. A systemic review of 102 studies demonstrated a median prevalence of hyperkalemia in hemodialysis patients of 21.6%. Some were taking concomitant potassium-sparing medications. The increased all-cause and cardiovascular mortalities were associated with the longer interval. The weakness of this review was that the definitions for hyperkalemia-associated mortality were not specified [39]. Seasonal variation can also influence hyperkalemia, with mid-week serum potassium values being higher in the summer months. Shortened dialysis periods to less than 4 h are also associated with a greater odds ratio of hyperkalemia (OR 2.568; 95% CI 1.045–6.313) [40].

Dietary manipulation, assuring adequate dialysis times, altering the dialysis days, and attentiveness to medications that potentiate hyperkalemia may help to control the serum potassium and prevent adverse events. A healthy plant-based diet (fruits, vegetables, nuts, and beans) has not been associated with hyperkalemia [41]. Potassium-based binders are now readily available and useful to control potassium levels. Further studies to determine evidence of their effectiveness in reducing mortality are needed. Therapy should be tailored to individual requirements [42, 43].

Hypokalemia ($K < 3.5$ mEq/L) is rare in hemodialysis patients but is often seen in patients on peritoneal dialysis. In hemodialysis patients, it generally reflects a decrease in total body potassium and may require dialysis on a higher potassium bath and sometimes potassium supplements. It can be associated with muscle weakness. In hemodialysis patients, it is most likely seen with poor nutritional intake or chronic diarrhea [44]. Six hundred twenty-four hemodialysis patients from a multicenter clinical trial were categorized by dialysis bath. Dialysis potassium baths of 1 mEq/L were associated with higher mortality than 2 or 3 mEq/L baths, particularly when the serum potassium was ≥5 mEq/L. [adjusted hazard ratio 2.87 (95% Confidence Level 1.51–5.46)] [45].

Inadequate Dialysis

Starting with Clyde Shields, the Boeing machinist who became the first chronic hemodialysis patient in March 1960, the frequency and duration of treatment times have varied. Shields was dialyzed 76 h at a time, but the duration was soon modified to 12–20 h twice a week. By October 1964, patients were dialyzing 6–8 h thrice weekly, and this became the standard by 1972 when Congress signed into law legislation that provided Medicare benefits to dialysis patients. In 1975, the National Institute of Health (NIH) sponsored the National Cooperative Dialysis Study (NCDS), using a mathematical relationship between urea equilibrium and the removal of solutes, the single pool Kt/*V* (spKt/*V*), to assess dialysis adequacy. The model was based on the dialyzer clearance rate of urea, K (mL/min), time (minutes), and the distribution volume of urea. Kt/*V* became the universal standard for assessing dialysis quality. Its use in the NCDS led the renal community to think that protein intake that fell to less than 0.8 was the cause of dialysis outcome failure. The protein catabolic rate (PCR) was shown to be a determinant of dialysis failure, with failure highest when the PCR fell below 0.8. The Kt/*V* was felt to be dependent on PCR. The study also suggested that elevated Kt/*V* rates did not improve dialysis outcomes. As a result of the NCDS, along with the development of high flux dialyzers, and the use of bicarbonate baths instead of acetate baths, dialysis times were shortened. By the late 1980s, the mortality rate in the USA was worse than that of other countries that had longer treatment times [46]. In 1993, it was demonstrated that raising the Kt/*V* to 1.4 was cost-effective and improved clinical outcomes [47]. The Hemodialysis Study (HEMO Study) was a large NIH trial that began in 1995 and ended in 2000. Hemodialysis patients were randomized between shorter and longer dialysis sessions. The equilibrated Kt/*V* (eKt/*V*) accounted for the blood rebound after dialysis and was generally 15–20% lower than the spKt/*V*. The study demonstrated that the shorter session patients with an spKt/*V* of 1.32 ± 0.09 and the high-dose group having an spKt/*V* of 1.71 ± 0.11 did not significantly differ in the risk of death. The study did demonstrate the benefit of high flux dialysis [48].

The current guidelines call for a minimum spKt/*V* of 1.20, but this adequacy parameter does not reflect the impact other molecules may have on patient well-being. Many of these molecules are also toxic, larger in size than urea, and have molecular weights in the 3000–30,000 range. Other toxins may be protein-bound. We are just beginning to explore toxins that are derived from the intestines. As therapy for kidney disease continues to evolve, we continue to question whether we are doing enough concerning renal replacement therapy [49, 50]. From a practical perspective, shortening treatment times to under 210 min is associated with a hazard ratio (HR) of 1.13 for sudden death. A Kt/*V* under 1.2 is associated with an HR for sudden death of 1.10 [31].

Conclusion

The complex process of using municipal water to create a solution that can be interfaced with extracorporeal blood to maintain the health of patients with end-stage kidney disease is one of the finest achievements in the history of medicine. Although errors and complications related to the procedure are rare, they can and do happen. This chapter described the procedure and highlights where pitfalls can occur and what precautions can be taken to minimize them.

References

1. Bray BD, Boyd J, Daly C, Doyle A, Donaldson K, Fox JG, et al. How safe is renal replacement therapy? A national study of mortality and adverse events contributing to the death of renal replacement therapy recipients. Nephrol Dial Transplant. 2014;29(3):681–7. https://doi.org/10.1093/ndt/gft197.
2. Reinhold RB. Dual failure in kidney machine blamed for 3 deaths in Dallas. New York: The New York Times; 1983.
3. Vick KE, Johnson CA. Aluminum-related osteomalacia in renal-failure patients. Clin Pharm. 1985;4(4):434–9.
4. Wills MR, Savory J. Water content of aluminum, dialysis dementia, and osteomalacia. Environ Health Perspect. 1985;63:141–7. https://doi.org/10.1289/ehp.8563141.
5. Chuang PH, Tsai KF, Wang IK, Huang YC, Huang LM, Liu SH, et al. Blood aluminum levels in patients with hemodialysis and peritoneal dialysis. Int J Environ Res Public Health. 2022;19(7):3885. https://doi.org/10.3390/ijerph19073885.
6. Michener JA. The source. New York: Random House; 1965.
7. Tipple MA, Shusterman N, Bland LA, McCarthy MA, Favero MS, Arduino MJ, et al. Illness in hemodialysis patients after exposure to chloramine contaminated dialysate. ASAIO Trans. 1991;37(4):588–91.
8. Calderaro RV, Heller L. Outbreak of hemolytic reactions associated with chlorine and chloramine residuals in hemodialysis water. Rev Saude Publica. 2001;35(5):481–6. https://doi.org/10.1590/s0034-89102001000500012.
9. Emenaker NJ, DiSilvestro RA, Nahman NS Jr, Percival S. Copper-related blood indexes in kidney dialysis patients. Am J Clin Nutr. 1996;64(5):757–60. https://doi.org/10.1093/ajcn/64.5.757.
10. Royer A, Sharman T. Copper toxicity. Treasure Island (FL): StatPearls Publishing; 2022.
11. Bland LA, Arnow PM, Arduino MJ, Bova J, McAllister SK. Potential hazards of deionization systems used for water purification in hemodialysis. Artif Organs. 1996;20(1):2–7. https://doi.org/10.1111/j.1525-1594.1996.tb04411.x.
12. Arnow PM, Bland LA, Garcia-Houchins S, Fridkin S, Fellner SK. An outbreak of fatal fluoride intoxication in a long-term hemodialysis unit. Ann Intern Med. 1994;121(5):339–44. https://doi.org/10.7326/0003-4819-121-5-199409010-00005.
13. Jack L. Lead poisoning: a historical perspective. 1985. **https://www.cdc.gov/fluoridation/basics/timeline.html**. Accessed 1985.

14. Huang W-H, Hsu C-W, Weng C-H, Lin-Tan D-T, Yen T-H. Negative relationship between erythropoietin dose and blood lead level in patients undergoing maintenance hemodialysis. Sci Rep. 2016;6(1):34313. https://doi.org/10.1038/srep34313.
15. Shalaby E, Abdelmawgoud H. MO894 Evaluations of toxic metals lead and mercury in regular hemodialysis smoker and nonsmoker patients by comparison with other healthy control subjects in an Egyptian population. Nephrol Dial Transplant. 2021;36(Supplement_1):19. https://doi.org/10.1093/ndt/gfab100.0019.
16. Heredia Martinez A, Rosa Diez G, Ferraris V, Coccia PA, Ferraris JR, Checa A, et al. Removal of nitrate and nitrite by hemodialysis in end-stage renal disease and by sustained low-efficiency dialysis in acute kidney injury. Nitric Oxide. 2020;98:33–40. https://doi.org/10.1016/j.niox.2020.02.004.
17. Yildirim I, Hur E, Magden K, İlikhan S, Engin H, Can M, et al. Serum sulphate levels in hemodialysis patients. Int J Nephrol. 2019;2019:1063514. https://doi.org/10.1155/2019/1063514.
18. Tonelli M, Wiebe N, Hemmelgarn B, Klarenbach S, Field C, Manns B, et al. Trace elements in hemodialysis patients: a systematic review and meta-analysis. BMC Med. 2009;7:25. https://doi.org/10.1186/1741-7015-7-25.
19. ANSI/AAMI ISO 23500-1:2019. Arlington, VA: Association for the Advancement of Medical Instrumentation; 2022.
20. Reason J. Managing the risks of organizational accidents. Burlington: Ashgate; 1997.
21. Ledebo I. Purification of dialysis fluid: historical background and perspective. Blood Purif. 2009;27(Suppl. 1):17–9. https://doi.org/10.1159/000213492.
22. Gotloib L, Servadio C. Microampere electrocution during haemodialysis—an unrecognised cause of sudden death. Proc Eur Dial Transplant Assoc. 1975;11:210–3.
23. Levin A, Goldstein MB. The benefits and side effects of ramped hypertonic sodium dialysis. J Am Soc Nephrol. 1996;7(2):242–6. https://doi.org/10.1681/asn.V72242.
24. Flythe JE, Tugman MJ, Narendra JH, Assimon MM, Li Q, Wang Y, et al. Effect of ultrafiltration profiling on outcomes among maintenance hemodialysis patients: a pilot randomized crossover trial. J Nephrol. 2021;34(1):113–23. https://doi.org/10.1007/s40620-020-00862-6.
25. Flythe JE, Mc Causland FR. Dialysate sodium: rationale for evolution over time. Semin Dial. 2017;30(2):99–111. https://doi.org/10.1111/sdi.12570.
26. Obialo C, John S, Bashir K. Iatrogenic hypernatremia in hemodialysis patients: a result erroneous online conductivity monitor and conductivity meter reading: hypernatremia and conductivity errors. Hemodial Int. 2017;21:E73–5. https://doi.org/10.1111/hdi.12546.
27. Yu C-H, Huang H-W, Sung J-M. Sudden coma and quadriplegia in a hemodialysis patient. Kidney360. 2020;1(9):1036–7. https://doi.org/10.34067/kid.0001622020.
28. Thornley-Brown D, Saha M. Dialysate content and risk of sudden cardiac death. Curr Opin Nephrol Hypertens. 2015;24(6):557–62. https://doi.org/10.1097/mnh.0000000000000177.
29. Bommer J, Locatelli F, Satayathum S, Keen ML, Goodkin DA, Saito A, et al. Association of predialysis serum bicarbonate levels with risk of mortality and hospitalization in the Dialysis Outcomes and Practice Patterns Study (DOPPS). Am J Kidney Dis. 2004;44(4):661–71.
30. Rhee CM, Chou JA, Kalantar-Zadeh K. Dialysis prescription and sudden death. Semin Nephrol. 2018;38(6):570–81. https://doi.org/10.1016/j.semnephrol.2018.08.003.
31. Pun PH, Lehrich RW, Honeycutt EF, Herzog CA, Middleton JP. Modifiable risk factors associated with sudden cardiac arrest within hemodialysis clinics. Kidney Int. 2011;79(2):218–27. https://doi.org/10.1038/ki.2010.315.
32. Flythe JE, Li NC, Lin SF, Brunelli SM, Hymes J, Lacson E Jr. Associates of cardiopulmonary arrest in the perihemodialytic period. Int J Nephrol. 2014;2014:961978. https://doi.org/10.1155/2014/961978.
33. Mustafa RA, Bdair F, Akl EA, Garg AX, Thiessen-Philbrook H, Salameh H, et al. Effect of lowering the dialysate temperature in chronic hemodialysis: a systematic review and meta-analysis. Clin J Am Soc Nephrol. 2016;11(3):442–57. https://doi.org/10.2215/cjn.04580415.
34. Eldehni MT, Odudu A, McIntyre CW. Randomized clinical trial of dialysate cooling and effects on brain white matter. J Am Soc Nephrol. 2015;26(4):957–65. https://doi.org/10.1681/asn.2013101086.

35. MyTEMP Writing Committee. Personalised cooler dialysate for patients receiving maintenance haemodialysis (MyTEMP): a pragmatic, cluster-randomised trial. Lancet. 2022;400(10364):1693–703. https://doi.org/10.1016/s0140-6736(22)01805-0.
36. Flythe JE, Kimmel SE, Brunelli SM. Rapid fluid removal during dialysis is associated with cardiovascular morbidity and mortality. Kidney Int. 2011;79(2):250–7. https://doi.org/10.1038/ki.2010.383.
37. Shibata S, Uchida S. Hyperkalemia in patients undergoing hemodialysis: its pathophysiology and management. Ther Apher Dial. 2021;26(1):3–14. https://doi.org/10.1111/1744-9987.13721.
38. Jadoul M, Thumma J, Fuller DS, Tentori F, Li Y, Morgenstern H, et al. Modifiable practices associated with sudden death among hemodialysis patients in the Dialysis Outcomes and Practice Patterns Study. Clin J Am Soc Nephrol. 2012;7(5):765–74. https://doi.org/10.2215/cjn.08850811.
39. Bem D, Sugrue D, Wilding B, Zile I, Butler K, Booth D, et al. The effect of hyperkalemia and long inter-dialytic interval on morbidity and mortality in patients receiving hemodialysis: a systematic review. Ren Fail. 2021;43(1):241–54. https://doi.org/10.1080/0886022x.2020.1871012.
40. Tsiagka D, Georgianos PI, Pikilidou MI, Vaios V, Roumeliotis S, Syrganis C, et al. Prevalence, recurrence and seasonal variation of hyperkalemia among patients on hemodialysis. Int Urol Nephrol. 2022;54(9):2327–34. https://doi.org/10.1007/s11255-022-03142-3.
41. González-Ortiz A, Xu H, Ramos-Acevedo S, Avesani CM, Lindholm B, Correa-Rotter R, et al. Nutritional status, hyperkalaemia and attainment of energy/protein intake targets in haemodialysis patients following plant-based diets: a longitudinal cohort study. Nephrol Dial Transplant. 2020;36(4):681–8. https://doi.org/10.1093/ndt/gfaa194.
42. Sanghavi S, Whiting S, Uribarri J. Potassium balance in dialysis patients. Semin Dial. 2013;26(5):597–603. https://doi.org/10.1111/sdi.12123.
43. Fishbane S, Charytan DM, Chertow GM, Ford M, Kovesdy CP, Pergola PE, et al. Consensus-based recommendations for the management of hyperkalemia in the hemodialysis setting. J Ren Nutr. 2021;32(4):e1–e14. https://doi.org/10.1053/j.jrn.2021.06.003.
44. Choi HY, Ha SK. Potassium balances in maintenance hemodialysis. Electrolyte Blood Press. 2013;11(1):9–16. https://doi.org/10.5049/ebp.2013.11.1.9.
45. Ferrey A, You AS, Kovesdy CP, Nakata T, Veliz M, Nguyen DV, et al. Dialysate potassium and mortality in a prospective hemodialysis cohort. Am J Nephrol. 2018;47(6):415–23. https://doi.org/10.1159/000489961.
46. Fadem S. Milestones in dialysis. Issues in dialysis. New York: Nova Science Publishers; 2012.
47. Hornberger JC. The hemodialysis prescription and cost effectiveness. Renal physicians association working committee on clinical guidelines. J Am Soc Nephrol. 1993;4(4):1021–7. https://doi.org/10.1681/asn.V441021.
48. Eknoyan G, Beck GJ, Cheung AK, Daugirdas JT, Greene T, Kusek JW, et al. Effect of dialysis dose and membrane flux in maintenance hemodialysis. N Engl J Med. 2002;347(25):2010–9. https://doi.org/10.1056/NEJMoa021583.
49. Daugirdas JT, Depner TA, Inrig J, Mehrotra R, Rocco MV, Suri RS, et al. KDOQI clinical practice guideline for hemodialysis adequacy: 2015 update. Am J Kidney Dis. 2015;66(5):884–930. https://doi.org/10.1053/j.ajkd.2015.07.015.
50. Vanholder R, Glorieux G, Eloot S. Once upon a time in dialysis: the last days of Kt/V? Kidney Int. 2015;88(3):460–5. https://doi.org/10.1038/ki.2015.155.

Cardiovascular and Hemodynamic Complications in Dialysis

2

Ana Flávia Moura, José A. Moura-Neto, Cibele Isaac Saad Rodrigues, Viviane Calice-Silva, and Roberto Pecoits-Filho

Introduction

Chronic kidney disease (CKD) is an important health issue, not only due to its high prevalence but also because it is closely associated with cardiovascular diseases (CVD), the leading cause of global mortality [1]. In CKD patients, hypertension (HTN) is the major cardiovascular complication, and its prevalence increases with declining kidney function.

There are currently around four million people on dialysis worldwide [2]. Considering the gap in renal replacement therapy, we can imagine that this number should be even higher. CVD mortality among dialysis patients is 20–50 times higher than in the general population [3]. In the United States, the prevalence of CVD in patients with CKD can reach 63%, depending on factors such as age-group [4]. This means a risk is about nine times higher than in the general population.

The estimated worldwide prevalence of patients with CKD is around 10% [5]. CVD and kidney disease are strongly associated, and impairment of one organ

A. F. Moura · J. A. Moura-Neto (✉)
Bahiana School of Medicine and Public Health, Salvador, Bahia, Brazil
e-mail: mouraneto@bahiana.edu.br

C. I. S. Rodrigues
Pontifical Catholic University of São Paulo, São Paulo, Brazil

Santa Lucinda Hospital (FUNDASP), Sorocaba, São Paulo, Brazil

V. Calice-Silva
Joinville Region University, Joinville, Santa Catarina, Brazil

Pro-Rim Foundation, Joinville, Santa Catarina, Brazil

R. Pecoits-Filho
Pontifical Catholic University of Parana, Curitiba, Brazil

Arbor Research Collaborative for Health, Ann Arbor, MI, USA

S. Z. Fadem et al. (eds.), *Complications in Dialysis*,
https://doi.org/10.1007/978-3-031-44557-6_2

causes dysfunction of the other. It is estimated that about 70–80% of patients on hemodialysis (HD) [6, 7] and 30–90% of patients on peritoneal dialysis (PD) [8, 9] have HTN. Stroke is also a significant global health issue; dialysis patients experience a tenfold higher incidence, with case fatality rates reaching 90% [10]. In the same way, 29–75% of patients on HD present left ventricular hypertrophy (LVH) [11].

Understanding the pathophysiological mechanisms involved in each prevalent condition is crucial for successful treatment. Dialysis patients have particularities that may make it difficult to choose the most appropriate medication or even require adjustments in dialysis therapy to achieve clinical compensation. This chapter intends to discuss the most prevalent cardiovascular complications among dialysis patients and the management of these conditions.

Blood Pressure and Dialysis Patients

HTN and chronic kidney disease (CKD) are seriously interrelated global public health problems. HTN is highly prevalent in end-stage renal disease (ESRD) patients undergoing dialysis [6]. It is estimated that about 70–80% of patients on HD [6, 7], and 30–90% of patients on PD [8, 9] have HTN, often characterized as resistant or refractory [12].

The risk of cardiovascular events, especially cardiovascular morbidity and mortality are 10–20 times higher in dialysis patients than in the general population.

Pathophysiology of Hypertension in Dialysis Patients

The pathophysiology of hypertension in dialysis patients has complex and multifactorial mechanisms and persists poorly understood.

Factors involved in the development of hypertension in dialysis patients can be seen in Fig. 2.1. Treatment of these patients aims to control sodium intake and volume overload and block the hyperactivity of vasopressor systems involved.

How and When to Measure Blood Pressure in Dialysis Patients for Diagnosis

Although blood pressure (BP) measurement is broadly available and performed in most clinical settings, including dialysis units, it still needs to be standardized, and practitioners frequently neglect the recommendations to prevent measurement errors [13]. Figure 2.2 summarizes the steps for proper patient preparation and office BP measurement.

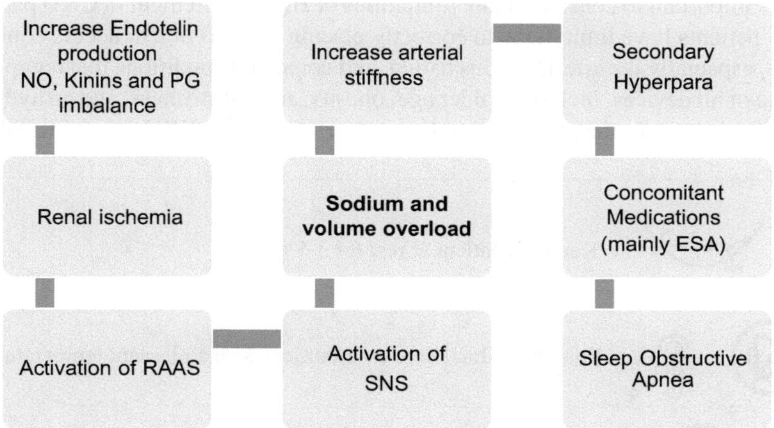

Fig. 2.1 Pathophysiology of hypertension in dialysis patients. *NO* nitric oxide, *PG* prostaglandins, *RAAS* renin–angiotensin–aldosterone system, *SNS* sympathetic nervous system, *Hyperpara* hyperparathyroidism, *ESA* erythropoiesis stimulating agents

Empowered patients who are well informed on how BP measurements should be performed at home or in a dialysis unit may be the best advocates for trustful BP measurements in routine clinical practice [14].

The preferred methods of BP measurement in HD patients have not been established, but most of the existent clinical studies have used pre-HD BP to determine target BP levels or investigate the outcomes of antihypertensive medications.

Regardless of whether BP is measured in the dialysis unit, at home (HBPM), or with ambulatory BP monitoring (ABPM), a proper technique is critical to certify as accurate an assessment as possible given the intrinsic variability of BP [14].

Meticulous guidance for BP measurement has been provided in the 2017 ACC/AHA BP guideline [15], the 2018 European Society of Cardiology/European Society of Hypertension (ESH) guidelines [16], a 2019 National Heart, Lung, and Blood Institute Working Group report [17], a 2019 AHA Scientific Statement [18] and the 2020 Brazilian Hypertension Guidelines [19].

BP measurements obtained outside of dialysis units should be performed to consistently diagnose hypertension among dialysis patients. Home BP monitoring is widely applied and strongly recommended by all guidelines for the diagnosis and management of HTN in the general population and chronic kidney disease (CKD) patients [15–19]. Out-of-dialysis-unit BP measurements have shown to be superior to conventional BP measurements as they are linearly associated with mortality [20].

ABPM is widely considered the "gold standard" method for diagnosing hypertension in patients receiving dialysis [21–24]. There is a high prevalence of sleep BP disturbances, non-dipping, and even nocturnal HTN in dialysis patients, which makes ABPM more compelling than in the general population [25].

It is important to consider many limitations of BP measurement in CKD patients. Many patients have limitations to correctly placing the cuff due to access considerations, especially the arteriovenous fistula, and comorbid conditions that complicate the use of all devices, including older age, obesity, arterial stiffness, and arrhythmias [26]. In many countries, there is another concern because ABPM is not available in

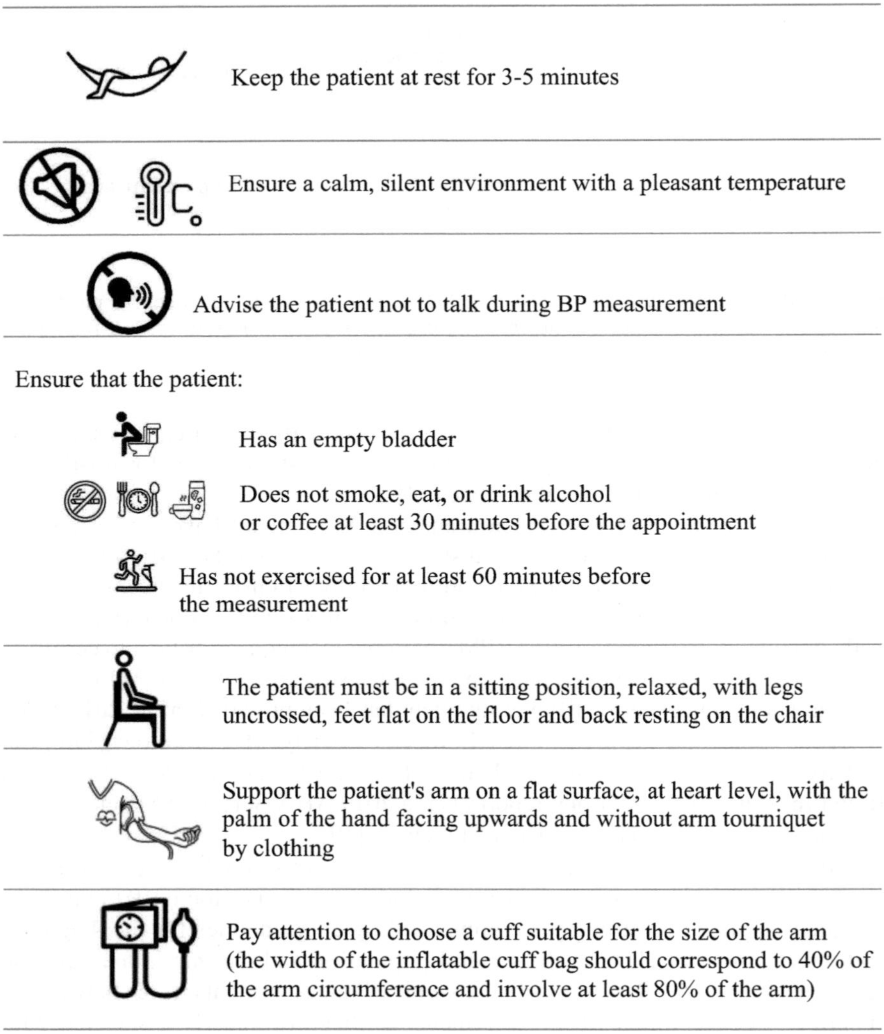

Fig. 2.2 Patient preparation and correct BP measurement in the office. *Applied to the auscultatory technique. *BP* blood pressure. (*Figure adapted from: In: Moura AF, Rodrigues CIS. Hipertensão Arterial: Manual Prático. Piracicaba (SP): Editora Balieiro; 2022.*)

Steps of Blood Pressure Measurement
Place the cuff, leaving no gaps, 2 to 3 cm above the cubital fossa, centralizing the middle of the inflatable bag over the brachial artery.
Estimate the level of systolic blood pressure*
Palpate the brachial artery in the cubital fossa and place the stethoscope bell or diaphragm without undue compression*
Rapidly inflate to 20-30 mmHg above the estimated systolic blood pressure*
Perform the deflation slowly (speed of 2 mmHg/second)*
Determine the systolic BP on auscultation of the first sound (Korotkoff phase I) and then slightly increase the deflation velocity*
Determine diastolic BP at the disappearance of sounds (Korotkoff phase V). Continue auscultation about 20-30 mmHg below the last sound to confirm its disappearance, and then proceed with rapid and complete deflation. If the beats persist until the zero level, determine the diastolic in the muffling of the sounds (Korotkoff phase IV) and write down systolic/diastolic/zero BP values, as can occur in children, pregnant women and in hyperkinetic states*

Fig. 2.2 (continued)

Table 2.1 Definition of hypertension in hemodialysis patients

• No recommendation can be made based on pre- or post-dialysis BP. When out-of-BP measurement is not available, the diagnosis can be based on office BP measurements taken in a mid-weekday free of hemodialysis, following all the steps of international guidelines. The average of three measurements with BP ≥140/90 mmHg can be used for diagnosing HTN in HD patients
• HBPM in HD patients: an average BP ≥135/85 mmHg for measurements taken twice/day, in a duplicate manner in the morning and in the evening, over 6 non-dialysis days (covering a period of 2 weeks). Measures should be performed as referred in guidelines
• ABPM in HD patients: an average BP ≥130/80 mmHg over 24-h monitoring during a mid-weekday free of hemodialysis. The preferred method, whenever possible, is extended 44-h ABPM, that is, covering a whole mid-week dialysis free interval

BP blood pressure, *HTN* hypertension, *ABPM* ambulatory blood pressure monitoring, *HBPM* home blood pressure monitoring

public health services, and the literature indicates that 44-h ABPM is probably the best method for dialysis patients.

Based on the evidence provided by a prospective cohort study, 44-h recording ABPM, or 1-week HBPM, has more prognostic power for target organ damage and mortality than conventional BP measurements [27].

The preferred definition of HTN in HD patients is presented in Table 2.1, and the preferred definition of HTN in PD patients is presented in Table 2.2.

Table 2.2 Definition of hypertension in peritoneal dialysis patients

• HBPM in PD patients: An average BP ≥135/85 mmHg for measurements taken twice/day, in a duplicate manner in the morning and in the evening, over 7 consecutive days Measures should be performed as referred in guidelines
• ABPM in PD patients: an average BP ≥130/80 mmHg over 24-h monitoring. The preferred method, whenever possible, is extended 44-h ABPM

BP blood pressure, *HTN* hypertension, *ABPM* ambulatory blood pressure monitoring, *HBPM* home blood pressure monitoring

Table 2.3 Blood pressure targets according to clinical practice guidelines

KDOQI 2005	Pre-dialysis BP <140/90 mmHg Post-dialysis BP <130/80 mmHg
KDOQI 2015 (update)	No target recommended (lack of good evidence)
ISPD 2015	BP <140/90 mmHg
EURECA-m, ERA—EDTA, ESH 2017	No target recommended (lack of good evidence)
KDIGO 2021	No target BP is recommended. KDIGO recommendations are specific for CKD population not-receiving dialysis
Brazilian HTN guidelines—2020	Individualization of treatment in renal replacement therapy, considering comorbidities, pharmacokinetics, and the cardioprotective effect of medications

KDOQI Kidney Disease Outcomes Quality Initiative, *EURECA-m* European Renal and Cardiovascular Medicine, *ISPD* International Society of Peritoneal Dialysis, *ERA EDTA* European Renal Association and European Dialysis and Transplant Association, *ESH* European Hypertension Society, *KDIGO* Kidney Diseases Improving Global Outcomes, *HTN* hypertension, *CKD* chronic kidney disease

Target Blood Pressure in Dialysis Patients

Most nephrologists rely on targets for HTN in dialysis patients that were inferred from the general population, which is inaccurate since dialysis patients have unique characteristics. Nonetheless, based on this rationale, the 2005 National Kidney Foundation Kidney Disease Outcomes and Quality Initiative (KDOQI) guidelines recommended aiming for pre-dialysis BP <140/90 mmHg and a post-dialysis BP <130/80 mmHg [28]. However, there is observational evidence that these BP levels are associated with higher mortality and may even be harmful.

In patients on dialysis, a high-risk population, the BP target is challenging and still controversial, considering that previous observational studies reported a U or reverse J-shaped association between BP and all-cause mortality, indicating higher mortality at low systolic BP [29]. Based on these studies, most guidelines recommend achieving a systolic BP >120 mmHg, which appears to have a protective effect on mortality among dialysis patients [30].

Accordingly, available clinical practice guidelines available do not recommend a target or otherwise use the pre-dialysis BP <140/90 mmHg (Table 2.3) based on expert opinion. For PD patients, most guidelines recommend BP <140/90 mmHg.

It's reasonable to advocate that BP goals should be individualized considering many factors like age, frailty, comorbidities (e.g., diabetes, coronary artery disease, stroke), dialysis type, dialysis vintage, interdialytic weight gain, intradialytic hypotension, and duration of HTN [29, 31].

Treating Hypertension in Dialysis Patients

A combination of pharmacological and non-pharmacological interventions should be employed to achieve better clinical outcomes in dialysis patients.

A key factor of BP in both HD and PD patients is sodium and body fluid volume. Individual patient BPs fluctuate in the pre-dialytic period, throughout a dialysis session, as well as between sessions [32]. Accordingly, the results of trials in non-end-stage renal disease (ESRD) patients cannot be extrapolated to patients with ESRD on dialysis. Therefore, ESRD patients have usually excluded from cardiovascular trials.

Restricting dietary salt and water intake is an evidence-based recommendation. High salt intake has been associated with high pre-dialysis systolic BP (SBP) and cardiovascular death [33]. It is a key point to maintain proper body fluid volume to manage hypertension in HD patients. For this purpose, providing education to patients in order to reduce dietary salt intake should be a first-line therapy. An increase in fluid volume can be monitored by body weight, and interdialytic weight gain should not exceed 0.8 kg/day.

In the Dry-weight (DW) Reduction in Hypertensive HD Patients (DRIP) randomized controlled trial (RCT), a 1-kg DW decrease at 8 weeks resulted in systolic and diastolic BP reductions by 6.6 and 3.3 mmHg, respectively [34]. It is a simple and effective way to improve BP control, despite the difficulties of using reliable parameters to establish a proper DW.

In two clinical trials, frequent HD significantly reduced BP and can be a good strategy to improve BP control when compared to conventional thrice weekly regimens [35, 36].

In PD patients, fluid removal strategies are different from those for HD patients. In this population, residual renal function contributes significantly to volume balance, and it should be frequently estimated. Therefore, the initial approach to hypertension in PD patients should always involve the evaluation of volume status and treatment of hypervolemia before any adjustment to the antihypertensive regimen. According to the International Society of Peritoneal Dialysis (ISPD), in spite of the utility of hypertonic glucose solutions for PD for volume removal, one should minimize glucose exposure in PD through salt restriction, use of diuretics among those with residual renal function (RRF), and when indicated, the use of glucose-sparing solutions to optimize volume control [30].

Two meta-analyses of randomized trials, published in 2009, suggest that controlling HTN with antihypertensive drugs is associated with reduced cardiovascular morbidity and mortality among dialysis patients [37, 38].

There is weak evidence to recommend one class of antihypertensive drug over another to dialysis patients, and only limited data from clinical trials have demonstrated some beneficial cardiovascular effects of RAAS inhibitors and β-adrenergic blockers in those patients. Table 2.4 brings together the main oral antihypertensives and their characteristics in terms of removal in dialysis.

Table 2.4 Antihypertensive drugs and their use in dialysis patients

Antihypertensive	Usual daily dose (mg)	Frequency of doses per day	Dose adjustment in CKD	Dialysis removal rate
Hydrochlorothiazide	25–50	1	No dose adjustment is necessary. Use not recommended if eGFR <30 mL/min	**HD:** Insignificant removal **PD:** Insignificant removal
Chlorthalidone	12.5–25	1	No dose adjustment is necessary. Use not recommended if eGFR <30 mL/min	**HD:** Insignificant removal **PD:** Insignificant removal
Indapamide	1.5–3.0	1	**GFR >50 mL/min:** No dose adjustment is necessary. **GFR <50 mL/min:** 1.25–2.5 mg/day	**HD:** Insignificant removal **PD:** Insignificant removal
Furosemide	20–240	1–3	**GFR >30 mL/min:** No dose adjustment is necessary. Higher doses required for GFR <30 mL/min	**HD:** Insignificant removal **PD:** Insignificant removal
Bumetanide	1–4	1–3	No dose adjustment is necessary	**HD:** Insignificant removal **PD:** Insignificant removal
Spironolactone	25–100	1–2	No dose adjustment is necessary. Use not recommended if eGFR <30 mL/min	**HD:** Insignificant removal **PD:** Insignificant removal
Amiloride	2.5–5	1	**GFR 10–50 mL/min:** 50% of the usual dose **GFR <10 mL/min:** Use not recommended	–
Amlodipine	2.5–10	1	No dose adjustment is necessary	**HD:** Insignificant removal **PD:** Insignificant removal
Felodipine	2.5–10	1	No dose adjustment is necessary	**HD:** Insignificant removal **PD:** Insignificant removal
Nifedipine	10–60	1–3	No dose adjustment is necessary	**HD:** Insignificant removal **PD:** Insignificant removal
Nitrendipine	10–30	1	No dose adjustment is necessary	**HD:** Insignificant removal **PD:** Insignificant removal
Lercanidipine	10–20	1	No dose adjustment is necessary	**HD:** Insignificant removal **PD:** Insignificant removal
Verapamil	120–360	1–2	No dose adjustment is necessary	**HD:** Insignificant removal **PD:** Insignificant removal
Diltiazem	80–240	1–2	No dose adjustment is necessary	**HD:** Insignificant removal **PD:** Insignificant removal

Captopril	25–150	2–3	**GFR 10-50 mL/min:** 75% of the usual dose every 12 h **GFR <10 mL/min:** 50% of the usual dose every 24 h	**HD:** Extra dose after HD **DP:** remoção insignificante
Enalapril	5–40	1–2	**GFR >30 mL/min:** No dose adjustment is necessary **GFR ≤30 mL/min:** starting 2.5 mg/day and slowly increase according to BP	**HD:** 20–50% removal rate. Extra dose of 2.5 mg after HD **DP:** Adjust dose to 25% of usual dose
Benazepril	10–40	1–2	**GFR >30 mL/min**: No dose adjustment is necessary **GFR ≤30 mL/min:** starting 5 mg/day and slowly increase according to BP	**HD:** Adjust dose to 25–50% of usual dose. No extra dose post-HD **DP:** Adjust dose to 25–50% of usual dose. No extra dose post-PD
Lisinopril	10–40	1	**RFG ≥30 mL/min:** No dose adjustment is necessary **GFR 10–30 mL/min:** starting 2.5–5 mg/day and slowly increase according to BP **GFR <10 mL/min:** consider substituting another drug (high risk of AE)	**HD:** 50% removal rate. Recommend use after HD on dialysis days or 10 mg thrice a week after HD, increasing the dose progressively according to BP **DP:** 2.5 mg/day and slowly increase according to BP
Fosinopril	10–40	1	No dose adjustment is necessary	**HD:** Insignificant removal **PD:** Insignificant removal
Ramipril	2.5–20	1–2	**GFR >40 mL/min:** No dose adjustment is necessary **GFR ≥40 mL/min:** 25% of the usual dose	**HD:** Insignificant removal **PD:** Insignificant removal
Perindopril	4–16	1	**GFR >80 mL/min:** No dose adjustment is necessary **GFR 30–80 mL/min:** starting 2 mg/day and slowly increase according to BP. Maximum dose 8 mg/day **GFR <30 mL/min:** Use not recommended	**HD:** Insignificant removal **PD:** Insignificant removal
Losartan	50–100	1–2	No dose adjustment is necessary	**HD:** Insignificant removal **PD:** Insignificant removal
Valsartan	80–320	1	No dose adjustment is necessary	**HD:** Insignificant removal **PD:** Insignificant removal
Irbesartan	150–300	1	No dose adjustment is necessary	**HD:** Insignificant removal **PD:** Insignificant removal
Candesartan	8–32	1	No dose adjustment is necessary	**HD:** Insignificant removal **PD:** Insignificant removal

(continued)

Table 2.4 (continued)

Antihypertensive	Usual daily dose (mg)	Frequency of doses per day	Dose adjustment in CKD	Dialysis removal rate
Olmesartan	20–40	1	No dose adjustment is necessary	**HD:** Insignificant removal **PD:** Insignificant removal
Telmisartan	20–80	1	No dose adjustment is necessary	**HD:** Insignificant removal **PD:** Insignificant removal
Propranolol	80–320	2–3	No dose adjustment is necessary	**HD:** Insignificant removal **PD:** Insignificant removal
Nadolol	40–160	1	**GFR >50 mL/min:** No dose adjustment is necessary **GFR 31–50 mL/min:** Dosing frequency: every 24–36 h **GFR 10–30 mL/min:** Dosing frequency: every 24–48 h **GFR <10 mL/min:** Dosing frequency: every 40–60 h	**HD:** Dosage use after HD **DP:** Dosing frequency: every 40–60 h
Pindolol	10–60	1	No dose adjustment is necessary	**HD:** Insignificant removal **PD:** Insignificant removal
Atenolol	50–100	1–2	**GFR >30 mL/min:** No dose adjustment is necessary **GFR 10–30 mL/min:** maximum dose 50 mg/day **GFR <10 mL/min:** maximum dose 25 mg/day	**HD:** removal rate 25–50%. Dosage use after HD **DP:** Insignificant removal. Maximum dose 25 mg/day
Metoprolol	50–200	1	No dose adjustment is necessary	**HD:** Insignificant removal **PD:** Insignificant removal
Bisoprolol	5–20	1	**GFR ≥40 mL/min:** No dose adjustment is necessary **GFR <40 mL/min:** starting 2.5 mg/day and slowly increase according to BP	**HD:** Insignificant removal **PD:** Insignificant removal
Nebivolol	2.5–10	1	**GFR <30 mL/min:** starting 2.5 mg/day and slowly increase according to BP	**HD:** Insignificant removal **PD:** Insignificant removal
Carvedilol	12.5–50	1–2	No dose adjustment is necessary	**HD:** Insignificant removal **PD:** Insignificant removal

Methyldopa	500–2000	1–3	**GFR >50 mL/min:** Dosing frequency: every 8 h **GFR 10–50 mL/min:** Dosing frequency: every 8–12 h **GFR <10 mL/min:** Dosing frequency: every 12–24 h	**HD:** removal rate up to 60%. Dosage use after HD **DP:** Dosing frequency: every 12–24 h
Clonidine	0.2–0.9	2	No dose adjustment is necessary **GFR <30 mL/min:** start low dose and slowly increase according to BP and AE	**HD:** Insignificant removal **PD:** Insignificant removal
Prazosin	1 a 20	2–3	No dose adjustment is necessary	**HD:** Insignificant removal **PD:** Insignificant removal
Doxazosin	1 a 16	1	No dose adjustment is necessary	**HD:** Insignificant removal **PD:** Insignificant removal
Hydralazine	50–200	2–3	No dose adjustment is necessary	**HD:** Insignificant removal **PD:** Insignificant removal
Aliskiren	150–300	1	No dose adjustment is necessary	**HD:** Insignificant removal **PD:** Insignificant removal

HD hemodialysis, *PD* peritoneal dialysis, *GFR* glomerular filtration rate, *AE* adverse effects, *BP* blood pressure
[a]Information for dose adjustment and dialysis removal based on UpToDate 2021 recommendations

RAAS Blockers

Angiotensin-converting enzyme inhibitors (ACEIs) or angiotensin AT_1 receptor blockers (ARBs) are not interchangeable for dialysis patients since there are significant pharmacological differences, especially the fact that most ARBs are not dialyzed during conventional HD. Inhibition of the RAS with ARBs has been recommended as the first-line BP-lowering therapy for dialysis patients due to their cardiovascular benefits in the general population. However, more randomized trials are needed to prove this recommendation [39]. In PD patients, these drug classes are considered first-line since they can retard the rate of loss of kidney function [30].

β-Blockers

Contrary to general and CKD populations, some clinical trial evidence proposes that among those on HD, β-blockers are more effective than drugs blocking RAAS in decreasing BP levels and protecting patients from cardiovascular morbidity and mortality. This recommendation is strongly supported by the HDPAL (Hypertension in Hemodialysis Treated with Atenolol or Lisinopril) 1-year trial. In this study, 200 HD patients with hypertension and left ventricular hypertrophy (LVH) were randomized to atenolol or lisinopril, each administered thrice a week after dialysis. Contrary to the primary hypothesis, the HDPAL trial showed no difference in the change of left ventricular mass index (LVMI) during follow-up, and patients in the atenolol group required less BP-lowering action than the lisinopril group. The superiority of atenolol is further supported by the premature termination of the HDPAL trial due to the excess risk of serious cardiovascular adverse events in the lisinopril group [40].

Long-Acting Dihydropyridine Calcium Channel Blockers (CCB)

The use of CCBs as add-on or combination therapy is sustained by their characteristics of potent and long-lasting BP-lowering efficacy and daily administration. They can successfully lower BP, even in the sodium volume-expanded state. CCBs are not removed during standard hemodialysis, and their pharmacokinetics are unchanged in ESRD [39]. In 2008, Tepel et al. studied the effects of amlodipine vs. placebo in hemodialysis patients. The conclusion was that this CCB reduces SBP and may have a beneficial effect on cardiovascular outcomes [41]. A more recent parallel-design, open-label single-center RCT compared bisoprolol vs. amlodipine. The results demonstrated that amlodipine was superior in reducing left ventricular mass and levels of asymmetric dimethylarginine (ADMA) despite similar BP reduction between groups [42].

Mineralocorticoids Receptor Antagonists (MRA)

Data for aldosterone blockade in chronic hemodialysis are scarce. Two RCTs, Spin-D (safety and cardiovascular efficacy of spironolactone in dialysis-dependent ESRD) [43] and MiREnda (Mineralocorticoid Receptor Antagonists in End-Stage Renal Disease) [44], observed the effects of spironolactone in patients on chronic hemodialysis. Both showed relative safety regarding hyperkalemia, but they failed to demonstrate progress in reducing cardiac diastolic function over

36 weeks or in left ventricular mass over 40 weeks with spironolactone use. Two double-blind large ongoing international RCTs will probably offer valuable clinical efficacy and safety data on the use of spironolactone 25 mg/day in HD patients: Aldosterone Antagonist Chronic Hemodialysis Interventional Survival Trial (ALCHEMIST) and Aldosterone Blockade for Health Improvement Evaluation in ESKD trial (ACHIEVE). These trials may bring to the medical community many answers, but not all, regarding efficacy and safety of MRA use in ESKD [45, 46]. Nonetheless, a recent meta-analysis suggests that finerenone confers significant renal and cardiovascular benefits in patients with CKD with higher risk of hyperkalemia with finerenone than placebo, but differences in adverse events were not significant [47].

Summary of main recommendations regarding blood pressure management

1. Counsel patients to take a low sodium diet of <2.0 g/day (approximates to <5 g NaCl/day)
2. Avoid dialysate Na^+ >140 mEq/L to reduce intradialytic weight gain and blood pressure (BP), which are associated with better outcomes. Lowering dialysate Na^+ can be tried in patients without intradialytic hypotension and should not be prolonged in a patient with intradialytic hypotension to avoid increased mortality risk [48]
3. Evidence-based recommendations are weak about choice of antihypertensive medication. Beta-blockers, angiotensin receptor blockers or ACE inhibitors, and dihydropyridine calcium channel blockers are all reasonable options
4. Fluid volume management is the most important recommendation to control HTN in HD patients [49]. Prolonged or more frequent HD may be essential for patients with high interdialytic weight gains or frequent intradialytic hypotension. For some patients, intermittent extra ultrafiltration sessions may be necessary to succeed and maintain euvolemia in those reluctant to accomplish prolonged or more frequent treatments on a regular basis

Hypotension During Hemodialysis Session

During hemodialysis, a significant number of patients experience an overall decline in BP [50]. It is yet unclear how to determine what an acceptable decline in intradialytic BP is and what might be considered intradialytic hypotension (IDH). In general, IDH is defined as systolic blood pressure (SBP) <90 mmHg or ≥20 mmHg drop on SBP during a hemodialysis session with symptoms such as abdominal pain, nausea, vomiting, cramping, dizziness, fainting, drowsiness [51].

The incidence of IDH varies between 6 and 27% in most cohort studies [52, 53]. IDH seems to be associated with poor long-term outcomes, such as increased mortality and risk of myocardial stunning [54, 55]. However, it is still unclear whether IDH can lead to poor outcomes or if it is just a marker of comorbidities that increases predisposition to IDH [51].

IDH can result from a reduction in blood volume, impaired cardiac function, and damaged constriction of resistance and capacitance vessels [56, 57]. Identifying these risks is the first step to preventing IDH and choosing the best way to treat it. The main causes associated with IDH are listed in Table 2.5.

Table 2.5 Main causes related to intradialytic hypotension

High interdialytic weight gain
Excessively low dry weight
Short dialysis weekly time
High dialysate temperature
Dialyzer reaction
Feeding during hemodialysis session
Use of antihypertensive medications (especially before dialysis)
Cardiac abnormalities (diastolic dysfunction; myocardial infarction; cardiac tamponade)
Anemia (especially in patients with cardiac disease)
Sepsis
Occult bleeding

How to Treat Hypotension in Hemodialysis?

Considering that IDH has a predictive power for fatal and non-fatal cardiovascular events, being attentive to the signs of hypotension is essential for the early implementation of measures and reestablishment of BP.

The first step to manage IDH is to immediately stop ultrafiltration and consider adoption of Trendelenburg position. The effect of Trendelenburg position on blood volume appears to be slight [58]. Some studies suggest an increase in central blood volume between 0.4 and 1.8% [59, 60]. In fact, more studies are necessary to confirm its efficacy. But, as it is a simple maneuver, it is widely performed in IDH treatment and should only be avoided in patients with potential associated risks. Stopping ultrafiltration usually results in a 2–2.3% increase in blood volume [60]. In addition, this measure will avoid further reduction of blood volume and facilitate blood volume replenishment [61]. Once BP is stabilized, restarting ultrafiltration should be considered.

In those patients with IDH refractory to Trendelenburg position and ultrafiltration stoppage, isotonic saline or colloid solutions should be infused to increase blood volume. In most randomized trials, isotonic saline and albumin solutions were found to be equally effective in the treatment of IDH [62, 63].

In most cases, stopping ultrafiltration and isotonic saline infusion is sufficient to reverse IDH. If the patient remains refractory to these measures, dialysis should be stopped, and the patient should be transferred to a hospital.

How to Prevent Hypotension in Hemodialysis?

For patients who present IDH as a frequent complication, some measures must be taken to prevent it. Regular assessment of dry body weight, proper dietary salt intake and interdialytic weight gain, individualization of the dialysis prescription, and avoidance of the use of antihypertensive drugs before sessions are the main steps.

Making the patient aware of the modifiable factors associated with IDH is perhaps the most important conduct to prevent IDH since some measures depend on the patient's compliance. Controlling interdialytic weight gain is the first step, and it is strictly linked with dietary salt and liquid intake [64]. A large interdialytic weight gain results in an increased ultrafiltration rate, leading to a higher reduction in blood volume and risk of IDH. In patients with residual renal function, diuretic therapy can help control interdialytic weight gain.

Dry body weight should be regularly assessed. Physical examination should always be the basis for patient evaluation. However, the physical examination is usually nonconclusive in identifying underhydration. Therefore, it is recommended to use a reliable assessment instrument, such as bioelectrical impedance spectroscopy (BIS), lung ultrasonography (US), and measurement of the inferior vena cava, whenever indicated [65, 66]. Several studies suggest that most unstable patients are normohydrated or underhydrated at the beginning of the dialysis session [67, 68], and that this is the main cause of IDH.

Although there is limited evidence about the effect of antihypertensive agents on IDH, most guidelines recommend not to give antihypertensive agents immediately before a dialysis session to patients with frequent IDH [69]. In addition, these patients should not eat immediately before or during the session. Avoiding eating during HD should be recommended particularly for those with diabetic autonomic neuropathy due to a higher risk of IDH [70]. In malnourished patients, restriction of intradialytic meals and supplements should be balanced against the nutritional needs of the patient. Studies suggest that restrictive in-center nutrition practices may interfere with the coverage of caloric requirements since these patients have at least three meals per week at dialysis units [71, 72].

Some adjustments to the dialysis prescription should be made to prevent IDH. The efficacy and safety of cool dialysate (35–36 °C) are proven in chronic HD patients, and it is a first-line option to prevent IDH [51]. Cool dialysis activates the sympathetic nervous system and induces vasoconstriction, decreasing the risk of IDH [73]. One meta-analysis including 484 patients showed that cool dialysate reduces the rate of IDH by 70% (95% CI 49–89) and increases intradialytic BP by 12 mmHg (95% CI 8–16) [74]. Cool dialysate is a simple measure and entails no additional costs to the session. Some patients describe unpleasant sensations, which can be controlled using individual pre-dialysis core body temperatures and reducing the dialysate temperature in 0.5 °C [51].

Reducing the ultrafiltration rate is another first-line option in the prevention of IDH. Longer sessions and frequent dialysis are the main measures to achieve such reduction. The Dialysis Outcomes and Practice Patterns Study (DOPPS) found that an ultrafiltration rate over 10 mL/h/kg is correlated with higher odds of IDH [odds ratio (OR) 1.30; *P* 0.045] [75]. Prolonging dialysis time allows the reduction of the ultrafiltration rate to safe levels. In the same way, increasing dialysis frequency results in a low interdialytic weight gain, therefore reducing the ultrafiltration rate as well [76].

Using high dialysate sodium concentration (>144 mmol/L) routinely, even as sodium profiling, is not recommended. Although sodium profiling can restore the osmotic gradient and plasma refill during hemodialysis, it results in higher all-cause and cardiovascular mortality [HR 1.36 (95% CI 1.14–1.63) and HR 1.34 (95% CI 1.04–1.73)] and higher risk of IDH [77]. It has fallen into disuse.

Despite midodrine being unregistered as a treatment for IDH in Europe, it should be considered in cases where major measures fail. Midodrine is an oral alpha-1 agonist, and its metabolite induces vasoconstriction. In general, it is prescribed 2.5–10 mg 30 min before the dialysis session. According to most studies, this use is effective and safe to prevent IDH. A study analyzed the effectiveness of midodrine compared to cool dialysis and found no difference between both therapies in BP response or incidence of IDH [78]. In addition, no additive effect of the combination of these therapies was observed [78]. The most common midodrine adverse effects are flushing, headache, scalp paresthesia, weakness, neck soreness, and heartburn. Data regarding long-term safety of midodrine use are lacking.

Other modifications in dialysate concentration can be prescribed to avoid IDH, although there is limited evidence about these measures

- Dialysate calcium concentration of 1.50 mmol/L should be considered: ionized calcium is directly related to myocardial contractility and inversely related to the mean arterial pressure during dialysis [79].
- Low magnesium dialysate (0.25 mmol/L) is not recommended, especially in combination with low-calcium dialysate [80].

Left Ventricular Hypertrophy (LVH) in Dialysis Patients

LVH Definition

Left ventricular hypertrophy (LVH) is defined as growth in left ventricular mass caused by increased cardiomyocyte size leading to an increase in wall thickness, cavity size, or both [81]. LVH can be a physiological adaptation to strenuous physical exercise, as in athletes, or it can be a pathological condition, which can be either genetic or secondary to LV overload, and its presentation can vary depending on the underlying pathology [81]. Physiological LVH is usually benign and regresses upon reduction/cessation of physical activity. Pathological LVH is a compensatory phenomenon, which may eventually become maladaptive and evolve toward progressive LV dysfunction and heart failure (HF) [81]. In addition to coronary microvascular dysfunction (CMD) and myocardial ischemia, which are present in most forms of pathological LVH, long-term pressure, volume overload status, or their combination, are also important factors leading to LVH and resulting in its eccentric or concentric form according to the compensatory mechanisms activated in the heart [82]. Furthermore, fibrotic infiltration is caused by distinct pathological processes, such as chronic inflammatory injury, metabolic disorders, and uremic toxicity. In patients with chronic kidney disease, these processes frequently coexist and generate an increase in LV mass while CKD progresses to the final stages [82].

LVH is one of the most common findings in the cardiovascular evaluation of patients starting dialysis, and its presence has been associated with poor prognosis. Based on observations from the HEMO study [11], approximately 80% of patients on hemodialysis presented cardiovascular diseases at the study baseline, with an LVH prevalence of 29–75% in this population. Many times, LVH is an occasional echocardiographic finding in patients with CKD as a result of a cardiological assessment due to signs and symptoms secondary to systemic hypertension, aortic stenosis, aortic or mitral regurgitation, hypertrophic cardiomyopathy, etc. [82]. The emerging evidence that non-atherosclerotic heart disease, particularly heart failure and LVH, plays a major role in increasing the risk of poor outcomes in end-stage kidney disease (ESKD) patients makes the LV evaluation in this population even more important [83–85].

Natural History of LVH in ESKD

The increased renal dysfunction occurring in the progression of CKD to pre-dialysis stages is also accompanied by an increase in LV mass, according to many longitudinal and cross-sectional studies [86, 87]. Around 70–80% of patients with CKD stages 4–5 have some manifestation of LVH before dialysis initiation. Fluid overload and increased arterial stiffness play an important role in LVH way before the start of dialysis therapy. Systolic arterial hypertension and elevated pulse pressure are strongly associated with LVH in patients with advanced CKD [88].

Also, there are important aspects of CKD complications involved in the pathophysiology of LVH in this population, such as anemia, mineral bone disease, hyperparathyroidism, hypervolemia, and an increase in levels of uremic toxin. CKD etiology can also be responsible for some cardiovascular manifestations. For example, patients with ADPKD frequently present many cardiovascular diseases, including hypertension, LVH, cardiac valvular abnormalities, and intracranial aneurysms. Cardiovascular complications are the leading cause of morbidity and mortality in this group of patients, secondary to its clinical presentation per se [86, 89].

Considering the hemodynamic factors related to renal replacement therapies (RRT), there is evidence in the literature that frequent nocturnal hemodialysis versus 3 times a week conventional HD improved left ventricular mass, reduced the need for blood pressure medications, improved some measures of mineral metabolism, and improved selected measures of quality of life in patients undergoing frequent nocturnal HD [87]. Also, in Frequent Hemodialysis Daily Trial (FHDT), frequent HD resulted in a significant reduction in LV mass (LVM 13.1 g; 95% CI 5.0–21.3 g; $p = 0.002$), LVM index (6.9 g/m^2; 95% CI 2.4–11.3 g/m^2; $p = 0.003$), and percent change in the geometric mean of LVM (7.0%; 95% CI 1.0–12.6; $p = 0.02$), being the more pronounced effect of frequent HD on LVM evident among patients with previous LVH at study baseline [90]. In the frequent HD group, changes in LVM were associated with changes in blood pressure (conventional hemodialysis: $R = 0.28$, $p = 0.01$; daily hemodialysis: $R = 0.54$, $p = 0.001$), and the magnitude of reduction in left and right ventricular end-diastolic volumes was accentuated among those patients with residual urine output [at least 100 mL/day (p value interaction = 0.02)]. It seems that effects on blood pressure and volume control may mediate this improvement, which may be the factors responsible for improvements in outcomes [90, 91]. There are also data to support the hypothesis that a reduction in the degree of LVH (but not a reversion to normal) can be achieved by aggressive fluid and BP control and perhaps by treatment of anemia, at least in certain circumstances [87].

Regarding kidney transplantation, previous exposure to the uremic milieu during the progression of CKD and the time spent in dialysis before transplantation may be responsible for persistent LVH observed in nearly half of patients after kidney transplantation [92, 93]. However, even though some studies have reported an improvement in cardiomyopathy after successful kidney transplantation [94, 95], recent clinical reports demonstrate that LVH may not regress, particularly in those patients in which renal function was not fully recovered [96].

Mechanisms of LVH in ESKD Patients

The mechanisms underlying left ventricular abnormalities in CKD are diverse and involve many aspects: (1) preload-related factors: volume overload, anemia, arterial-venous fistula resulting in myocardial cell lengthening and eccentric LV remodeling; (2) afterload-related factors: systemic arterial resistance (systolic and diastolic hypertension) and vascular compliance disturbances (vascular calcification) resulting in myocardial cell thickening and concentric LV remodeling; and (3) hemodynamic-independent factors such as oxidative stress, and inflammation, anemia, hyperphosphatemia, hyperparathyroidism, and hypovitaminosis D and FGF-23 elevation which play an important role in the earlier stage and increase cardiovascular risk as the disease progresses [88, 97, 98]. We have revised some of these aspects in detail below due to their prevalence and potential of action for treatment and prevention.

Chronic systemic hypertension leads to structural and functional changes in the heart that include LVH, fibrosis of the myocardial interstitium, and coronary angiopathy. Chronic arterial hypertension leads to increased wall stress both in the systemic arteries and in the LV. It results in LV systolic performance impairment and induces compensatory cardiomyocyte hypertrophy, increasing LV wall thickness to reduce wall stress following Laplace's law, in which LV geometry becomes more concentric [99, 100]. Also, neurohormonal stimuli occur secondary to HTN such as (a) increased sympathetic nervous system activity, (b) RAS system as a major regulator of blood pressure and hypertrophic response in hypertension and (c) angiotensin II stimulating sympathetic activity and aldosterone production, (d) aldosterone promoting endothelial dysfunction, vascular remodeling, oxidative stress, and inflammation through the mineralocorticoid receptor [101]. Other main pathways and signaling molecules of importance for the hypertrophic response to arterial hypertension include endothelin-1 and G proteins, microribonucleic acids (miRNAs), oxidative stress, heat shock proteins, calcium, and some kinases [102].

Anemia during the first year of renal replacement therapy was also associated with an increase in the prevalence of LVH (10 g/m^2 per 1.0 g of decline in hemoglobin) [103]. The impact of anemia on cardiomyopathy among CKD patients was recently evaluated in a clinical trial, including serial echocardiograms. In this study, anemia was an independent risk factor for diastolic heart failure even after adjustments for age, diabetes, and ischemic heart disease [103]. The treatment of severe anemia with erythropoietin and iron to increase hemoglobin levels seems to be beneficial for LVH, but the treatment of lesser degrees of anemia to even higher targets has not been proven to be beneficial for LVH [88]. Iron deficiency (ID) may also play a role in cardiovascular outcomes among CKD patients. Recent data from CKDOPPS have demonstrated that ID is associated with an increased risk of major cardiovascular events (MACE) and all-cause mortality [104]. Also, in the general population, patients with HF seem to benefit from ID correction regardless of the presence of anemia with less acute HF decompensation hospitalization events [105].

There is vast evidence in the literature that mineral metabolism disorders, including hyperphosphatemia, elevated parathyroid hormone (PTH) levels, and hypovitaminosis D, have been associated with LVH and myocardial hypertrophy in dialysis patients [106, 107]. However, the benefits of these aspects of CKD treatment on LVH and its consequences remain uncertain [88].

Two randomized trials, EVOLVE (Evaluation of Cinacalcet Hydrochloride Therapy to Lower Cardiovascular Events) and PRIMO (Paricalcitol Capsule Benefits in Renal Failure Induced Cardiac Morbidity), were unable to demonstrate benefits regarding the cardiovascular endpoints (death, myocardial infarction, unstable angina, heart failure, or peripheral vascular disease) analyzed and in terms of LVH improvement regardless of the reduction of cardiovascular-related hospitalizations [108, 109]. The negative results of those trials could be justified because CKD-MBD has different paths needing treatment, and all of these proposed medications' effects may be studied combined and in a different profile of patients, and followed up for longer periods to be able to demonstrate in real life the effects found in animal models. Other studies evaluated the cardiovascular effects of vitamin D, and it has been well-established that vitamin D has several biological effects on the heart, including cardiac cell contraction, proliferation, hypertrophy, and in the protein and collagen expression of cardiomyocytes [110]. Also, vitamin D plays a potential role in maintaining vascular tone and cardiac output. Thus its deficiency contributes to the development of heart failure among CKD patients [110, 111].

Recently, elevated FGF-23 concentrations were found to be associated with death, cardiovascular events, and kidney disease progression in patients with CKD. FGF receptors have been implicated in the pathogenesis of left ventricular (LV) hypertrophy, which predisposes left ventricular (LV) dysfunction, and is an important predictor of mortality in patients with CKD [112]. The HOST study (Homocysteine in Kidney and End-Stage Renal Disease Study) and a subset analysis of the CRIC (Chronic Renal Insufficiency Cohort) study demonstrated that higher FGF-23 concentration was an independent predictor of LV systolic dysfunction and increased LV mass index leading to a greater risk of eccentric and concentric LVH in CKD patients, respectively [113, 114]. A direct causal role for elevated FGF-23 in the pathogenesis of LVH has been demonstrated in animal models, with findings such as FGF-23 directly inducing pathological hypertrophy of isolated cardiomyocytes [114]. Thus, FGF-23 receptors blockers may be a potential way to improve LVH and dysfunction in CKD patients.

Despite scientific evidence showing that LV mass is a good predictor of cardiovascular outcomes and death in HD patients with LVH been widely taken as a representative endpoint for mortality [115, 116], a recent meta-analysis questioned the role of LVH as an effective surrogate in CKD patients because no clear association was found between intervention-induced LV mass regression and mortality [117]. Perhaps confounding factors related to the diagnosis of LVH by cardiovascular imaging may have contributed to contradictory results of this meta-analysis. Several imaging biomarkers have been used to reliably diagnose LVH in HD patients, but we know there are several intrinsic pitfalls in all of them.

Among CKD patients who develop LVH, serum levels of inflammatory biomarkers are significantly higher than those observed among patients without LVH [118]. The same relationship has been noted for C-reactive protein and N-terminal pro-B-type natriuretic peptide [119], suggesting a link between LV filling pressure and inflammation. It is also well known that CKD patients frequently have excessive activation of the renin–angiotensin–aldosterone system (RAS), potentially inducing myocardial fibrosis and hypertrophy. Activation of intra-cardiac RAS seems to be critically involved in overload status observed in CKD, but angiotensin II and aldosterone can also be involved in myocardial cell hypertrophy and fibrosis regardless of afterload [88]. Angiotensin II promotes growth in both fibroblasts and cardiac myocytes, contributing to cardiomyopathy in dialysis patients [120] while high aldosterone levels seem to be correlated with LVH regardless of hypertension in hemodialysis patients [121].

Also, some novel cellular mediator systems that translate hemodynamic and circulatory alterations to an increase in ventricular mass have brought attention to other pathways that produce or aggravate LVH. These potential cellular systems include VDR activation, calcineurin/nuclear factor of activated T cells, G-protein coupled receptor to angiotensin II and endothelin-1, and the mammalian target of rapamycin (mTOR) pathway [88]. The development of new, effective therapeutic strategies may be possible once these systems actions are better explained and comprehended.

Diagnosis of LVH

Currently, cardiac magnetic resonance imaging (CMRI) is considered the gold standard for measurement of LV mass, volume, and function, regardless of geometric assumptions [122] because CMRI offers very high spatial resolution and tissue contrast therefore being able to assess myocardial fibrosis [111]. However, in advanced CKD or ESKD populations, CMRI has been largely avoided due to the need of intravenous gadolinium contrast to detect myocardial fibrosis during the procedure. Gadolinium can cause nephrogenic systemic fibrosis [123, 124] in CKD, and its application should be avoided although the complication is rare. Another important aspect to be mentioned is that CMRI is a high-cost procedure, its availability is limited and it has some specific contraindications such as claustrophobia or cardiac implantable devices, therefore limiting its use in the clinical practice.

Cardiac tomography (CT) precisely measures LV mass and has the ability to quantify coronary calcium and coronary arterial stenosis through the application of iodinated contrast agents, which may affect residual renal function that is vital to CKD/ESKD patients. Having said that, echocardiography (ECHO) offers a reliable, non-invasive, rapidly available, and relatively inexpensive method to estimate LVM and it has been the main tool for LV mass assessment both in clinical practice and many research protocols. The accuracy of LVH assessment by ECHO among CKD patients depends on which technique is used, the timing of the test relative to the dialysis session, and the index used for the "normalization" of data generated [125]. LV mass estimates can derive from M-mode ECHO, two-dimensional (2D) ECHO, and real-time three-dimensional (3D) ECHO. Each method for LV mass measurement has its particular advantages, disadvantages, and value in specific situations. The serial monitoring of LV mass by ECHO is a potentially useful clinical tool in the evaluation of prognosis and success of interventions that may result in regression of LVH [125, 126].

Prevention and Treatment of LVH

Life modification strategies should be encouraged for all CKD/ESKD patients since the first consultation. All pathophysiological aspects related to LVH development in the CKD/ESKD population are important targets for treatment and prevention. Appropriate blood pressure control, anemia and iron deficiency management, mineral bone disorder treatments with correct control of phosphate, PTH, and vitamin D levels play an important role in CKD/ESKD management and may contribute to maintaining LV function and reducing LVM in these patients. Also, fluid volume management and the maintenance of a near euvolemic state are crucial to improving LVH.

Considering the inflammatory pathogenic mechanisms underlying LVH, it is suggested that measures to control oxidative and endoplasmic reticulum (ER) stress, support effective nitric oxide and hydrogen sulfide bioactivity, prevent a reduction in cardiomyocyte pH, and boost the production of protective hormones, such as fibroblast growth factor 21 (FGF-21), while suppressing fibroblast growth factor 23 (FGF-23) and marinobufagenin, may be helpful to prevent and control LVH. Examples of some of these agents include *N*-acetylcysteine, lipoic acid, ferulic acid, zinc, selenium, melatonin, tauroursodeoxycholic acid, berberine, citrulline, high-dose folate, cocoa flavanols, hawthorn extract, dietary nitrate, high-dose biotin, soy isoflavones, taurine, carnitine, magnesium orotate, EPA-rich fish oil, glycine, copper, and others. Also, the potential advantages of wholefood plant-based diets, moderation in salt intake, avoidance of phosphate additives, regular exercise training, and sauna sessions may lower inflammation [127].

Following this line of thought, studies have also reported that nut consumption is potentially beneficial in preventing cardiovascular diseases. The Kangbuk Samsung Health Study, which evaluated around 50,000 patients, demonstrated that among women nut consumption ≥2/week was associated with a decreased probability of

LVH. In this study, one serving dose of nuts (peanuts, pine nuts, and almonds) was defined as 15 g [128]. New drugs that are becoming available to the CKD population such as the sodium glucose cotransporter-2 inhibitors (iSGLT2) and selective mineralocorticoid receptor antagonists have produced a reduction in albuminuria, CKD progression risk, and cardiovascular outcomes, with some effects in improving LV function measured through ejection fraction as well [129, 130]. Also, in patients with T2D and LVH, dapagliflozin treatment significantly reduced LVM. This reduction in LVM was accompanied by reductions in systolic BP, body weight, visceral and subcutaneous adipose tissue, insulin resistance, and high-sensitivity C-reactive protein. This regression in LVM suggests that dapagliflozin may initiate reverse remodeling and changes in left ventricular structure that can contribute to its cardioprotective effects. This may increase the arsenal for treatment and impact the prevention of left ventricular hypertrophy among this population. These drugs have not yet been approved by the US FDA for use in dialysis patients in the USA.

Regarding LVH prevention, the dialysis modality and prescription must also be individualized according to patients' metabolic and volemic control needs. When prescribing dialysis, it is essential to consider their residual renal function, interdialytic weight gain, and the hemodynamic variations along ultrafiltration to reduce additional damage to the heart.

Heart Failure in ESKD Patients

As mentioned above, the HEMO study demonstrated a high percentage of ESKD patients in which hemodialysis (HD) patients are known to have one or more types of cardiovascular diseases such as coronary artery disease (CAD, 22–39%), heart failure (HF, 20–40%), atrial fibrillation (AF, 11–27%), and left ventricular hypertrophy (LVH, 29–75%) at the initiation of renal replacement therapy (RRT) [131]. Although CAD, peripheral and cerebral vascular disease represent a significant burden to ESKD patients, non-atherosclerotic heart disease also plays a significant role in the high cardiovascular morbimortality in ESKD [85, 132–134].

Heart failure (HF) is one of the most common causes of hospitalization and death in ESRD patients [135]. In general, the pathogenesis of HF in these patients can be divided into two categories: HF related to traditional risk factors as seen in the general population, such as older age, diabetes mellitus, hypertension, obesity, and smoking, and HF-related to non-traditional risk factors associated with the underlying kidney disease itself, such as uremia, inflammation, anemia, vascular calcification due to mineral bone disease, and others [136, 137]. In contrast to earlier stages of CKD, when traditional risk factors play a significant role, many studies have shown that as CKD progresses, the kidney-disease-related, non-traditional risk factors become more prominent and contribute to HF development [138, 139] (Table 2.6).

The mechanisms involved in HF development in the general population are well-established. They are related to previous ischemic events and those

Table 2.6 Risk factor of ischemic heart disease in chronic kidney disease and end-stage renal disease population

Risk factors for atheromatous ischemic heart disease in CKD/ESRD
Uremia-related risk factors
Atherogenic lipid profiles and dyslipidemia
Derangement of platelet function with high levels of prothrombotic factors
Increased oxidative stress
Hyperhomocysteinemia
Abnormal divalent ion metabolism
Disturbances of glucose metabolism including advanced glycation end-products
Inflammation, with dysregulation in proinflammatory cytokines

Traditional risk factors
Age
Gender
Hypertension
Diabetes mellitus
Smoking
Left ventricular hypertrophy
Dyslipidemia
Fibrinogen
Menopause

Source: Adapted from The kidney-Brenner and the Framingham Risk Score

secondary to arterial hypertension, volume overload, and genetic cardiomyopathies [140]. In the CKD population, several mechanisms are usually at play simultaneously. They are linked to the secondary manifestations of kidney disease itself, such as mineral metabolism disorders, which increases vascular calcification and the risk of myocardial infarction, anemia and its treatment, which can interfere in blood pressure control, fluid overload resulting in an increased preload to the heart as well as systemic and tissue inflammation which plays a role in left ventricular remodeling [141].

The association between HF and coronary artery disease (CAD) leading to ischemic HF (I-HF) is well understood. However, ESKD patients often present with non-ischemic HF (NI-HF), similar clinical features but different in etiology. Furthermore, as said, ischemic and non-ischemic pathogenetic factors will often be present simultaneously in ESKD patients. Nonetheless, the non-ischemic component of HF potentially contributes to the overall mortality risk in ESKD patients in a significant way.

The incidence, severity, and outcomes of HF in patients undergoing dialysis are poorly characterized and potentially undertreated. The New York Heart Association (NYHA) classification system for heart failure is based on a grading of dyspnea relative to the intensity of physical activity, which does not seem to be the optimal parameter to evaluate in ESRD patients who are constantly fluid-overloaded [136]. In the same way, the identification of patients with heart failure secondary or not to ischemic cardiac events in CKD population is difficult because what generally is seen is a combined manifestation of systolic heart failure and diastolic heart failure, secondary to LVH, previous myocardial ischemia, and non-hemodynamic effects of uremic cardiomyopathy [142, 143].

Echocardiography is essential in diagnosing and determining cardiac dysfunction (LVH, diastolic and systolic dysfunction) and prognosis. However, it does not show the details regarding myocardial tissue composition, which could help determine whether the myocardial fibrosis aspect is secondary to ischemia or uremia effect [111, 144]. Therefore, the determination of what is causing HF in CKD/ESKD patients (I-HF, uremic cardiomyopathy, or both) becomes essential, considering the potentially modifiable risk factors and predictors secondary to renal disease and RRT.

As discussed above, there are many hemodynamic and non-hemodynamic mechanisms in which CKD and RRT (especially HD) affect the heart functioning over time, leading to a higher risk of cardiovascular disease in this population compared to non-CKD patients.

Currently, ischemic or not, cardiac disease management in renal patients is based on guidelines developed for the general population, disregarding all the critical aspects caused by kidney impairment. Many studies have been performed to generate better knowledge about how CKD/ESKD patients behave to the treatment of the traditional and non-traditional risk factors and how much it could improve outcomes in this group of patients [85, 132, 145]. However, there is still a lot to be done. The more is known about cardiac diseases in CKD/ESRD patients, and the more potential therapeutic paths are opened to generate more complete strategies and treatments that will bring better survival and quality of life. These must be the goal of those who work taking care of them.

Acute Myocardial Infarction in Dialysis Patients

The prevalence of acute myocardial infarction (AMI) among dialysis patients is significantly higher than in the general population [146]. Several studies confirm the high prevalence of advanced chronic kidney disease (CKD) among patients with AMI [146–148]. About 50% of deaths and 30% of hospitalizations of patients on hemodialysis (HD) are attributable to cardiovascular causes [149, 150].

In recent decades, important therapeutic improvements (including coronary reperfusion) have occurred in the general population, considerably reducing the incidence of AMI and mortality from this cause [151, 152]. Despite the apparent improvement, the results obtained with the general population cannot be extrapolated to the dialysis population.

The incidence of AMI among dialysis patients peaked in 2002 (80.8 and 78.5 per 1000 patient-years among hemodialysis and peritoneal dialysis patients, respectively) and has been declining ever since (73.1 and 66.9 per 1000 patient-years, respectively, in 2011), likely reflecting the success of population-based preventive strategies [153].

A recent study evaluated AMI mortality in 42,933 dialysis patients, using data from the US Renal Data System. This study concluded that between 1993 and 2008 for all patients with AMI, in-hospital mortality rates decreased (31.9% in 1993, 18.8% in 2008; $p < 0.001$) [153]. Entretanto, proportional increases occurred in patient groups aged ≥75 years (23% and 31%, respectively; $P < 0.001$), of black race (25% and 31%, respectively; $P < 0.001$), with end-stage renal disease due to diabetes (42% and 55%, respectively; $P < 0.001$), and with non-STEMI (42.2% and 80.7%, respectively) [149].

Secondary prevention therapy, based on the prescription of antiplatelets, β-blockers, statins, and renin–angiotensin–aldosterone system inhibitors is recommended by the main guidelines for the general population [154, 155]. However, there are still few studies evaluating the benefits of these drugs in patients on dialysis after an episode of AMI. A recent analysis showed that patients with CKD remain underrepresented in most of cardiovascular disease clinical trials [156].

A study including 1471 incidents HD patients to examine the association of guideline-recommended medications (antiplatelets, β-blockers, statins, and renin–angiotensin–aldosterone system inhibitors) with all-cause mortality after AMI and they found that using evidence-based medications for secondary prevention after AMI reduces the risk of all-cause mortality in HD patients [157].

Another randomized trial evaluated 777 patients with advanced kidney disease and moderate or severe ischemia on the stress test to be treated with an initial invasive strategy (coronary angiography or revascularization) added to medical therapy or an initial conservative strategy consisting of medical therapy only, with performing angiography for those in whom medical therapy has failed. This study found that the invasive strategy was associated with a higher incidence of stroke than the conservative strategy (hazard ratio, 3.76; 95% CI 1.52–9.32; $P = 0.004$) and with a higher incidence of death or initiation of dialysis (hazard ratio, 1.48; 95% CI 1.04–2.11; $P = 0.03$) [158].

More studies on the use of drugs for secondary prevention of IM, as well as invasive procedures, are needed to clarify the benefits and risks of these therapies in the dialysis population.

Stroke in Dialysis Patients

Stroke is the third leading cause of death worldwide [159]. In patients with chronic kidney disease, the risk of cardiovascular events is higher compared to the general population [160]. In some cases, this risk can be 10 times higher [161], and normally frequency and time of hemodialysis session, dialyzer, and interdialytic weight gain interfere with the risk of cardiovascular events [161].

In dialysis patients, the risk of stroke is higher in the first 6 months of dialysis. Because of the high incidence of stroke in this population, neurological disorders such as severe or frequent headache, convulsive attacks, anisocoria, dysarthria, and

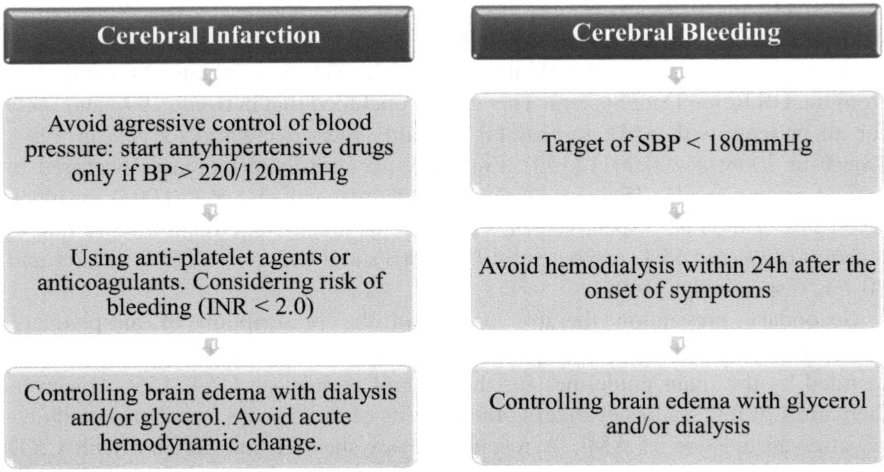

Fig. 2.3 Recommendations for the management of acute phase of stroke in dialysis patients according to JSDT guidelines. *BP* blood pressure, *SBP* systolic blood pressure, *INR* international normalized ratio, *JSDT* Japanese Society for Dialysis Therapy

aphasia should be investigated. Most of the times this can be diagnosed by computed tomography (CT), magnetic resonance imaging (MRI), or MRI angiography. It is worth noting that the use of gadolinium should be avoided in patients on dialysis due to the risk of nephrogenic systemic fibrosis [162].

During the acute phase of cerebral infarction, permissive hypertension is recommended to prevent an increase in the ischemia area. Antihypertensive drugs should be avoided unless SBP >220 mmHg or DBP >120 mmHg or thrombolytic therapy is indicated (BP <180/105 mmHg). When reduction of blood pressure is necessary, it must be slow with a target level around 85% of the previous value. Hemodialysis should be avoided on the day of the event since acute hemodynamic change can worsen the condition. Antiplatelet agents (aspirin, clopidogrel, ticagrelor) or anticoagulants (heparin, warfarin, apixaban, argatroban) can be used for secondary prevention within 1 month. If the use of anticoagulants during the acute phase is needed, the risk of bleeding should be considered and it is recommended to keep INR <2.0 [163].

Regarding cerebral bleeding, during the acute phase, systolic blood pressure should be kept under 180 mmHg. For secondary prevention, the recommended target of blood pressure is around 140/90 mmHg. Hemodialysis should be avoided within the first 24 h of the event due to the risk of increasing hematoma size. In the case of brain edema, glycerol should be the first-line treatment, and hemodialysis may be an option, preferably after 24 h of onset [163]. Figure 2.3 summarizes the main recommendations for managing the acute phase of stroke in dialysis patients.

Conclusion

CVD and kidney disease are strongly associated, and impairment of one organ causes dysfunction of the other. Hypertension, IDH, AMI, HF, stroke, and LVH are highly prevalent cardiovascular complications among dialysis patients. Understanding how to manage these conditions is crucial since dialysis patients have specific demands regarding medications and dialysis prescription.

References

1. Institute for Health Metrics and Evaluation (IHME). GBD compare | VizHub. VizHub. 2018. http://vizhub.healthdata.org/gbd-compare.
2. Moura-Neto JA, Divino-Filho JC, Ronco C. Nephrology worldwide: the vision, the project, and the mission. In: Moura-Neto JA, Divino-Filho JC, Ronco C, editors. Nephrology worldwide. Basel: Springer Nature Switzerland AG; 2021. p. 1–9.
3. Hou FF. Cardiovascular risk in Chinese patients with chronic kidney diseases: where do we stand? Chin Med J. 2005;118:883–6.
4. Gaita D, Mihaescu A, Schiller A. Of heart and kidney: a complicated love story. Eur J Prev Cardiol. 2012;21:840–6.
5. United Nations Department of Economic and Social Affairs, Population Division. World Population Prospects 2022: Summary of Results. UN DESA/POP/2022/TR/NO. 3. 2022.
6. Agarwal R, Nissenson AR, Batlle D, Coyne DW, Trout JR, Warnock DG. Prevalence, treatment, and control of hypertension in chronic hemodialysis patients in the United States. Am J Med. 2003;115:291–7.
7. Agarwal R. Epidemiology of interdialytic ambulatory hypertension and the role of volume excess. Am J Nephrol. 2011;34:381–90.
8. Ortega LM, Materson BJ. Hypertension in peritoneal dialysis patients: epidemiology, pathogenesis, and treatment. J Am Soc Hypertens. 2011;5:128–36.
9. Cocchi R, Degli Esposti E, Fabbri A, Lucatello A, Sturani A, Quarello F, et al. Prevalence of hypertension in patients on peritoneal dialysis: results of an Italian multicentre study. Nephrol Dial Transplant. 1999;14:1536–40.
10. Power A. Stroke in dialysis and chronic kidney disease. Blood Purif. 2013;36(3–4):179–83. https://doi.org/10.1159/000356086.
11. Cheung AK, Sarnak MJ, Yan G, Berkoben M, Heyka R, Kaufman A, et al. Cardiac diseases in maintenance hemodialysis patients: results of the HEMO study. Kidney Int. 2004;65(6):2380–9.
12. Horowitz B, Miskulin D, Zager P. Epidemiology of hypertension in CKD. Adv Chronic Kidney Dis. 2015;22(2):88–95. https://doi.org/10.1053/j.ackd.2014.09.004.
13. Rahman M, Griffin V, Kumar A, et al. A comparison of standardized versus "usual" blood pressure measurements in hemodialysis patients. Am J Kidney Dis. 2002;39:1226–30.
14. Drawz PE, Beddhu S, Kramer HJ, Rakotz M, Rocco MV, Whelton PK. Blood pressure measurement: a KDOQI perspective. Am J Kidney Dis. 2020;75(3):426–34. https://doi.org/10.1053/j.ajkd.2019.08.030.
15. Whelton PK, Carey RM, Aronow WS, et al. 2017 ACC/AHA/AAPA/ABC/ACPM/AGS/APhA/ASH/ASPC/NMA/PCNA guideline for the prevention, detection, evaluation, and management of high blood pressure in adults: executive summary: a report of the American College of Cardiology/American Heart Association task force on clinical practice guidelines. J Am Coll Cardiol. 2018;71(19):2199–269.
16. Williams B, Mancia G, Spiering W, et al. 2018 ESC/ESH guidelines for the management of arterial hypertension. Eur Heart J. 2018;39(33):3021–104.

17. Muntner P, Einhorn PT, Cushman WC, et al. Blood pressure assessment in adults in clinical practice and clinic-based research: JACC scientific expert panel. J Am Coll Cardiol. 2019;73(3):317–35.
18. Muntner P, Shimbo D, Carey RM, et al. Measurement of blood pressure in humans: a scientific statement from the American Heart Association. Hypertension. 2019;73(5):e35–66.
19. Barroso WKS, Rodrigues CIS, Bortolotto LA, Mota-Gomes MA, Brandão AA, Feitosa ADM, et al. Brazilian guidelines of hypertension—2020. Arq Bras Cardiol. 2021;116(3):516–658.
20. Mallamaci F, Torino C, Sarafidis P, Ekart R, Loutradis C, Siamopoulos K, Del Giudice A, Aucella F, Morosetti M, Raptis V, Bikos A, Papagianni A, Balafa O, Pappas E, Tripepi R, Marino C, Tripepi G, Ferro C, Malyszko J, Dekker FW, Jager KJ, London GM, Zoccali C. Treatment-resistant hypertension in the hemodialysis population: a 44-h ambulatory blood pressure monitoring-based study. J Hypertens. 2020;38(9):1849–56. https://doi.org/10.1097/HJH.0000000000002448.
21. Agarwal R, Flynn J, Pogue V, et al. Assessment and management of hypertension in patients on dialysis. J Am Soc Nephrol. 2014;25:1630–46.
22. Parati G, Ochoa JE, Bilo G, et al. Hypertension in chronic kidney disease part 1: out-of-office blood pressure monitoring: methods, thresholds, and patterns. Hypertension. 2016;67:1093–101.
23. Agarwal R. Pro: Ambulatory blood pressure should be used in all patients on hemodialysis. Nephrol Dial Transplant. 2015;30:1432–7.
24. Sarafidis PA, Rumjon A, Macdougall IC. Ambulatory blood pressure monitoring: an invaluable tool comes of age for patients with chronic kidney disease? Am J Nephrol. 2012;35:238–41.
25. Parati G, Ochoa JE, Bilo G, et al. Hypertension in chronic kidney disease part 2: role of ambulatory and home blood pressure monitoring for assessing alterations in blood pressure variability and blood pressure profiles. Hypertension. 2016;67:1102–10.
26. Jardine AG, Agarwal R. Con: Ambulatory blood pressure measurement in patients receiving haemodialysis: a sore arm and a waste of time? Nephrol Dial Transplant. 2015;30:1438–41.
27. Agarwal R, Brim NJ, Mahenthiran J, Andersen MJ, Saha C. Out-of-hemodialysis-unit blood pressure is a superior determinant of left ventricular hypertrophy. Hypertension. 2006;47(1):62–8.
28. K/DOQI. K/DOQI clinical practice guidelines for cardiovascular disease in dialysis patients. Am J Kidney Dis. 2005;45(4):16–153. https://doi.org/10.1053/j.ajkd.2005.01.019.
29. Jhee JH, Park J, Kim H, et al. The optimal blood pressure target in different dialysis populations. Sci Rep. 2018;8:14123. https://doi.org/10.1038/s41598-018-32281-w.
30. Wang AYM, Brimble KS, Brunier G, et al. ISPD cardiovascular and metabolic guidelines in adult peritoneal dialysis patients part I—assessment and management of various cardiovascular risk factors. Perit Dial Int. 2015;35:379–87. https://doi.org/10.3747/pdi.2014.00279.
31. Robinson BM, Tong L, Zhang J, Wolfe RA, Goodkin DA, Greenwood RN, Kerr PG, Morgenstern H, Li Y, Pisoni RL, Saran R, Tentori F, Akizawa T, Fukuhara S, Port FK. Blood pressure levels and mortality risk among hemodialysis patients in the dialysis outcomes and practice patterns study. Kidney Int. 2012;82(5):570–80. https://doi.org/10.1038/ki.2012.136.
32. Kuipers J, Usvyat LA, Oosterhuis JK, et al. Variability of predialytic, intradialytic, and postdialytic blood pressures in the course of a week: a study of Dutch and US maintenance hemodialysis patients. Am J Kidney Dis. 2013;62(4):779–88. https://doi.org/10.1053/j.ajkd.2013.03.034.
33. Mc Causland FR, Waikar SS, Brunelli SM. Increased dietary sodium is independently associated with greater mortality among prevalent hemodialysis patients. Kidney Int. 2012;82(2):204–11. https://doi.org/10.1038/ki.2012.42.
34. Agarwal R, Alborzi P, Satyan S, Light RP. Dry-weight reduction in hypertensive hemodialysis patients (DRIP): a randomized, controlled trial. Hypertension. 2009;53(3):500–7. https://doi.org/10.1161/HYPERTENSIONAHA.108.125674.
35. Group TFT. In-center hemodialysis six times per week versus three times per week. N Engl J Med. 2010;363:2287–300.

36. Zimmerman DL, Ruzicka M, Hebert P, Fergusson D, Touyz RM, Burns KD. Short daily versus conventional hemodialysis for hypertensive patients: a randomized cross-over study. PLoS One. 2014;9(5):1–8. https://doi.org/10.1371/journal.pone.0097135.
37. Agarwal R, Sinha AD. Cardiovascular protection with antihypertensive drugs in dialysis patients: systematic review and meta-analysis. Hypertension. 2009;53:860–6.
38. Heerspink HJ, Ninomiya T, Zoungas S, et al. Effect of lowering blood pressure on cardiovascular events and mortality in patients on dialysis: a systematic review and meta-analysis of randomised controlled trials. Lancet. 2009;373:1009–15.
39. Sarafidis PA, Persu A, Agarwal R, Burnier M, de Leeuw P, Ferro CJ, Halimi J-M, Heine GH, Jadoul M, Jarraya F, Kanbay M, Mallamaci F, Mark PB, Ortiz A, Parati G, Pontremoli R, Rossignol P, Ruilope L, Van der Niepen P, Vanholder R, Verhaar MC, Wiecek A, Wuerzner G, London GM, Zoccali C. Hypertension in dialysis patients: a consensus document by the European Renal and Cardiovascular Medicine (EURECA-m) working group of the European Renal Association–European Dialysis and Transplant Association (ERA-EDTA) and the Hypertension and the Kidney working group of the European Society of Hypertension (ESH)*. Nephrol Dial Transplant. 2017;32(4):620–40. https://doi.org/10.1093/ndt/gfw433.
40. Agarwal R, Sinha AD, Pappas MK, et al. Hypertension in hemodialysis patients treated with atenolol or lisinopril: a randomized controlled trial. Nephrol Dial Transplant. 2014;29:672–81.
41. Tepel M, Hopfenmueller W, Scholze A, Maier A, Zidek W. Effect of amlodipine on cardiovascular events in hypertensive haemodialysis patients. Nephrol Dial Transplant. 2008;23(11):3605–12. https://doi.org/10.1093/ndt/gfn304.
42. Youssef AM, Elghoneimy HA, Helmy MW, Abdelazeem AM, El-Khodary NM. Effect of amlodipine versus bisoprolol in hypertensive patients on maintenance hemodialysis: a randomized controlled trial. Medicine (Baltimore). 2021;100(51):e28322. https://doi.org/10.1097/MD.0000000000028322.
43. Charytan DM, Himmelfarb J, Ikizler TA, Raj DS, Hsu JY, Landis JR, Anderson AH, Hung AM, Mehrotra R, Sharma S, Weiner DE, Williams M, DiCarli M, Skali H, Kimmel PL, Kliger AS, Dember LM. Hemodialysis Novel Therapies Consortium: safety and cardiovascular efficacy of spironolactone in dialysis-dependent ESRD (SPin-D): a randomized, placebo-controlled, multiple dosage trial. Kidney Int. 2019;95:973–82.
44. Hammer F, Malzahn U, Donhauser J, Betz C, Schneider MP, Grupp C, Pollak N, Störk S, Wanner C, Krane V. MiREnDa Study Group: a randomized controlled trial of the effect of spironolactone on left ventricular mass in hemodialysis patients. Kidney Int. 2019;95:983–91.
45. Agarwal A, Cheung AK. Mineralocorticoid receptor antagonists in ESKD. Clin J Am Soc Nephrol. 2020;15(7):1047–9. https://doi.org/10.2215/CJN.13221019.
46. Moura-Neto JA, Ronco C. Finerenone and chronic kidney disease outcomes in type 2 diabetes. N Engl J Med. 2021;384(11):e42. https://doi.org/10.1056/NEJMc2036175.
47. Zhang MZ, Bao W, Zheng QY, Wang YH, Sun LY. Efficacy and safety of finerenone in chronic kidney disease: a systematic review and meta-analysis of randomized clinical trials. Front Pharmacol. 2022;13:819327. https://doi.org/10.3389/fphar.2022.819327.
48. Dunlop JL, Vandal AC, Marshall MR. Low dialysate sodium levels for chronic haemodialysis. Cochrane Database Syst Rev. 2019;1:Cd011204.
49. Hecking M, Moissl U, Genser B, et al. Greater fluid overload and lower interdialytic weight gain are independently associated with mortality in a large international hemodialysis population. Nephrol Dial Transplant. 2018;33(10):1832–42.
50. Dinesh K, Kunaparaju S, Cape K, Flythe JE, Feldman HI, Brunelli SM. A model of systolic blood pressure during the course of dialysis and clinical factors associated with various blood pressure behaviors. Am J Kidney Dis. 2011;58:794–803.
51. Kooman J, Basci A, Pizzarelli F, Canaud B, Haage P, Fouque D, et al. EBPG guideline on haemodynamic instability. Nephrol Dial Transplant. 2007;22(Suppl 2):ii22–44. https://doi.org/10.1093/ndt/gfm019.
52. Daugirdas JT. Dialysis hypotension: a hemodynamic analysis. Kidney Int. 1991;39:233–46.

53. al Muhanna FA, Saeed I, al Muelo S, Larbi E, Rubaish A. Disease profile, complications and outcome in patients on maintenance haemodialysis at King Faisal University Hospital, Saudi Arabia. E Afr Med J. 1999;76:664–7.
54. Tisler A, Akocsi K, Borbas B, et al. The effect of frequent or occasional dialysis-associated hypotension on survival of patients on maintenance haemodialysis. Nephrol Dial Transplant. 2003;18:2601–5.
55. Hung SY, Hung YM, Fang HC, et al. Cardiac troponin I and creatine kinase isoenzyme MB in patients with intradialytic hypotension. Blood Purif. 2004;22:338–43.
56. Nette RW, van den Dorpel MA, Krepel HP, et al. Hypotension during hemodialysis results from an impairment of arteriolar tone and left ventricular function. Clin Nephrol. 2005;63:276–83.
57. Zoccali C, Tripepi G, Mallamaci F, Panuccio V. The heart rate response pattern to dialysis hypotension in haemodialysis patients. Nephrol Dial Transplant. 1997;12:519–23.
58. Sibbald WJ, Paterson NA, Holliday RL, Baskerville J. The Trendelenburg position: hemodynamic effects in hypotensive and normotensive patients. Crit Care Med. 1979;7:218–24.
59. Bivins HG, Knopp R, dos Santos PA. Blood volume distribution in the Trendelenburg position. Ann Emerg Med. 1985;14:641–3.
60. Coll E, Valles M, Torguet P, Bronsoms J, Mate G, Mauri JM. Evaluation of plasma volume variation during different hemodialysis maneuvers. Nefrologia. 2004;24:463–9.
61. Aronoff GR. The effect of treatment time, dialysis frequency, and ultrafiltration rate on intradialytic hypotension. Semin Dial. 2017;30(6):489–91. https://doi.org/10.1111/sdi.12625.
62. Knoll GA, Grabowski JA, Dervin GF, O'Rourke K. A randomized, controlled trial of albumin versus saline for the treatment of intradialytic hypotension. J Am Soc Nephrol. 2004;15:487–92.
63. van der Sande FM, Kooman JP, Barendregt JN, Nieman FH, Leunissen KM. Effect of intravenous saline, albumin, or hydroxyethyl starch on blood volume during combined ultrafiltration and hemodialysis. J Am Soc Nephrol. 1999;10:1303–8.
64. Maduell F, Navarro V. Assessment of salt intake in hemodialysis. Nefrologia. 2001;21:71–7.
65. Gullapudi VRL, Kazmi I, Selby NM. Techniques to improve intradialytic haemodynamic stability. Curr Opin Nephrol Hypertens. 2018;27:413–9.
66. Ekinci C, Karabork M, Siriopol D, et al. Effects of volume overload and current techniques for the assessment of fluid status in patients with renal disease. Blood Purif. 2018;46:34–47.
67. Pizzarelli F, Dattolo P, Piacenti M, Morales MA, Cerrai T, Maggiore Q. Non-invasive monitoring of hemodynamic parameters during hemodialysis. Int J Artif Organs. 1995;18:499–503.
68. Kinet JP, Soyeur D, Balland N, Saint-Remy M, Collignon P, Godon JP. Hemodynamic study of hypotension during hemodialysis. Kidney Int. 1982;21:868–76.
69. Sherman RA, Casale P, Cody R, Horton MW. Effect of predialysis verapamil on intradialytic blood pressure in chronic hemodialysis patients. ASAIO Trans. 1990;36:67–9.
70. Fotiadou E, Georgianos PI, Chourdakis M, Zebekakis PE, Liakopoulos V. Eating during the hemodialysis session: a practice improving nutritional status or a risk factor for intradialytic hypotension and reduced dialysis adequacy? Nutrients. 2020;12(6):1703. https://doi.org/10.3390/nu12061703.
71. Kalantar-Zadeh K, Tortorici AR, Chen JL, Kamgar M, Lau WL, Moradi H, Rhee CM, Streja E, Kovesdy CP. Dietary restrictions in dialysis patients: is there anything left to eat? Semin Dial. 2015;28:159–68.
72. Piccoli GB, Lippi F, Fois A, Gendrot L, Nielsen L, Vigreux J, Chatrenet A, D'Alessandro C, Cabiddu G, Cupisti A. Intradialytic nutrition and hemodialysis prescriptions: a personalized stepwise approach. Nutrients. 2020;12:785.
73. Toth-Manikowski SM, Sozio SM. Cooling dialysate during in-center hemodialysis: beneficial and deleterious effects. World J Nephrol. 2016;5:166–71.
74. Mustafa RA, Bdair F, Akl EA, et al. Effect of lowering the dialysate temperature in chronic hemodialysis: a systematic review and meta-analysis. Clin J Am Soc Nephrol. 2016;11:442–57.

75. Saran R, Bragg-Gresham JL, Levin NW, et al. Longer treatment time and slower ultrafiltration in hemodialysis: associations with reduced mortality in the DOPPS. Kidney Int. 2006;69:1222–8.
76. Flythe JE, Kimmel SE, Brunelli SM. Rapid fluid removal during dialysis is associated with cardiovascular morbidity and mortality. Kidney Int. 2011;79(2):250–7. https://doi.org/10.1038/ki.2010.383.
77. Dasgupta I, Thomas GN, Clarke J, et al. Associations between hemodialysis facility practices to manage fluid volume and intradialytic hypotension and patient outcomes. Clin J Am Soc Nephrol. 2019;14:385–93.
78. Cruz DN, Mahnensmith RL, Brickel HM, Perazella MA. Midodrine and cool dialysate are effective therapies for symptomatic intradialytic hypotension. Am J Kidney Dis. 1999;33:920–6.
79. Kyriazis J, Stamatiadis D, Mamouna A. Intradialytic and interdialytic effects of treatment with 1.25 and 1.75 mmol/L of calcium dialysate on arterial compliance in patients on hemodialysis. Am J Kidney Dis. 2000;35:1096–103.
80. Kyriazis J, Kalogeropoulou K, Bilirakis L, et al. Dialysate magnesium level and blood pressure. Kidney Int. 2004;66:1221–31.
81. Lazzeroni D, Rimoldi O, Camici PG. From left ventricular hypertrophy to dysfunction and failure. Circ J. 2016;80(3):555–64.
82. Gersh BJ, Maron BJ, Bonow RO, Dearani JA, Fifer MA, Link MS, et al. 2011 ACCF/AHA guideline for the diagnosis and treatment of hypertrophic cardiomyopathy: executive summary: a report of the American College of Cardiology Foundation/American Heart Association task force on practice guidelines. J Am Coll Cardiol. 2011;58(25):2703–38.
83. Wanner C, Krane V, Marz W, Olschewski M, Asmus HG, Kramer W, et al. Randomized controlled trial on the efficacy and safety of atorvastatin in patients with type 2 diabetes on hemodialysis (4D study): demographic and baseline characteristics. Kidney Blood Press Res. 2004;27(4):259–66.
84. Investigators ET, Chertow GM, Block GA, Correa-Rotter R, Drueke TB, Floege J, et al. Effect of cinacalcet on cardiovascular disease in patients undergoing dialysis. N Engl J Med. 2012;367(26):2482–94.
85. Sharp Collaborative Group. Study of Heart and Renal Protection (SHARP): randomized trial to assess the effects of lowering low-density lipoprotein cholesterol among 9438 patients with chronic kidney disease. Am Heart J. 2010;160(5):785–94 e10.
86. Liut F, Izzi C, Dallera N, Scolari F. ADPKD and heart. G Ital Nefrol. 2017;34(Suppl 69):119–30.
87. Culleton BF, Walsh M, Klarenbach SW, Mortis G, Scott-Douglas N, Quinn RR, et al. Effect of frequent nocturnal hemodialysis vs conventional hemodialysis on left ventricular mass and quality of life: a randomized controlled trial. JAMA. 2007;298(11):1291–9.
88. Glassock RJ, Pecoits-Filho R, Barberato SH. Left ventricular mass in chronic kidney disease and ESRD. Clin J Am Soc Nephrol. 2009;4(Suppl 1):S79–91.
89. Paoletti E, Bellino D, Cassottana P, Rolla D, Cannella G. Left ventricular hypertrophy in nondiabetic predialysis CKD. Am J Kidney Dis. 2005;46(2):320–7.
90. Chan CT, Greene T, Chertow GM, Kliger AS, Stokes JB, Beck GJ, et al. Determinants of left ventricular mass in patients on hemodialysis: Frequent Hemodialysis Network (FHN) Trials. Circ Cardiovasc Imaging. 2012;5(2):251–61.
91. Chan CT, Greene T, Chertow GM, Kliger AS, Stokes JB, Beck GJ, et al. Effects of frequent hemodialysis on ventricular volumes and left ventricular remodeling. Clin J Am Soc Nephrol. 2013;8(12):2106–16.
92. Rigatto C, Parfrey P. Therapy insight: management of cardiovascular disease in the renal transplant recipient. Nat Clin Pract Nephrol. 2006;2(9):514–26.
93. Pecoits-Filho R, Calice-Silva V. Unchain the heart: impact of left ventricular myocardial hypertrophy regression in kidney transplant outcomes. Nephrol Dial Transplant. 2016;31(7):1025–6.

94. Parfrey PS, Harnett JD, Foley RN, Kent GM, Murray DC, Barre PE, et al. Impact of renal transplantation on uremic cardiomyopathy. Transplantation. 1995;60(9):908–14.
95. Rigatto C, Foley RN, Kent GM, Guttmann R, Parfrey PS. Long-term changes in left ventricular hypertrophy after renal transplantation. Transplantation. 2000;70(4):570–5.
96. Patel RK, Mark PB, Johnston N, McGregor E, Dargie HJ, Jardine AG. Renal transplantation is not associated with regression of left ventricular hypertrophy: a magnetic resonance study. Clin J Am Soc Nephrol. 2008;3(6):1807–11.
97. Diez J, Laviades C. Hypertensive heart disease in the patient with chronic kidney disease. Nefrologia. 2008;28(2):135–42.
98. Lopez B, Gonzalez A, Hermida N, Laviades C, Diez J. Myocardial fibrosis in chronic kidney disease: potential benefits of torasemide. Kidney Int Suppl. 2008;111:S19–23.
99. Cramariuc D, Gerdts E. Epidemiology of left ventricular hypertrophy in hypertension: implications for the clinic. Expert Rev Cardiovasc Ther. 2016;14(8):915–26.
100. Aurigemma GP, Silver KH, Priest MA, Gaasch WH. Geometric changes allow normal ejection fraction despite depressed myocardial shortening in hypertensive left ventricular hypertrophy. J Am Coll Cardiol. 1995;26(1):195–202.
101. Briet M, Barhoumi T, Mian MOR, Coelho SC, Ouerd S, Rautureau Y, et al. Aldosterone-induced vascular remodeling and endothelial dysfunction require functional angiotensin type 1a receptors. Hypertension. 2016;67(5):897–905.
102. Cacciapuoti F. Molecular mechanisms of left ventricular hypertrophy (LVH) in systemic hypertension (SH)-possible therapeutic perspectives. J Am Soc Hypertens. 2011;5(6):449–55.
103. Foley RN, Parfrey PS, Harnett JD, Kent GM, Murray DC, Barre PE. The impact of anemia on cardiomyopathy, morbidity, and mortality in end-stage renal disease. Am J Kidney Dis. 1996;28(1):53–61.
104. Guedes M, Muenz DG, Zee J, Bieber B, Stengel B, Massy ZA, Mansencal N, Wong MMY, Charytan DM, Reichel H, Waechter S, Pisoni RL, Robinson BM, Pecoits-Filho R, CKDopps Investigators. Serum biomarkers of iron stores are associated with increased risk of all-cause mortality and cardiovascular events in nondialysis CKD patients, with or without anemia. J Am Soc Nephrol. 2021;32(8):2020–30.
105. Ponikowski P, Kirwan BA, Anker SD, McDonagh T, Dorobantu M, Drozdz J, Fabien V, Filippatos G, Göhring UM, Keren A, Khintibidze I, Kragten H, Martinez FA, Metra M, Milicic D, Nicolau JC, Ohlsson M, Parkhomenko A, Pascual-Figal DA, Ruschitzka F, Sim D, Skouri H, van der Meer P, Lewis BS, Comin-Colet J, von Haehling S, Cohen-Solal A, Danchin N, Doehner W, Dargie HJ, Motro M, Butler J, Friede T, Jensen KH, Pocock S, Jankowska EA, AFFIRM-AHF Investigators. Ferric carboxymaltose for iron deficiency at discharge after acute heart failure: a multicentre, double-blind, randomised, controlled trial. Lancet. 2020;396(10266):1895–904.
106. Bucharles S, Barberato SH, Stinghen AE, Gruber B, Meister H, Mehl A, et al. Hypovitaminosis D is associated with systemic inflammation and concentric myocardial geometric pattern in hemodialysis patients with low iPTH levels. Nephron Clin Pract. 2011;118(4):c384–91.
107. Wolf M, Shah A, Gutierrez O, Ankers E, Monroy M, Tamez H, et al. Vitamin D levels and early mortality among incident hemodialysis patients. Kidney Int. 2007;72(8):1004–13.
108. Moe SM, Thadhani R. What have we learned about chronic kidney disease-mineral bone disorder from the EVOLVE and PRIMO trials? Curr Opin Nephrol Hypertens. 2013;22(6):651–5.
109. Pritchett Y, Jemiai Y, Chang Y, Bhan I, Agarwal R, Zoccali C, et al. The use of group sequential, information-based sample size re-estimation in the design of the PRIMO study of chronic kidney disease. Clin Trials. 2011;8(2):165–74.
110. Achinger SG, Ayus JC. The role of vitamin D in left ventricular hypertrophy and cardiac function. Kidney Int Suppl. 2005;95:S37–42.
111. Pecoits-Filho R, Bucharles S, Barberato SH. Diastolic heart failure in dialysis patients: mechanisms, diagnostic approach, and treatment. Semin Dial. 2012;25(1):35–41.
112. Kendrick J, Cheung AK, Kaufman JS, Greene T, Roberts WL, Smits G, et al. FGF-23 associates with death, cardiovascular events, and initiation of chronic dialysis. J Am Soc Nephrol. 2011;22(10):1913–22.

113. Sharma S, Joseph J, Chonchol M, Kaufman JS, Cheung AK, Rafeq Z, et al. Higher fibroblast growth factor-23 concentrations associate with left ventricular systolic dysfunction in dialysis patients. Clin Nephrol. 2013;80(5):313–21.
114. Faul C, Amaral AP, Oskouei B, Hu MC, Sloan A, Isakova T, et al. FGF23 induces left ventricular hypertrophy. J Clin Invest. 2011;121(11):4393–408.
115. McCullough PA, Chan CT, Weinhandl ED, Burkart JM, Bakris GL. Intensive hemodialysis, left ventricular hypertrophy, and cardiovascular disease. Am J Kidney Dis. 2016;68(5S1):S5–S14.
116. Barberato SH, Bucharles SG, Barberato MF, Pecoits-Filho R. Association between clinical and Doppler echocardiographic parameters with sudden death in hemodialysis patients. Arq Bras Cardiol. 2016;107(2):124–30.
117. Badve SV, Palmer SC, Strippoli GFM, Roberts MA, Teixeira-Pinto A, Boudville N, et al. The validity of left ventricular mass as a surrogate end point for all-cause and cardiovascular mortality outcomes in people with CKD: a systematic review and meta-analysis. Am J Kidney Dis. 2016;68(4):554–63.
118. Cottone S, Nardi E, Mule G, Vadala A, Lorito MC, Riccobene R, et al. Association between biomarkers of inflammation and left ventricular hypertrophy in moderate chronic kidney disease. Clin Nephrol. 2007;67(4):209–16.
119. Ortega O, Gallar P, Munoz M, Rodriguez I, Carreno A, Ortiz M, et al. Association between C-reactive protein levels and N-terminal pro-B-type natriuretic peptide in pre-dialysis patients. Nephron Clin Pract. 2004;97(4):c125–30.
120. Vlahakos DV, Hahalis G, Vassilakos P, Marathias KP, Geroulanos S. Relationship between left ventricular hypertrophy and plasma renin activity in chronic hemodialysis patients. J Am Soc Nephrol. 1997;8(11):1764–70.
121. Sato A, Funder JW, Saruta T. Involvement of aldosterone in left ventricular hypertrophy of patients with end-stage renal failure treated with hemodialysis. Am J Hypertens. 1999;12(9 Pt 1):867–73.
122. Marwick TH, Gillebert TC, Aurigemma G, Chirinos J, Derumeaux G, Galderisi M, et al. Recommendations on the use of echocardiography in adult hypertension: a report from the European Association of Cardiovascular Imaging (EACVI) and the American Society of Echocardiography (ASE). J Am Soc Echocardiogr. 2015;28(7):727–54.
123. Graham-Brown MP, March DS, Churchward DR, Stensel DJ, Singh A, Arnold R, et al. Novel cardiac nuclear magnetic resonance method for noninvasive assessment of myocardial fibrosis in hemodialysis patients. Kidney Int. 2016;90(4):835–44.
124. Rutherford E, Talle MA, Mangion K, Bell E, Rauhalammi SM, Roditi G, et al. Defining myocardial tissue abnormalities in end-stage renal failure with cardiac magnetic resonance imaging using native T1 mapping. Kidney Int. 2016;90(4):845–52.
125. Barberato SH, Pecoits-Filho R. Echocardiographic alterations in patients with chronic kidney failure undergoing hemodialysis. Arq Bras Cardiol. 2010;94(1):140–6.
126. Calice-Silva, Moura-Neto J, Divino-Filho JC, Ronco C, et al. Left ventricular hypertrophy, nephrology worldwide. 1st ed. Springer; 2021.
127. Park SK, Oh CM, Kang JG, Seok HS, Jung JY. The association between left ventricular hypertrophy and consumption of nuts, including peanuts, pine nuts, and almonds. Nutr Metab Cardiovasc Dis. 2021;31(1):76–84.
128. Wheeler DC, Stefánsson BV, Jongs N, Chertow GM, Greene T, Hou FF, McMurray JJV, Correa-Rotter R, Rossing P, Toto RD, Sjöström CD, Langkilde AM, Heerspink HJL, DAPA-CKD Trial Committees and Investigators. Effects of dapagliflozin on major adverse kidney and cardiovascular events in patients with diabetic and non-diabetic chronic kidney disease: a prespecified analysis from the DAPA-CKD trial. Lancet Diabetes Endocrinol. 2021;9(1):22–31.
129. Agarwal R, Filippatos G, Pitt B, Anker SD, Rossing P, Joseph A, Kolkhof P, Nowack C, Gebel M, Ruilope LM, Bakris GL, FIDELIO-DKD and FIGARO-DKD Investigators. Cardiovascular and kidney outcomes with finerenone in patients with type 2 diabetes and chronic kidney disease: the FIDELITY pooled analysis. Eur Heart J. 2022;43(6):474–84.

130. Brown AJM, Gandy S, McCrimmon R, Houston JG, Struthers AD, Lang CC. A randomized controlled trial of dapagliflozin on left ventricular hypertrophy in people with type two diabetes: the DAPA-LVH trial. Eur Heart J. 2020;41(36):3421–32.
131. Cheung AK, et al. Cardiac diseases in maintenance hemodialysis patients: results of the HEMO Study. Kidney Int. 2004;65(6):2380–9.
132. Wanner C, et al. Randomized controlled trial on the efficacy and safety of atorvastatin in patients with type 2 diabetes on hemodialysis (4D study): demographic and baseline characteristics. Kidney Blood Press Res. 2004;27(4):259–66.
133. EVOLVE Trial Investigators, et al. Effect of cinacalcet on cardiovascular disease in patients undergoing dialysis. N Engl J Med. 2012;367(26):2482–94.
134. Harnett JD, et al. Congestive heart failure in dialysis patients: prevalence, incidence, prognosis and risk factors. Kidney Int. 1995;47(3):884–90.
135. National Institute of Diabetes and Digestive and Kidney Diseases. United States Renal Data System, annual data report: epidemiology of kidney disease in the United States. Bethesda: National Institutes of Health; 2014.
136. Chawla LS, et al. Proposal for a functional classification system of heart failure in patients with end-stage renal disease: proceedings of the acute dialysis quality initiative (ADQI) XI workgroup. J Am Coll Cardiol. 2014;63(13):1246–52.
137. Bansal N, et al. A longitudinal study of left ventricular function and structure from CKD to ESRD: the CRIC study. Clin J Am Soc Nephrol. 2013;8(3):355–62.
138. Kottgen A, et al. Reduced kidney function as a risk factor for incident heart failure: the atherosclerosis risk in communities (ARIC) study. J Am Soc Nephrol. 2007;18(4):1307–15.
139. Pocock SJ, et al. Predicting survival in heart failure: a risk score based on 39,372 patients from 30 studies. Eur Heart J. 2013;34(19):1404–13.
140. Hasenfuss G, Mann DL. Pathophysiology of heart failure. In: Braunwald E, editor. Braunwald's heart disease: a textbook of cardiovascular medicine. Philadelphia: Elsevier Saunders; 2015. p. 454–72.
141. Malik J, et al. Mechanisms of chronic heart failure development in end-stage renal disease patients on chronic hemodialysis. Physiol Res. 2009;58(5):613–21.
142. Hakeem A, Bhatti S, Chang SM. Screening and risk stratification of coronary artery disease in end-stage renal disease. JACC Cardiovasc Imaging. 2014;7(7):715–28.
143. London GM, Parfrey PS. Cardiac disease in chronic uremia: pathogenesis. Adv Ren Replace Ther. 1997;4(3):194–211.
144. Herzog CA, et al. Cardiovascular disease in chronic kidney disease. A clinical update from kidney disease: improving global outcomes (KDIGO). Kidney Int. 2011;80(6):572–86.
145. Feldman HI, et al. The chronic renal insufficiency cohort (CRIC) study: design and methods. J Am Soc Nephrol. 2003;14(7 Suppl 2):S148–53.
146. Shroff GR, Frederick PD, Herzog CA. Renal failure and acute myocardial infarction: clinical characteristics in patients with advanced chronic kidney disease, on dialysis, and without chronic kidney disease. A collaborative project of the United States Renal Data System/National Institutes of Health and the National Registry of Myocardial Infarction. Am Heart J. 2012;163:399–406.
147. Herzog CA, Littrell K, Arko C, Frederick PD, Blaney M. Clinical characteristics of dialysis patients with acute myocardial infarction in the United States: a collaborative project of the United States Renal Data System and the National Registry of Myocardial Infarction. Circulation. 2007;116:1465–72.
148. Iseki K, Fukiyama K. Long-term prognosis and incidence of acute myocardial infarction in patients on chronic hemodialysis. The Okinawa Dialysis Study Group. Am J Kidney Dis. 2000;36:820–5.
149. Shroff GR, Li S, Herzog CA. Trends in mortality following acute myocardial infarction among dialysis patients in the United States over 15 years. J Am Heart Assoc. 2015;4:e002460.
150. Herzog CA, Ma JZ, Collins AJ. Poor long-term survival after acute myocardial infarction among patients on long-term dialysis. N Engl J Med. 1998;339:799–805.

151. Fox KA, Steg PG, Eagle KA, Goodman SG, Anderson FA Jr, Granger CB, Flather MD, Budaj A, Quill A, Gore JM, GRACE Investigators. Decline in rates of death and heart failure in acute coronary syndromes, 1999–2006. JAMA. 2007;297:1892–900.
152. Yeh RW, Sidney S, Chandra M, Sorel M, Selby JV, Go AS. Population trends in the incidence and outcomes of acute myocardial infarction. N Engl J Med. 2010;362:2155–65.
153. National Institute of Diabetes and Digestive and Kidney Diseases. U.S. Renal Data System. USRDS 2013 annual data report: atlas of chronic kidney disease and end-stage renal disease in the United States, vol. 2. Bethesda: National Institutes of Health; 2013. p. 252.
154. Smith SC Jr, Benjamin EJ, Bonow RO, et al. AHA/ACCF secondary prevention and risk reduction therapy for patients with coronary and other atherosclerotic vascular disease: 2011 update: a guideline from the American Heart Association and American College of Cardiology Foundation. Circulation. 2011;124:2458–73.
155. Amsterdam EA, Wenger NK, Brindis RG, et al. 2014 AHA/ACC guideline for the management of patients with non-ST-elevation acute coronary syndromes: executive summary: a report of the American College of Cardiology/American Heart Association task force on practice guidelines. Circulation. 2014;130:2354–94.
156. Maini R, Wong DB, Addison D, et al. Persistent underrepresentation of kidney disease in randomized, controlled trials of cardiovascular disease in the contemporary era. J Am Soc Nephrol. 2018;29:2782–6.
157. Lin TY, Hsieh TH, Hung SC. Association of secondary prevention medication use after myocardial infarction with mortality in hemodialysis patients. Clin Kidney J. 2022;15(11):2135–43. https://doi.org/10.1093/ckj/sfac170.
158. Matsushita K, van der Velde M, Astor BC, et al. Association of estimated glomerular filtration rate and albuminuria with all-cause and cardiovascular mortality in general population cohorts: a collaborative meta-analysis. Lancet. 2010;375:2073–81.
159. Levey A. Chronic kidney disease. Lancet. 2012;379:165–80.
160. Toyoda K, Fujii K, Fujimi S, et al. Stroke in patients on maintenance hemodialysis: a 22-year single-center study. Am J Kidney Dis. 2005;45:1058–66.
161. Daftari Besheli L, Aran S, Shaqdan K, Kay J, Abujudeh H. Current status of nephrogenic systemic fibrosis. Clin Radiol. 2014;69(7):661–8. https://doi.org/10.1016/j.crad.2014.01.003.
162. Hirakata H, Japanese Society for Dialysis Therapy, et al. Japanese Society for Dialysis Therapy guidelines for management of cardiovascular diseases in patients on chronic hemodialysis. Ther Apher Dial. 2012;16(5):387–435. https://doi.org/10.1111/j.1744-9987.2012.01088.x.
163. Bangalore S, Maron DJ, O'Brien SM, Fleg JL, Kretov EI, Briguori C, Kaul U, Reynolds HR, Mazurek T, Sidhu MS, Berger JS, Mathew RO, Bockeria O, Broderick S, Pracon R, Herzog CA, Huang Z, Stone GW, Boden WE, Newman JD, Ali ZA, Mark DB, Spertus JA, Alexander KP, Chaitman BR, Chertow GM, Hochman JS, ISCHEMIA-CKD Research Group. Management of coronary disease in patients with advanced kidney disease. N Engl J Med. 2020;382(17):1608–18. https://doi.org/10.1056/NEJMoa1915925.

Dementia, Dwindles, Depression, Nonadherence, and Symptom Burden in End-Stage Kidney Disease

3

Angelina R. Edwards

Introduction

Holistic care of patients with end-stage kidney disease requires a careful assessment of metabolic parameters and dialysis adequacy and the assessment and management of physical and emotional well-being. Given their advanced age and comorbidities, ESKD patients suffer a disproportionate degree of dementia and cognitive decline compared to their age-matched cohorts with normal renal function. Patient-reported stressors encountered during dialysis are similar to those experienced by other patients with chronic medical illnesses. Symptom burden is high among ESKD and often leads to challenges with adherence to treatment and dialysis. This chapter will focus on these critical elements, providing an overview of incidence, associations, treatment options, and suggestions for future initiatives.

Cognitive Dysfunction in End-Stage Renal Disease

Cognitive impairment, including dementia, increases with declining renal function and manifests as executive function, orientation, and attention deficiencies. The incidence of dementia in patients with renal impairment is estimated at 10–30% in young- and middle-aged and upwards of 30–55% in the elderly. It is poorly recognized and under-reported [1]. Incidence increases among patients on dialysis. Observations from the Chronic Renal Insufficiency Cohort showed a significant decline in executive function within 2 years of dialysis initiation [2]. Cognitive and

A. R. Edwards (✉)
Division of Kidney Diseases, Hypertension and Transplantation, Department of Medicine, Houston Methodist Hospital, Houston, TX, USA
e-mail: aredwards@houstonmethodist.org

S. Z. Fadem et al. (eds.), *Complications in Dialysis*,
https://doi.org/10.1007/978-3-031-44557-6_3

functional impairment is a surrogate of frailty and is independently associated with increased mortality [3].

Mechanisms that Lead to Cognitive Decline

Various factors lead to cognitive decline in dialysis patients and can be divided into non-kidney-associated factors, chronic kidney disease-specific factors, and dialysis-specific factors.

Non-kidney-associated risk factors for cognitive decline include cardiovascular disease and age. Patients with renal impairment have a disproportionately high burden of cardiovascular disease owing to the high prevalence of comorbidities, including diabetes, hypertension, and hyperlipidemia. Small vessel disease in particular leads to increased cerebrovascular disease and ischemic dementia. Comorbidities of diabetes, hypertension, and hyperlipidemia lead to increased CVD events, including myocardial infarction and cerebrovascular accidents. Older age is the most common cause of cognitive decline. The burden of ESKD is not equally distributed across the age spectrum, and patients older than 65 make up a disproportionately high percentage of those initiating dialysis. Societal guidelines do not specify whom to screen, but the elderly and those with prior cerebrovascular events should be prioritized, with testing performed biannually (Fig. 3.1) [4].

Both reduced renal function and microalbuminuria are independent risk factors for cognitive impairment [5–7]. A cohort study of the Systolic Blood Pressure Intervention Trial-Memory and Cognition in Decreased Hypertension (SPRINT-MIND) assessed over 2800 patients with cardiovascular disease and chronic kidney disease [8]. Patients were screened with neurocognitive testing. Those with higher degrees of albuminuria scored worse on global cognitive testing, executive function, and memory. In a subset of patients who underwent Magnetic Resonance Imaging (MRI), those with albuminuria had higher white matter volume abnormalities and

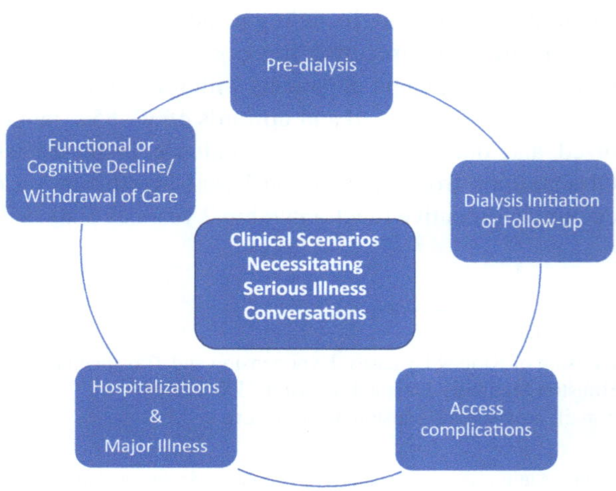

Fig. 3.1 [4]: Recommendations on withholding or withdrawing dialysis

subsequent cerebral atrophy, suggesting that loss of cognitive fitness is likely related to abnormal brain perfusion and ischemic injury.

Retention of uremic toxins and phosphates is a known contributor of cognitive decline and encephalopathy [9]. Impaired tubular secretion and retention of organic solutes contribute to cognitive impairment even in early stages of CKD [10]. While routine renal replacement therapy has eliminated the most severe manifestations of uremic encephalopathy, there are thousands of other metabolites of renal failure that are not cleared. Even in the era of high-flux dialyzers, clearance of middle molecules such as tumor necrosis factor and interleukin-6 is reduced, leading to chronic inflammation, oxidative stress, atherosclerosis, and vascular calcification. Reduced clearance of protein-bound metabolites such as *p*-cresol sulfate and hippurate carries neuronal toxicity and is associated with cognitive impairment.

Dialysis-related factors that contributed to cognitive decline are mainly related to hemodynamic changes during hemodialysis treatments. Intradialytic hypotension can lead to a significant decline in cerebral perfusion, hastening cognitive dysfunction [11]. Diminished vascular tone from atherosclerosis is often noted in ESKD patients, but the circulatory stress of hemodialysis results in decreased systemic blood pressure. The impact of osmotic shifts and volume removal on cerebral blood flow while on dialysis have been clearly demonstrated using transcranial doppler ultrasound. Reduced cerebral perfusion is associated with a decline in global cognitive scores.

Screening for Cognitive Decline

Cognitive decline usually manifests earlier in the course of renal dysfunction, is exacerbated during the post-dialysis period, and is often unrecognized and underappreciated [12]. Because of this, routine testing for global cognitive deficits is recommended every 6 months in ESRD patients. The modified mini-mental state examination has been validated in ESKD patients and offers a robust yet lengthy assessment of global cognitive function, including visual-spatial, recall and memory, along with multi-stage commands. The montreal cognitive assessment is a one-page screening of cognition and has recently been validated in the ESKD population and found to be a sensitive tool for detecting mild cognitive decline. Deficits in the cognitive domains of executive function, orientation, and attention are the most frequently observed.

Approach to Management of Cognitive Decline

Early interventions to aggressively minimize albuminuria in the early stages of kidney disease may prove beneficial for slowing the incidence of cognitive dysfunction, and intense blood pressure control preserves cerebral perfusion and cognitive fitness [13, 14]. Efforts to control CVD risk factors and to reduce intradialytic hypotension may slow cognitive decline. Small observational studies show cooling dialysate results in improved hemodynamic tolerability and less brain white matter injury [15]. Ongoing randomized controlled studies will assess utility and feasibility of sustained dialysate cooling and improvement of cognitive decline [16].

Early recognition is key [12]. If initial screens are positive, additional neurocognitive assessment, including referral to a neurologist is advised. Reversible causes of cognitive dysfunction should be excluded, including vitamin B12 deficiency and thyroid abnormalities. If focal deficits are present, neuroimaging is recommended.

Polypharmacy is an independent risk factor for cognitive decline [17]. End-stage kidney disease patients have the highest number of medications of all chronically ill patients and are subject to drug-related side effects and higher adverse drug events due to impaired clearance [18]. De-prescribing practices should be adopted in a multidisciplinary approach, and non-medical interventions should be sought for symptom management.

There is a high incidence of cognitive impairment and frailty in ESKD patients, and both are highly associated with adverse health outcomes [12, 19]. Physical inactivity parallels frailty and the majority of ESKD are sedentary. Physical exercise programs are safe and effective, and numerous studies have shown the benefit of home-based and intradialytic exercise programs in combating frailty and improving cognitive function [20]. Exercise therapy leads to enhanced cerebral blood flow, increased brain volume in the prefrontal and hippocampal area, increased neurotrophic factors, and decreased inflammation. This can lead to increased brain plasticity and executive function [21]. Novel strategies to increase physical activity include tai chi, intradialytic yoga, electrical stimulation of muscle, and virtual reality gaming [22]. Despite the numerous benefits of exercise, broad-scale implementation in dialysis units remains low, and patient adherence is poor. With the recent establishment of the global renal exercise work group, future research will focus on prioritizing high-quality clinical studies and supporting patients and clinicians with evidence-based guidance on exercise interventions.

Pharmacologic interventions and treatment recommendations are lacking due to limited data as a consequence of CKD and ESKD patients being largely excluded from these studies [4]. Given the multi-variable contributors to dementia in CKD, one unifying treatment is not available. As cognitive decline sets in, patients are less capable of engaging in meaningful discussions. Ideally, management must focus on early discussion with the patient and family to align treatment goals both now and in the future. A conservative approach to kidney care is a consideration, particularly in those who have made their wishes clear or who have such advanced stages of dementia where dialysis would prove futile.

Kidney Supportive Care

In a shared-decision model, a serious illness conversation guide facilitates the clinician to become acquainted with the patient's awareness of prognosis and disease state, factors that impact treatment decision-making and goals of care (Table 3.1) [23, 24].

Table 3.1 (Ariadne Labs, 2015): Recommended dialogue using the Serious Illness Conversation Guide

Patient-tested dialogue for Serious Illness Conversations for Withdrawing Dialysis
Set Up: *"I understand you have been thinking about whether you should continue dialysis. Would it be ok for us to talk more about your goals and preferences, so we can think about this together?*
Assess: "*What is your understanding of what it means to stop dialysis?"*
Share: *"I want to share with you my understanding now. What, if any, information about what lies ahead would you like me to share?*
Explore: *What are your most important goals if you stop dialysis and are approaching the end of your life?* *What are your fears and worries as you are considering stopping dialysis?* *What things continue to give you strength as you look to the future?* *What functions are most important for you to continue after stopping dialysis?* *If you stop dialysis, what areas of your comfort and wellbeing need to be prioritized?* *Have you discussed your thoughts of stopping dialysis with your family?*
Close: "In summary, we covered a lot of important points and I heard that _____ is really important for you. I recommend that we _____. How does this plan seem to you? I will do everything I can to help you. You will not alone. These are my recommendations…"

Table 3.2 Patient characteristics that warrant Serious Illness Conversations in Advanced Kidney Disease [23–25]

Patient characteristics
CKD stage 4 or 5, any age
CKD stage 3b, over age 80
CKD stage 3b, with diabetes mellitus type 2 and/or hypertension, over age 70
CKD stage 3b, any age, with advanced end-organ disease including heart failure with NYHA III or IV, end stage liver disease, MELD >17, severe COPD
CKD stage 3b, any age, with metastatic cancer

CKD chronic kidney disease, *NYHA* New York Heart Association, *MELD* model for end-stage liver disease

Over 90% of patients express a desire to have these conversations with their nephrologist but less than 10% do. Providers often avoid these conversations over concerns it will contribute to patient anxiety and hopelessness but studies do not support this [25]. Through these dialogues, the patient is gently guided by the physician to grasp the extent of their medical condition and should be performed throughout the continuum of care of chronic kidney disease and at major health events (see Table 3.2).

The executive summary of the KDIGO Controversies Conference on Supportive Care in CKD provides guidance to practitioners as they help patients cope with the challenges of living and dying with CKD [26]. Consistent use of Health-Related Quality of Life (HRQL) surveys, such as the Edmonton Symptom Assessment System Revised Renal, the Palliative Care Outcome Scale-Renal, and the Dialysis Symptom Index allows early identification of patients with worrisome symptoms and even those in their last days of life [27–30].

If a patient is not yet on dialysis, a conservative kidney management approach with non-dialysis and non-transplant care should be considered, with emphasis on quality of life, symptom-focused therapy, and advanced care planning [31]. Given the high prevalence of geriatric syndromes, including frailty, multidisciplinary care in conjunction with geriatrics and palliative care is preferred. Limited studies of those managed with conservative measures showed patients survived for many years and experienced a sustained quality of life until late into their illness course [32]. The use of acute care services was high and points to the high variability of practice patterns of conservative kidney management. Furthermore, non-dialytic management of advanced CKD is underutilized in the United States due to inadequate training, misperceptions that conservative care equates with absence of care, and financial systems that fail to incentivize supportive care [33]. Attempts to align the patient's wishes with appropriate care services would lead to considerable improvement to access to these conservative treatment options and substantial cost-savings. Many have proposed that the Advancing American Kidney Health Initiative should include actionable principles of supportive care for those that forego conventional dialysis and make the case for conservative kidney management being considered equivalent to a home modality [34].

Advanced Care Planning

According to the 2019 United States Renal Data System (USRDS) Annual Data Report, mortality rates among those with ESKD are twice as high as those with heart failure and three times higher than those with cancer [35]. The intensity of end-of-life care among dialysis patients is higher than cancer patients or patients with 4 or more comorbidities, with 30% dying within 30 days of dialysis initiation [36]. At any age, those treated with dialysis have approximately one-third the life expectancy observed in the general public. Surprisingly, less than half of all ESKD patients have an advanced directive addressing preferences for cardiopulmonary resuscitation (CPR) and have completed a Medical Orders for Life-Sustaining Treatment Form [37]. Ideally, advanced directives should be a part of advanced care planning, a holistic, evidence-based practice that decreases suffering. This improves HRQL by incorporating patients' values and life goals into care decisions, while engaging health surrogates and family members [38]. This process of shared decision-making and renal supportive care best addresses the complex needs of this population. Barriers to advance care planning include deficiencies in communication, challenges in estimating prognosis, and inadequate transition care teams. Patients are hesitant to engage their family members in these aspects of care. The USRDS Study of Treatment Preferences (USTATE) showed that only 30% of patients have discussed their wishes for end-of-life care with their family members, and the majority of family members are unaware of their loved-ones preferences regarding life-sustaining measures including CPR and ventilator use [35]. The majority (62%) of family members who were identified as surrogate decision makers had spoken with the patient about treatment preferences and the kinds of health situations that would make life not worth living. Moreover, two-thirds of family members surveyed thought that the patient would prefer to die at home or at the home of a relative but less than 30% had discussed transition to hospice or stopping dialysis [35].

Across the board, hospice use within the ESKD population remains low due to lack of advanced care planning, professional training, and reimbursement challenges for hospice care [39]. Furthermore, deficiencies in communication, challenges estimating prognosis and inadequate transition care teams equate with a lack of advanced care planning [38]. Advanced care planning must involve educated personnel and a structured, multidisciplinary approach. Effective tools should be created and adopted to provide skills-based training for dialysis social workers and nurses, which focus on patient preference, cultural sensitivity, spirituality, family and caregiver assessment, and care coordination [40, 41].

Withdrawal of Dialysis

Elective withdrawal of dialysis is common among patients with ESKD and is often made in the context of hospitalizations or acute medical complications [42]. However, there is a rising trend of discontinuation of dialysis in the non-acute setting, particularly in those who fail to thrive on dialysis and the elderly. One-third of medicare beneficiaries with ESKD reside in nursing homes near the end of life and experience a substantial decline in functional status and clinical frailty [43]. Higher mortality rates are seen in those with comorbidities, such as cardiovascular disease, where the survival advantage of dialysis, particularly in those over the age of 75 years old, is substantially reduced compared to young patients [36]. Roughly 30% of patients will electively discontinue dialysis in the first year of initiation, with 1 in 7 dying within the first 6 months from elective withdrawal [44]. In the United States, those who elect to withdraw dialysis are usually white females. In fact, the observation that ethnic minorities usually have better survival rates on dialysis is largely attributable to the higher frequency of dialysis discontinuation among whites [45]. The Renal Physicians Association (RPA) and the American Society of Nephrology (ASN) proposed 4 scenarios where consideration to withhold or withdraw dialysis is appropriate [46].

The approach to withdrawal of dialysis varies across the world. Patients in low-income countries often elect to stop dialysis due to limited financial resources [47]. Dialysis funding is offered for a time-limited period in some countries, and dialysis rationing is reserved only for those who are eligible for transplant. This is in contrast to those in high-income countries where choice-driven dialysis withdrawal prioritizes patient autonomy and shared decision-making.

Dialysis withdrawal consists of two parts: the initial decision process to withdraw from treatment and the care approach following withdrawal. The average time to death with dialysis withdrawal is usually 10 days but can extend up to 3 weeks. The process must consider the cultural, religious, and ethical-legal concerns of the patient and support the patient and family. Complexities in implementation include lengthy conversations with multiple stakeholders and heightened emotions. While no standardized approach exists to accommodate the multitude of clinical scenarios, multidisciplinary team discussions and the transition to kidney supportive care allow collaborative discussions to achieve shared goals of care. Providing the patient and family adequate end-of-life care and bereavement support are invaluable during this difficult time. Linkage with hospice and additional community support is also helpful.

Psychological Factors that Impact ESRD Patients

Incidence and Prevalence of Psychological Disorders

In the ESKD population, a broad range of psychiatric illnesses can be encountered, including dementia, depression, anxiety, schizophrenic disorders, and substance abuse. Individuals with comorbid mental illness have poorer outcomes with a higher risk of treatment nonadherence, worse quality of life, hospitalizations, hospital length of stay, and death [48]. Additionally, hospitalizations with psychiatric diagnoses are common in ESKD patients and are associated with significantly higher mortality compared to those hospitalized without a psychiatric diagnosis [49]. Although psychiatric illnesses are common, the true prevalence is difficult to determine, given the variability of screening methods and definitions, the overlap of symptoms from uremia and medication-related side effects, and inconsistent reporting [50]. Depression is the most common psychiatric illness in the ESKD population, with interview-defined prevalence up to 25% and self-reported prevalence up to 45% among dialysis patients [51]. Depressive syndromes are categorized as dysthymia, minor depression, and major depression. A diagnosis of depression based on DSM-IV criteria requires persistence of symptoms for at least 2 weeks that significantly impair function (see Table 3.3) [52].

Several patient health questionnaires evaluating depression have been validated in the ESKD and the older ESKD population [53, 54]. Depression may have atypical presentations therefore, coexistent cognitive impairment, substance abuse, and suicide risk should be assessed. Substance abuse and illicit drug use are known to cause and exacerbate renal disease. Of ESKD patients under the age of 40, approximately 4% suffer from illicit drug dependence and are 4–9 times more likely to die

Table 3.3 [52]: Major depression requires 5 or more symptoms with significant impairment in daily function, for at least 2 weeks

DSM-IV diagnostic criteria for depression	
1. Depressed mood	6. Loss of energy
2. Anhedonia	7. Reduced concentration
3. Change in sleep	8. Thoughts of worthlessness or guilt
4. Change in appetite or weight	9. Thoughts of death or suicide
5. Change in psychomotor activity	

Minor depression requires 2–4 symptoms, including depressed mood or anhedonia, with significant impairment in daily function, for at least 2 weeks. Dysthymia requires 3–4 symptoms, including depressed mood with impaired function for at least 2 years from drug overdose [55]. As for suicidality among ESKD patients, White or Asian men, over the age of 75, struggling with substance abuse and recent hospitalizations for mental illness are significantly more likely to commit suicide then persons in the general population [56]. For both substance abuse and suicidality, risk should be ascertained and immediate targeted interventions pursued to prevent premature mortality.

Management of Depression in ESKD

No established guidelines exist for treating depression in adults with ESKD. The initial choice of therapy should be based on treatment history, coexisting medical conditions, and patient preferences. Despite the high prevalence of depression in dialysis patients and patient prioritization of efficacy in treatments, evidence for the use of antidepressants is limited and inconclusive [57]. The efficacy and safety of depression treatments have only been assessed in small trials in ESKD patients [58]. Although selective serotonin reuptake inhibitors (SSRIs) are the best-studied antidepressant in ESKD patients, only 40–65% of patients respond to treatment. Adverse effects are similar in type and frequency as reported in the general population. Notable concerns of SSRI use in ESKD are observed increased risk of hip fractures, regardless of dose or duration, and QT-prolongation in older adults with a subsequent higher risk of sudden cardiac death [59, 60]. Tricyclic antidepressants (TCAs) are not considered first-line therapy in patients with ESKD due to cardiac conduction problems and orthostatic hypotension. If pharmacotherapy is initiated, a low doses should be used and clinical response and side effects should be assessed frequently during the first 3–4 weeks, with a minimum of 8–12 weeks of treatment prior to declaration of treatment failure [61]. A treatment effect should be assessed at 12 weeks to avoid prolonged ineffective medication. Lack of a treatment effect should also prompt screening for concomitant anxiety. Up to 44% of dialysis-dependent patients have an anxiety disorder, and if symptoms persist despite a full therapeutic trial of antidepressants, a psychiatry evaluation should be pursued.

Non-pharmacologic treatment with psychosocial interventions has also been assessed. A Cochrane review by Natale et al. showed moderate certainty evidence that cognitive behavioral therapy (CBT) improves depressive symptoms [62]. The cognitive model suggests that health threats and triggers lead to chronic maladaptive responses of altered feelings, emotions, thoughts, and behaviors (see Fig. 3.2) [63]. Through CBT, patients are equipped to interpret, process, and manage these threats. Additionally, small-group CBT rather than individualized psychotherapy improved depression severity, quality of life domains, fluid restriction, and treatment adherence and lead to reduced suicidality [64, 65]. Cognitive behavior therapy offers an additional treatment option with reduced adverse side effects compared to SSRIs [66]. Additional interventions to treat depression include addressing family discord, barriers to social interactions, and marital tension [67,

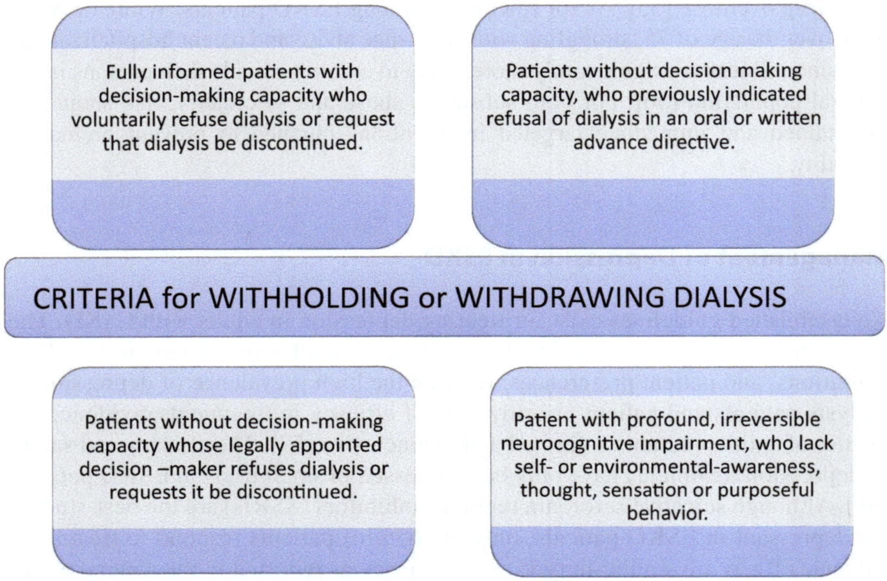

Fig. 3.2 [46]: Clinical practice guideline, recommendations on withholding or withdrawing dialysis

68]. Assessing social support and providing caregiver burnout are also vital in assessment of depression [69].

Exercise is another adjunct for management of depression. While high-quality evidence is lacking, multiple small studies have shown the benefit of short-term exercise programs in reducing depressive symptoms. Given the benefits of exercise in reducing fatigue and combating frailty, exercise should be considered for management of mild to moderate depression [70, 71].

Symptom Burden in End-Stage Kidney Disease

Patients with ESKD experience a wide array of symptoms, some of which are shared across multiple chronic conditions and others that are specific to renal failure (see Table 3.4) [72].

Severity of symptoms is high at baseline and worsens over time. Symptom burden correlates with rates of depression and lower quality of life [73]. Based on the Charlson Comorbidity Index (CCI), symptom burden in ESKD is similar to that experienced by inpatient and outpatient oncology patients. The science of symptoms seeks to understand the experience of the patient, assess the extent to which those symptoms are related to the underlying pathophysiology of chronic disease, and develop targeted treatments. Symptom burden is common in ESKD, with over 50% of patients experiencing fatigue, chronic pain, and pruritis. Over 40% report challenges with sleeplessness (see Fig. 3.3).

Table 3.4 [72]: Commonly encountered debilitating symptoms in end stage kidney disease

Symptom burden in end stage kidney disease
Chronic pain, particularly musculoskeletal pain
Pruritus
Restless legs syndrome
Sleeplessness
Fatigue

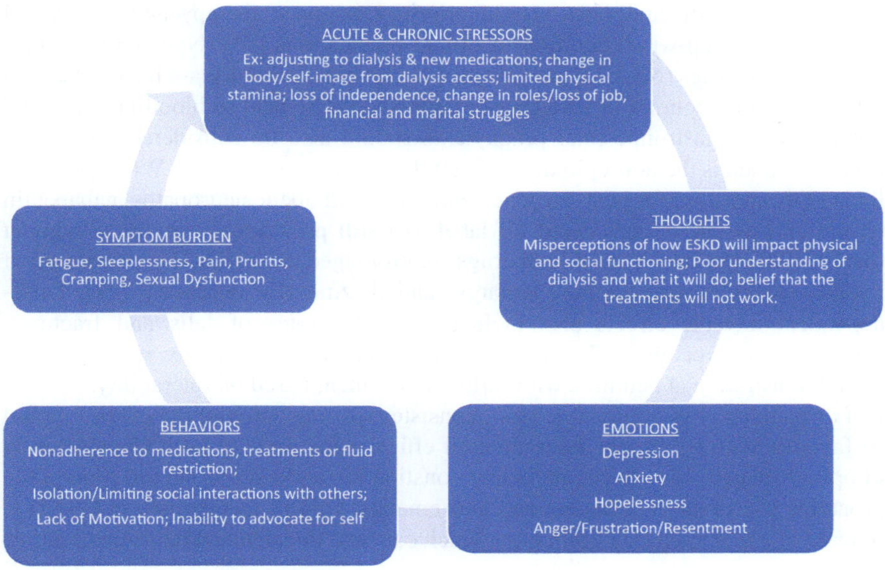

Fig. 3.3 [73]: Cognitive model of ESKD—Interconnected relationship of challenges encountered on dialysis

Chronic Pain

Chronic non-cancer pain is common in patients with CKD and ESKD and is associated with significant disability and lower health-related quality of life. Pain is difficult to control, with over 80% of patients rating their pain as moderate to severe. The etiology of pain is predominantly musculoskeletal, specifically from the effects of arthritis (osteoarthritis or inflammatory arthritis), osteoporosis, renal osteodystrophy, and osteomyelitis [74]. Other contributors include neuropathic pain, dialysis-procedure related pain (access-pain), peripheral vascular disease, carpal tunnel syndrome, pain associated with polycystic kidney, calciphylaxis, or trauma [75]. Chronic pain leads to increased depressive symptoms, more frequent ER visits and hospitalizations, treatment nonadherence (shortened or missed treatments), and rates of dialysis withdrawal.

Assessment of pain can be done using multidimensional intensity scales that have been validated in the ESKD population, including the McGill Pain

Questionnaire, the Brief Pain Inventory, and the Edmonton Symptom Assessment System Revised Renal [76]. Assessment of intensity, chronicity, and type of pain directs management and treatment goals, recognizing that with chronic pain, the goal is controlling pain to a tolerable level for acceptable function and quality of life rather than complete alleviation of pain. Most patients express a pain intensity goal of less than 3 out of 10, and the use of the World Health Organization (WHO) three-step analgesic ladder provides a well validated, staged approach to treat pain in the ESKD population (see Fig. 3.4) [77].

Management of analgesics should prioritize adjuvant therapy and non-opioid options with "step-wise" addition of opioid medications [76]. Non-steroidal anti-inflammatory drugs (NSAIDS) are avoided in chronic kidney disease but can be used for time-limited courses in ESKD. Attention should be paid to blood pressure and volume status; gastrointestinal prophylaxis should also be considered. In ESKD, acetaminophen is the non-opioid, non-NSAID medication of choice. While pregabalin is FDA approved for post-herpetic neuralgia and diabetic neuropathy, gabapentin is not, and its use is considered off-label, but still provides an important adjunct therapy [78]. The half-lives of both drugs are prolonged in ESKD. The monitoring of toxicity, including myoclonus, lethargy, and dizziness is necessary [79]. Dose-dependent adverse effects also include increased rates of falls and fractures. Therefore, dose recommendation is to start low and up-titrate slowly, with preferential administration at bedtime, with further adjustment based on tolerability.

For patients with predictable pain, consistent dosing "around the clock" should be favored, with a frequent assessment of efficacy and toxicity [80]. Consideration of opioid-related side effects, including constipation and nausea, should prompt the proactive use of stool softeners and anti-emetics. Opioid metabolism in ESKD is blunted due to decreased elimination which can lead to enhanced build-up of active

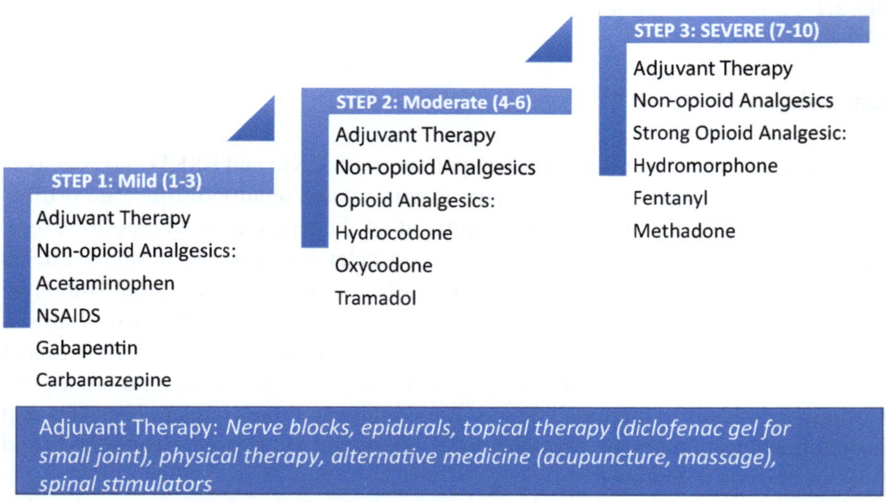

Fig. 3.4 [77]: Step-wise approach to pharmacological management of pain in patients with ESKD

metabolites and enhanced toxicity. Considerations of dialysis clearance can confound analgesic effect, particularly during dialysis treatments. Opioids with a predictable pharmacokinetic and analgesic profile in ESKD include hydromorphone, fentanyl, methadone, and buprenorphine. Therapies to be avoided include morphine, codeine, hydrocodone, and extended-release tramadol, as active metabolites accumulate with impaired renal clearance, leading to CNS depression, hypotension, and respiratory arrest. Given the complex nature of these therapies, referral to a pain management specialist trained in the assessment of opioid abuse or misuse, administration, and prescribing is recommended.

Pruritus

Uremic pruritis is a debilitating and burdensome symptom that affects over 40% of ESKD patients [81]. It leads to decreased quality of life, sleeplessness, missed dialysis treatments, morbidity, and mortality. Itching is non-dermatomal, and other dermatologic manifestations (bullous lesions, rash, ulcerations) are absent. Distribution is generalized, symmetric, and involves large areas of distribution. Symptoms are unrelenting; most patients endorse daily struggles with pruritus. The pathophysiology of pruritus is not fully understood and is likely an interplay of multiple factors. Possible contributors include factors unique to renal dysfunction such as dryness of the stratum corneum, uremia, chronic inflammation from renal dysfunction, and overactivity of μ-opioid receptors. More importantly, it is not driven by histamine release; while anti-histamines are the most commonly prescribed treatment by nephrologists for pruritis. Their use should be limited due to lack of efficacy and significant side-effect profile, particularly drowsiness and confusion. Furthermore, no proven data has shown a correlation of low phosphorous diet and reduced rates of itching. Also, dialysis optimization with increased clearance does not correlate with improved itching. Management focuses on maintaining moisture of the skin with emollients, with frequent repeat application throughout the day. Various pharmacotherapy has been suggested but none has proven effective except gabapentin [82]. Recent studies of difelikefalin, a selective κ-opioid receptor agonist showed rapid and sustained efficacy in itching and is the first therapy approved by the US FDA for CKD-related pruritis [83, 84].

Restless Legs Syndrome, Sleep Disturbance, and Muscle Cramps

Restless leg syndrome (RLS) is the urge to move during periods of activity and is relieved by movement [81]. It affects up to 70% of dialysis patients and is associated with iron deficiency anemia, diabetic peripheral neuropathy, and the use of antidepressants (SSRIs, TCAs). It is associated with poor quality of life and depression. Iron supplementation, enhanced exercise, and intradialytic exercise have shown benefits in RLS [85]. Pharmacotherapy with dopamine agonists like pramipexole or ropinirole can reduce symptoms and are well tolerated.

Sleep disturbance is common in ESKD, with up to 50% of patients reporting challenges in sleep initiation, sleep latency, and experience early morning awakenings [81]. Sleeplessness correlates highly with reduced HRQL metrics. Non-kidney-related comorbidities that impact sleep include congestive heart failure, obstructive sleep apnea (OSA), and dementia. Factors such as caffeine intake and stimulant medications lead to inefficient sleep. While several knowledge gaps remain, kidney-specific parameters impacting sleep include a blunted surge of melatonin in the evening hours in ESKD patients and associated restless leg syndrome and pruritis [86]. It is unclear if variation in dialysis modality impacts sleep. While no proven treatment is recommended, interventions should focus on non-pharmacologic interventions including optimizing concomitant OSA, minimizing daytime napping, and establishing basic sleep hygiene.

Muscle cramps also impact sleep quality in addition to overall wellness and activities of daily living [86]. Understanding of the pathophysiology of muscle cramps is limited. Fluid and electrolyte shifts, in part, can contribute to muscle cramps, but other considerations include heightened muscle fatigue, nutritional and vitamin deficiencies, and impaired oxygen delivery. Muscle fatigue is commonly encountered in the ESKD population, particularly in elderly patients with decreased physical capacity, frailty, and deconditioning. Patient-reported improvement in cramps include use of spicy substances such as pickle juice and mustard. Limited data also shows a role for gabapentin. Perception of dehydration-related cramps often leads to reduced dialysis adherence with reduced treatment duration and subsequent challenges from under-dialysis. While more research is needed, the current treatment focus includes objective ultrafiltration goals and reversing muscle fatigue through structured exercise programs.

Fatigue

Over 60% of patients with ESKD report fatigue. Increasingly associated with chronic medical illnesses, fatigue is a debilitating syndrome associated with renal failure and leads to increased mortality [87]. Self-reported exhaustion, weakness, tiredness, and lack of energy are descriptive terms used by patients with fatigue. It is often associated with depression, sleep disturbance, and other distressing symptoms of ESKD. While no standard assessment has been validated in patients with CKD or ESKD, the Functional Assessment of Chronic Illness Therapy (FACIT) questionnaire is a useful tool, assessing not only fatigue but other health-related quality of life domains [88]. Multiple factors have been implicated in fatigue, including decreased oxygen delivery with associated anemia, altered cardiovascular response to exertion, and subsequent metabolic acidosis from lactic acidosis [89]. As a whole, oxygen delivery is blunted due to perturbations of oxygen convection, conduction, and utilization [90]. Anemia commonly contributes to fatigue and is associated with decreased arterial oxygen-carrying capacity. For every 1 g/dL drop in hemoglobin, there is a 20% increased risk of fatigue [91]. The expected hyperdynamic cardiovascular response to anemia is blunted in ESKD patients, likely due to underlying systolic and diastolic heart failure and use of beta blockers. Skeletal muscle and vascular recruitment is blunted in patients with CKD due to comorbid peripheral vascular disease and reduction in muscle vitality from uremia [89]. Downstream impact includes protein catabolism and sarcopenia, decreased strength and physical performance, and impaired cardiovascular fitness.

Interventions are targeted at improving other associations of fatigue, including uremia and inflammation, managing depression, appropriately correcting anemia, addressing sleep disturbance, and increasing physical reserve [90].

Conclusion

Management of dementia, depression, and symptomatology of ESKD remains a daunting task but can be successfully obtained through consistent assessments, early interventions, and reliance on multidisciplinary care teams. Unmet needs include improved understanding of the causes, uniformed approaches to management, and implementation of effective treatment strategies that are acceptable to patients. Early engagement with patients and caregivers will allow advanced care planning and avoid unnecessary interventions that are burdensome. In addition, future research efforts must focus on evidence-based therapies for common symptoms encountered in renal failure.

References

1. Kurella Tamura M, Yaffe K. Dementia and cognitive impairment in ESRD: diagnostic and therapeutic strategies. Kidney Int. 2011;79:14–22.
2. Kurella Tamura M, Vittinghoff E, Hsu C-Y, et al. Loss of executive function after dialysis initiation in adults with chronic kidney disease. Kidney Int. 2017;91:948–53.
3. Song Y-H, Cai G-Y, Xiao Y-F, Chen X-M. Risk factors for mortality in elderly haemodialysis patients: a systematic review and meta-analysis. BMC Nephrol. 2020;21:377.
4. Drew DA, Weiner DE, Sarnak MJ. Cognitive impairment in CKD: pathophysiology, management, and prevention. Am J Kidney Dis. 2019;74:782–90.
5. Weiner DE, Bartolomei K, Scott T, Price LL, Griffith JL, Rosenberg I, Levey AS, Folstein MF, Sarnak MJ. Albuminuria, cognitive functioning, and white matter hyperintensities in homebound elders. Am J Kidney Dis. 2009;53:438–47.
6. Kurella Tamura M, Gaussoin SA, Pajewski NM, et al. Kidney disease, intensive hypertension treatment, and risk for dementia and mild cognitive impairment: the systolic blood pressure intervention trial. J Am Soc Nephrol. 2020;31:2122–32.
7. Bikbov B, Soler MJ, Pešić V, et al. Albuminuria as a risk factor for mild cognitive impairment and dementia-what is the evidence? Nephrol Dial Transplant. 2021;37:ii55–62.
8. Weiner DE, Gaussoin SA, Nord J, et al. Cognitive function and kidney disease: baseline data from the systolic blood pressure intervention trial (SPRINT). Am J Kidney Dis. 2017;70:357–67.
9. Lim YJ, Sidor NA, Tonial NC, Che A, Urquhart BL. Uremic toxins in the progression of chronic kidney disease and cardiovascular disease: mechanisms and therapeutic targets. Toxins (Basel). 2021;13:142.
10. Lidgard B, Bansal N, Zelnick LR, et al. Association of proximal tubular secretory clearance with long-term decline in cognitive function. J Am Soc Nephrol. 2022;33:1391–401.
11. Wolfgram DF. Intradialytic cerebral hypoperfusion as mechanism for cognitive impairment in patients on hemodialysis. J Am Soc Nephrol. 2019;30:2052–8.

12. Kallenberg MH, Kleinveld HA, Dekker FW, van Munster BC, Rabelink TJ, van Buren M, Mooijaart SP. Functional and cognitive impairment, frailty, and adverse health outcomes in older patients reaching ESRD—a systematic review. Clin J Am Soc Nephrol. 2016;11:1624–39.
13. Kurella Tamura M, Gaussoin S, Pajewski NM, et al. Kidney disease, hypertension treatment, and cerebral perfusion and structure. Am J Kidney Dis. 2022;79:677–687.e1.
14. Dolui S, Detre JA, Gaussoin SA, et al. Association of intensive vs standard blood pressure control with cerebral blood flow: secondary analysis of the SPRINT MIND randomized clinical trial. JAMA Neurol. 2022;79:380–9.
15. Eldehni MT, Odudu A, McIntyre CW. Randomized clinical trial of dialysate cooling and effects on brain white matter. J Am Soc Nephrol. 2015;26:957–65.
16. Dasgupta I, Odudu A, Baharani J, et al. Evaluation of the effect of cooled haemodialysis on cognitive function in patients suffering with end-stage kidney disease (E-CHECKED): feasibility randomised control trial protocol. Trials. 2020;21:820.
17. Battistella M, Ng P. Addressing polypharmacy in outpatient dialysis units. Clin J Am Soc Nephrol. 2021;16:144–6.
18. Pai AB, Cardone KE, Manley HJ, St. Peter WL, Shaffer R, Somers M, Mehrotra R. Medication reconciliation and therapy management in dialysis-dependent patients: need for a systematic approach. Clin J Am Soc Nephrol. 2013;8:1988–99.
19. McAdams-DeMarco MA, Tan J, Salter ML, Gross A, Meoni LA, Jaar BG, Kao W-HL, Parekh RS, Segev DL, Sozio SM. Frailty and cognitive function in incident hemodialysis patients. Clin J Am Soc Nephrol. 2015;10:2181–9.
20. Howden EJ, Coombes JS, Strand H, Douglas B, Campbell KL, Isbel NM. Exercise training in CKD: efficacy, adherence, and safety. Am J Kidney Dis. 2015;65:583–91.
21. Chu NM, McAdams-DeMarco MA. Exercise and cognitive function in patients with end-stage kidney disease. Semin Dial. 2019;32:283–90.
22. Chang J-H, Koo M, Wu S-W, Chen C-Y. Effects of a 12-week program of Tai Chi exercise on the kidney disease quality of life and physical functioning of patients with end-stage renal disease on hemodialysis. Complement Ther Med. 2017;30:79–83.
23. Mandel EI, Bernacki RE, Block SD. Serious illness conversations in ESRD. Clin J Am Soc Nephrol. 2017;12:854–63.
24. Ariadne Labs Serious Illness Conversation Guide. In: © 2015 Ariadne Labs: A Joint Center for Health Systems Innovation and Dana-Farber Cancer Institute. https://www.ariadnelabs.org. Accessed 10 Feb 2022.
25. Thamcharoen N, Nissaisorakarn P, Cohen RA, Schonberg MA. Serious illness conversations in advanced kidney disease: a mixed-methods implementation study. BMJ Support Palliat Care. 2021.
26. Davison SN, Levin A, Moss AH, et al. Executive summary of the KDIGO controversies conference on supportive care in chronic kidney disease: developing a roadmap to improving quality care. Kidney Int. 2015;88:447–59.
27. Yarlas AS, White MK, Yang M, Saris-Baglama RN, Bech PG, Christensen T. Measuring the health status burden in hemodialysis patients using the SF-36® health survey. Qual Life Res. 2011;20:383–9.
28. Wen J, Jin X, al Sayah F, Short H, Ohinmaa A, Davison SN, Walsh M, Johnson JA. Mapping the Edmonton symptom assessment system-revised: renal to the EQ-5D-5L in patients with chronic kidney disease. Qual Life Res. 2022;31:567–77.
29. Murphy EL, Murtagh FEM, Carey I, Sheerin NS. Understanding symptoms in patients with advanced chronic kidney disease managed without dialysis: use of a short patient-completed assessment tool. Nephron Clin Pract. 2008;111:c74–80.
30. Weisbord SD, Fried LF, Arnold RM, Rotondi AJ, Fine MJ, Levenson DJ, Switzer GE. Development of a symptom assessment instrument for chronic hemodialysis patients: the dialysis symptom index. J Pain Symptom Manag. 2004;27:226–40.
31. Davison SN, Tupala B, Wasylynuk BA, Siu V, Sinnarajah A, Triscott J. Recommendations for the care of patients receiving conservative kidney management. Clin J Am Soc Nephrol. 2019;14:626–34.

32. Wong SPY, Rubenzik T, Zelnick L, Davison SN, Louden D, Oestreich T, Jennerich AL. Long-term outcomes among patients with advanced kidney disease who forgo maintenance dialysis. JAMA Netw Open. 2022;5:e222255.
33. Zarantonello D, Rhee CM, Kalantar-Zadeh K, Brunori G. Novel conservative management of chronic kidney disease via dialysis-free interventions. Curr Opin Nephrol Hypertens. 2021;30:97–107.
34. Gelfand SL, Mandel EI, Mendu ML, Lakin JR. Palliative care in the Advancing American Kidney Health Initiative: a call for inclusion in kidney care delivery models. Am J Kidney Dis. 2020;76:877–82.
35. 2021 United States Renal Data System. 2021 USRDS Annual Data Report: Epidemiology of kidney disease in the United States. In: National Institutes of Health, National Institute of Diabetes and Digestive and Kidney Diseases. 2021. https://adr.usrds.org/. Accessed 10 Sept 2022.
36. Wachterman MW, O'Hare AM, Rahman O-K, Lorenz KA, Marcantonio ER, Alicante GK, Kelley AS. One-year mortality after dialysis initiation among older adults. JAMA Intern Med. 2019;179:987.
37. Amro OW, Ramasamy M, Strom JA, Weiner DE, Jaber BL. Nephrologist-facilitated advance care planning for hemodialysis patients: a quality improvement project. Am J Kidney Dis. 2016;68:103–9.
38. Goff SL, Unruh ML, Klingensmith J, Eneanya ND, Garvey C, Germain MJ, Cohen LM. Advance care planning with patients on hemodialysis: an implementation study. BMC Palliat Care. 2019;18:64.
39. Berzoff J, Kitsen J, Klingensmith J, Cohen LM. Advance care planning training for renal social workers. J Soc Work End Life Palliat Care. 2020;16:5–18.
40. Rodriguez de Sosa G, Nicklas A, Thamer M, Anderson E, Reddy N, Stevelos J, Germain MJ, Unruh ML, Lupu DE. Implementing advance care planning for dialysis patients: HIGHway project. BMC Palliat Care. 2022;21:129.
41. Kurella Tamura M, Holdsworth L, Stedman M, et al. Implementation and effectiveness of a learning collaborative to improve palliative care for seriously ill hemodialysis patients. Clin J Am Soc Nephrol. 2022;17:1495–505.
42. Roberts MJ, Johansen KL, Copeland TP, McCulloch CE, Coufal S, Ku E. Factors associated with dialysis discontinuation outside of the acute care setting. Kidney360. 2021;2:331–5.
43. Kurella Tamura M, Montez-Rath ME, Hall YN, Katz R, O'Hare AM. Advance directives and end-of-life care among nursing home residents receiving maintenance dialysis. Clin J Am Soc Nephrol. 2017;12:435–42.
44. Wetmore JB, Roetker NS, Gilbertson DT, Liu J. Early withdrawal and non-withdrawal death in the months following hemodialysis initiation: a retrospective cohort analysis. Hemodial Int. 2019;23:261–72.
45. Agunbiade A, Dasgupta A, Ward MM. Racial/ethnic differences in dialysis discontinuation and survival after hospitalization for serious conditions among patients on maintenance dialysis. J Am Soc Nephrol. 2020;31:149–60.
46. Galla JH. Clinical practice guideline on shared decision-making in the appropriate initiation of and withdrawal from dialysis. J Am Soc Nephrol. 2000;11:1340–2. https://doi.org/10.1681/ASN.V1171340.
47. Chen JHC, Lim WH, Howson P. Changing landscape of dialysis withdrawal in patients with kidney failure: implications for clinical practice. Nephrology (Carlton). 2022;27:551–65.
48. Lacson E, Bruce L, Li N-C, Mooney A, Maddux FW. Depressive affect and hospitalization risk in incident hemodialysis patients. Clin J Am Soc Nephrol. 2014;9:1713–9.
49. Kimmel PL, Fwu C-W, Abbott KC, Moxey-Mims MM, Mendley S, Norton JM, Eggers PW. Psychiatric illness and mortality in hospitalized ESKD dialysis patients. Clin J Am Soc Nephrol. 2019;14:1363–71.

50. Wilk AS, Hu J-C, Chehal P, Yarbrough CR, Ji X, Cummings JR. National estimates of mental health needs among adults with self-reported CKD in the United States. Kidney Int Rep. 2022;7:1630–42.
51. Palmer S, Vecchio M, Craig JC, et al. Prevalence of depression in chronic kidney disease: systematic review and meta-analysis of observational studies. Kidney Int. 2013;84:179–91.
52. Elizabeth A, O'Connor P. Screening for depression in adults and older adults in primary care an updated systematic review. Rockville: Agency for Healthcare Research and Quality (US); 2009.
53. Hedayati SS, Minhajuddin AT, Toto RD, Morris DW, Rush AJ. Validation of depression screening scales in patients with CKD. Am J Kidney Dis. 2009;54:433–9.
54. Lacson E, Xu J, Lin S-F, Dean SG, Lazarus JM, Hakim RM. A comparison of SF-36 and SF-12 composite scores and subsequent hospitalization and mortality risks in long-term dialysis patients. Clin J Am Soc Nephrol. 2010;5:252–60.
55. Grubbs V, Vittighoff E, Grimes B, Johansen KL. Mortality and illicit drug dependence among hemodialysis patients in the United States: a retrospective cohort analysis. BMC Nephrol. 2016;17:56.
56. Kurella M, Kimmel PL, Young BS, Chertow GM. Suicide in the United States end-stage renal disease program. J Am Soc Nephrol. 2005;16:774–81.
57. Palmer SC, Natale P, Ruospo M, Saglimbene VM, Rabindranath KS, Craig JC, Strippoli GFM. Antidepressants for treating depression in adults with end-stage kidney disease treated with dialysis. Cochrane Database Syst Rev. 2016;2016(5):CD004541.
58. Susan Hedayati S, Yalamanchili V, Finkelstein FO. A practical approach to the treatment of depression in patients with chronic kidney disease and end-stage renal disease. Kidney Int. 2012;81:247–55.
59. Vangala C, Niu J, Montez-Rath ME, Yan J, Navaneethan SD, Winkelmayer WC. Selective serotonin reuptake inhibitor use and hip fracture risk among patients on hemodialysis. Am J Kidney Dis. 2020;75:351–60.
60. Assimon MM, Brookhart MA, Flythe JE. Comparative cardiac safety of selective serotonin reuptake inhibitors among individuals receiving maintenance hemodialysis. J Am Soc Nephrol. 2019;30:611–23.
61. Ma TK-W, Li PK-T. Depression in dialysis patients. Nephrology. 2016;21:639–46.
62. Natale P, Palmer SC, Ruospo M, Saglimbene VM, Rabindranath KS, Strippoli GF. Psychosocial interventions for preventing and treating depression in dialysis patients. Cochrane Database Syst Rev. 2019;12(12):CD004542. https://doi.org/10.1002/14651858.CD004542.pub3.
63. Hudson JL, Moss-Morris R, Game D, Carroll A, Chilcot J. Improving Distress in Dialysis (iDiD): a tailored CBT self-management treatment for patients undergoing dialysis. J Ren Care. 2016;42:223–38.
64. Duarte PS, Miyazaki MC, Blay SL, Sesso R. Cognitive–behavioral group therapy is an effective treatment for major depression in hemodialysis patients. Kidney Int. 2009;76:414–21.
65. Cukor D, ver Halen N, Asher DR, Coplan JD, Weedon J, Wyka KE, Saggi SJ, Kimmel PL. Psychosocial intervention improves depression, quality of life, and fluid adherence in hemodialysis. J Am Soc Nephrol. 2014;25:196–206.
66. Mehrotra R, Cukor D, Unruh M, et al. Comparative efficacy of therapies for treatment of depression for patients undergoing maintenance hemodialysis. Ann Intern Med. 2019;170:369.
67. Krespi MR. Psychosocial interventions to improve outcomes among dialysis patients. Semin Dial. 2018;31:65–71.
68. Daneker B, Kimmel PL, Ranich T, Peterson RA. Depression and marital dissatisfaction in patients with end-stage renal disease and in their spouses. Am J Kidney Dis. 2001;38:839–46.
69. Low J, Smith G, Burns A, Jones L. The impact of end-stage kidney disease (ESKD) on close persons: a literature review. NDT Plus. 2008;1:67–79.
70. Chopra P, Ayers CK, Antick JR, Kansagara D, Kondo K. The effectiveness of depression treatment for adults with ESKD: a systematic review. Kidney360. 2021;2:558–85.
71. Ghafourifard M, Mehrizade B, Hassankhani H, Heidari M. Hemodialysis patients perceived exercise benefits and barriers: the association with health-related quality of life. BMC Nephrol. 2021;22:94.

72. Weisbord SD, Carmody SS, Bruns FJ, Rotondi AJ, Cohen LM, Zeidel ML, Arnold RM. Symptom burden, quality of life, advance care planning and the potential value of palliative care in severely ill haemodialysis patients. Nephrol Dial Transplant. 2003;18:1345–52.
73. Weisbord SD, Fried LF, Arnold RM, Fine MJ, Levenson DJ, Peterson RA, Switzer GE. Prevalence, severity, and importance of physical and emotional symptoms in chronic hemodialysis patients. J Am Soc Nephrol. 2005;16:2487–94.
74. Davison SN. Pain in hemodialysis patients: prevalence, cause, severity, and management. Am J Kidney Dis. 2003;42:1239–47.
75. Raouf M, Bettinger J, Wegrzyn EW, Mathew RO, Fudin JJ. Pharmacotherapeutic management of neuropathic pain in end-stage renal disease. Kidney Dis. 2020;6:157–67.
76. Davison SN. Clinical pharmacology considerations in pain management in patients with advanced kidney failure. Clin J Am Soc Nephrol. 2019;14:917–31.
77. Barakzoy AS, Moss AH. Efficacy of the World Health Organization analgesic ladder to treat pain in end-stage renal disease. J Am Soc Nephrol. 2006;17:3198–203.
78. Raouf M, Atkinson T, Crumb M, Fudin J. Rational dosing of gabapentin and pregabalin in chronic kidney disease. J Pain Res. 2017;10:275–8.
79. Ishida JH, McCulloch CE, Steinman MA, Grimes BA, Johansen KL. Opioid analgesics and adverse outcomes among hemodialysis patients. Clin J Am Soc Nephrol. 2018;13: 746–53.
80. Koncicki HM, Unruh M, Schell JO. Pain management in CKD: a guide for nephrology providers. Am J Kidney Dis. 2017;69:451–60.
81. Scherer JS, Combs SA, Brennan F. Sleep disorders, restless legs syndrome, and uremic pruritus: diagnosis and treatment of common symptoms in dialysis patients. Am J Kidney Dis. 2017;69:117–28.
82. Hercz D, Jiang SH, Webster AC. Interventions for itch in people with advanced chronic kidney disease. Cochrane Database Syst Rev. 2020;12(12):CD011393. https://doi.org/10.1002/14651858.CD011393.pub2.
83. Topf J, Wooldridge T, McCafferty K, et al. Efficacy of difelikefalin for the treatment of moderate to severe pruritus in hemodialysis patients: pooled analysis of KALM-1 and KALM-2 phase 3 studies. Kidney Med. 2022;4:100512.
84. Fishbane S, Jamal A, Munera C, Wen W, Menzaghi F. A phase 3 trial of difelikefalin in hemodialysis patients with pruritus. N Engl J Med. 2020;382:222–32.
85. Kambampati S, Wasim S, Kukkar V, Awad VM, Malik BH. Restless leg syndrome in the setting of patients with end-stage renal disease on hemodialysis: a literature review. Cureus. 2020;12(8):e9965. https://doi.org/10.7759/cureus.9965.
86. Flythe JE, Hilliard T, Lumby E, et al. Fostering innovation in symptom management among hemodialysis patients: paths forward for insomnia, muscle cramps, and fatigue. Clin J Am Soc Nephrol. 2019;14:150–60.
87. Jhamb M, Pike F, Ramer S, Argyropoulos C, Steel J, Dew MA, Weisbord SD, Weissfeld L, Unruh M. Impact of fatigue on outcomes in the hemodialysis (HEMO) study. Am J Nephrol. 2011;33:515–23.
88. Webster K, Cella D, Yost K. The functional assessment of chronic illness therapy (FACIT) measurement system: properties, applications, and interpretation. Health Qual Life Outcomes. 2003;1:79.
89. Wilund KR, Thompson S, Viana JL, Wang AY-M. Physical activity and health in chronic kidney disease. Contrib Nephrol. 2021;199:43–55.
90. Gregg LP, Bossola M, Ostrosky-Frid M, Hedayati SS. Fatigue in CKD. Clin J Am Soc Nephrol. 2021;16:1445–55.
91. Gregg LP, Jain N, Carmody T, Minhajuddin AT, Rush AJ, Trivedi MH, Hedayati SS. Fatigue in nondialysis chronic kidney disease: correlates and association with kidney outcomes. Am J Nephrol. 2019;50:37–47.

Hemodialysis Infectious Complications

4

Ibironke W. Apata, Matthew J. Arduino, and Shannon Novosad

Introduction

Hemodialysis, a life-saving procedure, places patients at risk of acquiring infections. In the United States, more than 500,000 receive hemodialysis; 98% receive treatment in one of the 7500 outpatient dialysis facilities across the country, and 2% receive hemodialysis at home [1]. Outpatient dialysis facilities usually have an open-room layout, allowing for multiple patients to receive hemodialysis concurrently in one, large room. Hemodialysis requires direct access into the bloodstream via vascular access, including central venous catheters (catheters), arteriovenous grafts (AVG), or arteriovenous fistulas (AVF). The hemodialysis procedure, vascular access, and facility layout provide several opportunities for the development of healthcare-acquired infections (HAIs) and transmission of pathogens via the environment (e.g., shared air), devices including catheters, shared equipment and supplies, environmental surfaces, and the hands of healthcare personnel (HCP) or other patients [2, 3]. In addition, patients with end-stage renal disease (ESRD), including those on chronic hemodialysis, have impaired immune function, including neutrophil function, cellular immunity, and complement activation, placing them at increased risk of developing infections [4, 5].

I. W. Apata (✉)
Division of Healthcare Quality Promotion, Centers for Disease Control and Prevention, Atlanta, GA, USA

Division of Renal Medicine, Emory University School of Medicine, Atlanta, GA, USA
e-mail: iba2@cdc.gov

M. J. Arduino · S. Novosad
Division of Healthcare Quality Promotion, Centers for Disease Control and Prevention, Atlanta, GA, USA

S. Z. Fadem et al. (eds.), *Complications in Dialysis*,
https://doi.org/10.1007/978-3-031-44557-6_4

Bacterial bloodstream infections (BSIs), infections from viral bloodborne pathogens, and respiratory infections contribute to the burden of infections among patients on hemodialysis. Infections in the hemodialysis population are associated with significant morbidities such as hospitalizations, increased mortality, and additional healthcare costs. According to national data from the United States Renal Data System (USRDS), infections were the second leading cause of hospitalizations among hemodialysis patients. Hospitalization rates from infections were relatively stable from 2010 to 2019; however in 2020, hospitalization rates from infections increased, likely from COVID-19-related hospitalizations [1]. Outbreaks of bloodstream infections and bloodborne pathogens in outpatient dialysis facilities have underscored the vulnerability of hemodialysis patients (and dialysis HCP) to HAIs, the impact of breaches in infection control practices on patient outcomes, and opportunities for improved practices and interventions [3].

Studies have repeatedly demonstrated that infections can be prevented in the hemodialysis setting, even on a large scale, with the collaboration of public health organizations and dialysis stakeholders. For example, with the implementation of CDC recommendations to prevent hepatitis B virus (HBV) transmission in the hemodialysis setting, HBV transmission in outpatient dialysis facilities has been rare for over two decades [6]. Further, national efforts to improve uptake of CDC recommendations to prevent BSIs among dialysis patients likely played a role in decreasing rates of BSIs and sepsis among hemodialysis patients [7]. Finally, the COVID-19 pandemic demonstrated how dialysis stakeholders could work together to rapidly develop and implement infection prevention and control strategies for SARS-CoV-2 infections [8, 9]. In spite of the progress made, infections remain the second leading cause of death among hemodialysis patients. Continued efforts in public health, research, innovation, and education are needed to promote hemodialysis patient safety.

A comprehensive review of all infections in patients on hemodialysis is beyond the scope of this chapter. We will discuss prevention of infections and infectious complications with a particular emphasis on the role of infection prevention for vascular access-related infections, bloodborne pathogen infections such as HBV, hepatitis C virus (HCV) and human immune deficiency virus (HIV), respiratory infections including influenza and COVID-19, and hemodialysis water systems.

Best Practices and Standard Precautions

Standard precautions include infection control procedures and practices that should be used for all patient care. In this section, we highlight some of the best practices and precautions to prevent transmission of infections in the hemodialysis setting. A summary of infection control recommendations is provided in Table 4.1.

Table 4.1 Recommended infection control practices for hemodialysis units

Care of all patients[a]
• **Hand hygiene**
• Hand hygiene should be performed
– Before and after having direct contact with a patient's intact skin
– Before performing an aseptic task (e.g., placing an indwelling device) or handling invasive medical devices
– After contact with blood, body fluids or excretions, mucous membranes, non-intact skin, or wound dressings
– After contact with inanimate objects (including medical equipment) in the immediate vicinity of the patient
– If hands will be moving from a contaminated-body site to a clean-body site during patient care
– After glove removal
• Wear disposable gloves when caring for the patient or touching the patient's equipment at the dialysis station; remove gloves and perform hand hygiene between each patient or station
• **Environmental cleaning and disinfection**
• Items taken into the dialysis station should be disposed of or cleaned and disinfected before taken to a common clean area or used on another patient
– Non-disposable items taken to the patient treatment station that cannot be cleaned or disinfected (e.g., adhesive tape) should be discarded after use
– Unused medications (including multi-dose vials) or supplies (syringes, alcohol swabs, etc.) taken to the patient's station should be used only for that patient and should not be returned to a common clean area or used on other patients
• Clean and disinfect the dialysis station (chair, side tables, machine, IV pole, etc.) between patients
– Start cleaning only when patient has left the station and only admit new patient after cleaning and disinfection are completed
– Give special attention to cleaning control panels on the dialysis machine and other surfaces that are frequently touched and potentially contaminated with patient's blood
– Discard all fluid, and clean and disinfect all surfaces and containers associated with the prime waste (including buckets attached to the machines). Allow prime buckets to air dry after disinfection and before use
• Do not reuse dialyzers or blood tubing. Place all used dialyzers and tubing in a leak-proof container for transport to disposal area
• If external transducer protectors (venous or arterial) are utilized, they should be changed between each patient treatment, when they become wet[a], and should not be reused. The redundant internal transducer protectors do not need to be changed routinely between patients. If the external transducer protectors have blood breakthrough, the internal transducer protector should be assessed for contamination before dialyzing another patient with the same machine
• **Medication preparation and injection safety**
• Single-dose medications are preferred. When multi-dose medication vials are used (including vials containing diluents), they should be assigned to a single patient whenever possible
• Prepare individual patient doses of medications in a clean (centralized) area away from dialysis stations and deliver separately to each patient. Do not carry multi-dose medication vials from station to station
– Discard single-dose vials after use and store multi-dose vials appropriately
• Do not use common medication carts to deliver medications to patients. Do not carry medication vials, syringes, alcohol swabs, or supplies in pockets
• Perform hand hygiene and using aseptic technique when preparing medication
• Disinfect the septum of the vial with alcohol and use a new needle and a new syringe to withdraw medication
• Do not handle or store used supplies, equipment, blood samples, or biohazard containers in or adjacent to areas where medications are handled
• Perform hand hygiene, putting on new, clean gloves, scrubbing the injection port with antiseptic and using aseptic technique when administering medications
• Prepare injectable medications in a designated clean workspace that is free of obvious contamination sources (e.g., blood, body fluids, contaminated equipment, tap water). This workspace should be clearly separated from the patient treatment area and ideally in a separate room

(continued)

Table 4.1 (continued)

Care of Hepatitis B surface antigen-positive (HBsAg-positive) patients
• Follow infection control practices recommended for all hemodialysis patients • Dialyze HBsAg-positive patients in a separate room using separate machines, equipment, instruments, and supplies • Staff members caring for HBsAg-positive patients should not care for HBV susceptible patients at the same time (e.g., during same shift or during patient change over)
Vaccinations
Hepatitis B vaccine • Vaccinate all susceptible patients against hepatitis B[b] • Test foranti-HBs 1–2 months after the last dose – If anti-HBs is <10 mIU/mL (or the lab-specific level that represents immunity), consider patient susceptible, repeat the vaccine series, and retest for anti-HBs[c] – If anti-HBs is ≥10 mIU/mL (or the lab-specific level that represents immunity), consider immune and retest annually Give booster dose of vaccine if anti-HBs declines to <10 mIU/mL and continues to retest annually[d] • Vaccinate all susceptible patient care staff and follow standard recommendations for post-vaccination testing of staff Influenza vaccine • Annual vaccination for all patients • Annual vaccination for all staff Pneumococcal vaccine • All patients should be vaccinated with pneumococcal vaccines per current guidelines[e] COVID-19 vaccine • All patients should receive COVID-19 vaccine per current guidelines[f] • All staff should receive COVID-19 vaccine per current guidelines[f]

HBsAg hepatitis B surface antigen, *anti-HBs* antibody to HBsAg

[a]Adapted from CDC's recommendations for preventing transmission of infections among chronic hemodialysis patients https://www.cdc.gov/mmwr/preview/mmwrhtml/rr5005a1.htm

[b]Vaccination is recommended for all pre-end-stage renal disease patients before they become dialysis dependent

[c]If patient has not mounted an adequate antibody response after the repeat vaccine series, consider the patient susceptible and test HBsAg monthly

[d]Retesting immediately after the booster dose is not necessary

[e]Schedule depends on the vaccination status of patients and is available on CDC website (https://www.cdc.gov/vaccines/hcp/acip-recs/vacc-specific/pneumo.html) [10]

[f]https://www.cdc.gov/coronavirus/2019-ncov/vaccines/stay-up-to-date.html

Hand Hygiene

Hand hygiene is a critical aspect of infection prevention. Several outbreaks have been linked to the transmission of infections via the hands of healthcare workers [11]. There are multiple opportunities when hand hygiene should be performed during a single dialysis session. Staff hand hygiene practices should be evaluated at regular intervals, and feedback should be provided to staff on their performance [12]. Nephrologists and other clinicians rounding in their dialysis facilities should also adhere to appropriate hand hygiene practices. Ensuring hand sanitizers are available and easily accessible (close to dialysis stations) can foster good hand hygiene practices. CDC has several audit tools that can help to assess and trend staff practices over time [13].

Environmental Cleaning and Disinfection

Environmental cleaning (i.e., the physical removal of foreign and organic material such as microorganisms, blood, secretions etc., from surfaces) and disinfection (i.e., a thermal or chemical process for inactivating microorganisms on inanimate objects) is a fundamental infection prevention intervention. It is well documented that environmental contamination in healthcare settings plays a role in the transmission of HAIs [14]. Outbreaks linked to environmental contamination, and improper environmental cleaning and disinfection have been documented in dialysis [11, 15]. CDC has several tools to guide environmental cleaning and audit environmental cleaning practices in dialysis facilities [13].

Medication Preparation and Injection Safety

Adhering to best practices for preparing and administering injectable medications reduces both the spread of bloodborne viruses and BSIs [16]. Medications should be prepared in an aseptic manner in a dedicated area and administered using aseptic technique. Both single-use and multidose vials should always be used according to the manufacturer's recommendations. Notably, single-use medications should not be punctured more than once, and multidose medications should be assigned to a single patient whenever possible.

CDC recommends: (a) preparing medications in a separate room (preferred) or, if a separate room is not available, in an area removed from the patient treatment area and designated for medications; (b) performing hand hygiene and using aseptic technique when preparing medication; (c) disinfecting the septum of the vial with alcohol and using a new needle and a new syringe to withdraw medication; (d) discarding single-dose vials after use and storing multidose vials appropriately; (e) not handling or storing used supplies, equipment, blood samples, or biohazard containers in or adjacent to areas where medications are handled; (f) delivering medications separately to each patient and not using common carts within the patient treatment area to prepare or distribute medications; and (g) performing hand hygiene, putting on new, clean gloves, scrubbing the injection port with antiseptic and using aseptic technique when administering medications [17]. CDC has audit tools for dialysis injection safety to assess staff practices [13].

Bacterial Infections

This section addresses vascular access-related infections including BSIs, antibiotic resistant organisms, and antibiotic stewardship.

Vascular Access Infections (VAIs)

Case Presentation

A 45-year-old female with a history of poorly controlled hypertension and ESRD on hemodialysis presents to the hospital with mental status changes and right-hand weakness. Her dialysis access includes a right internal jugular tunneled dialysis catheter and left upper extremity AVF. The dialysis catheter and the arteriovenous fistula (AVF) were placed 6 months ago. The AVF has been used for the past 6 weeks without any issues. The patient missed her appointment to have the catheter removed 10 days ago. Her presentation vitals are as follows: temperature 38 °C, blood pressure 110/70 mmHg, heart rate 110 beats/min, respiratory rate 12 breaths/min. Her physical examination is remarkable for a grade 3/6 holosystolic murmur in the left lower sternal border, soiled dialysis catheter dressing with purulent drainage at the exit site, and erythema and tenderness along the catheter tunnel. Her AVF site is unremarkable (good thrill; no erythema, tenderness, or area of fluctuance or induration). She is alert and oriented to person only. She has a right-hand wrist drop.

Hospital course: Head CT was done, revealing multiple areas of infarcts suggestive of an embolic source. The neurology team was consulted. Two sets of blood cultures were drawn. Following this, intravenous vancomycin and cefepime were initiated. Twenty-four hours later, Gram-positive cocci in clusters were isolated from the blood cultures. A transthoracic echocardiogram was performed revealing a mobile vegetation on the mitral valve. On hospital day 2, the Gram-positive cocci were identified as methicillin-resistant *Staphylococcus aureus*. Vancomycin was continued, and cefepime was discontinued. Her mental status improved to her baseline, but she continued to have right-hand weakness.

Introduction, Clinical Presentation, and Complications

VAIs are infections related to hemodialysis access including non-tunneled catheters, tunneled catheters, and permanent dialysis access (AVF and AVG). VAIs consist, primarily, of bacterial infections resulting in local infections (e.g., catheter exit-site infection, catheter tunnel infections, cellulitis, abscesses at AVG/AVF) or a systemic BSI. VAIs are associated with increased morbidity including pain, access loss, hospitalization, access-related procedures and surgeries, and mortality. Patients with local access-related infections can present with symptoms or signs of local infections such as pain, erythema, or purulent drainage at the access site. Systemic infections, including BSIs, may present with fevers, chills, tachycardia, or malaise. BSIs may progress to complicated or metastatic infections such as endocarditis, embolic strokes, and spinal infections (e.g., spinal epidural abscesses). Depending on the site of metastasis, patients can present with varying signs and symptoms such as back pain, heart failure, or a new murmur. It is important that clinicians are vigilant and maintain a high index of suspicion for VAIs as early recognition and diagnosis can improve patient outcomes.

Pathogenesis

Understanding the pathogenesis of VAIs can highlight target sites for interventions, innovations, and strategies to prevent these infections. Catheter-related infections, a subset of VAIs, comprise the majority of VAIs. Organisms can contaminate the catheter by either (1) colonization of the outside of the catheter at insertion or via the catheter exit, typically by skin organisms, (2) colonization of the lumen of the catheter via the hub from hands or contaminated infusates, or (3) hematogenous seeding of the catheter from an infected focus (e.g., prosthetic joint). Biofilm formation on the catheter has been recognized as an important player in the development of catheter-related infections. Biofilm is a matrix of extracellular polymeric substances released by bacteria that adhere to the catheter and can evade the innate immune system. Bacteria in the biofilm can result in bloodstream infections. AVF/AVG VAIs can occur from the introduction of bacteria during cannulation, contaminated infusates, hematogenous seeding of the AVF/AVF from another nidus of infection, and colonization of the cannulation track or AVF/AVG [18].

VAIs can be from endogenous pathogens (i.e., invasion by an organism or bacteria on or in the patient) or exogenous pathogens (i.e., acquired from external sources such as contaminated infusates or devices). Exogenous pathogens have been implicated in outbreaks attributed to equipment and practices such as dialyzer reuse, contaminated water systems, and contaminated medications [11, 16, 19].

Surveillance

To monitor and characterize BSIs and VAIs in hemodialysis over time, CDC and Centers for Medicare and Medicaid Services (CMS) have promoted "The National Healthcare Safety Network (NHSN) Dialysis Event" module. The Dialysis Event module is a component of the larger NHSN surveillance system, which tracks HAIs across the United States [20]. Outpatient hemodialysis facilities in the U.S. are eligible to participate. Data collected from the Dialysis Event module are used to measure dialysis facility performance as part of CMS' ESRD Quality Incentive Program (QIP) [21]. In essence, facilities are financially incentivized to participate, and as a result almost all outpatient dialysis facilities report to NHSN. While CDC, CMS, and public health organizations can use the data to identify areas for improvement and measure the impact of quality improvement efforts on a national level, individual facilities can track facility-level performance in real-time and compare performance to other facilities.

The Dialysis Event module uses a standardized data collection form to capture three types of dialysis events from outpatients treated in the facility: (1) positive blood culture, (2) intravenous antimicrobial start, and (3) pus, redness, or increased swelling at the vascular access site [22]. These events serve as indicators of BSIs and/or local VAIs. It is important to note that definitions of infections for NHSN may not be the same as clinical definitions. For example, all positive blood cultures are reportable whether they are considered contaminants or clinically insignificant. Underreporting of dialysis events is a challenge to BSI and VAI surveillance in the hemodialysis setting. Outpatient dialysis facilities may sometimes be unaware of dialysis events that are captured in the hospital, potentially contributing to underreporting of dialysis events [23]. Improved communication between hospitals and outpatient dialysis facilities is essential to BSI surveillance efforts.

Epidemiology

The bulk of VAIs are caused by Gram-positive organisms. *Staphylococcus aureus* (32–53% of cases) accounts for the majority of VAIs, followed by coagulase-negative Staphylococci (20–32% of cases), Gram-negative bacilli (10–18%), other Gram-positive cocci (10–12%, e.g., enterococci), and fungi (<1%) [23–25]. Among BSIs, *S. aureus* remains the most commonly reported pathogen; in 2014, 40% of the *S. aureus* isolated from blood were resistant to methicillin [23].

From 2014 to 2019, BSIs in patients on outpatient hemodialysis decreased approximately 40%. The BSI pooled mean rates per 1000 patient-months across access types in 2019 were 0.17 for AVF, 0.32 for AVG, and 1.21 for catheters (including tunneled and non-tunneled), indicating that while substantial progress has been made in the prevention of BSI the differential risk among access types remains [26]. While hemodialysis catheters allow for immediate use and do not require surgery, they are associated with substantially higher rates of VAI, BSI, and access-related BSI (ARBSI) compared to other vascular access types. In addition to having a lower risk of infectious complications compared to other vascular access types, AVFs have a longer lifespan and require fewer interventions following maturation [27]. Consequently, AVFs are widely considered the preferred access type; national organizations have recommended AVFs, and national efforts have promoted AVFs over other access types [28]. However, the majority of incident hemodialysis patients (i.e., patients initiating hemodialysis in a given year) continue to initiate hemodialysis with a catheter. The USRDS reports that among patients initiating hemodialysis in 2018, 81% of patients used a catheter, 16% used an AVF, and 3% used an AVG at hemodialysis initiation [1]. The percentage of patients initiating hemodialysis with a catheter (with or without a maturing AVF or AVG) was relatively unchanged between 2009 (82.4%) and 2019 (81.8%). Among prevalent patients receiving hemodialysis in December 2019, 81% were using permanent vascular access [i.e., AVF (65%) or AVG (17%)]; 19% were using a catheter [1].

There are numerous barriers to performing permanent vascular access planning and placement in advance of hemodialysis initiation [29–31]. For example, many patients lack pre-ESRD insurance because Medicare ESRD program benefits do not extend to individuals with advanced chronic kidney disease (CKD), and a subset of patients who initiate dialysis in a hospital after experiencing a sudden decline in renal function may have had little opportunity for pre-dialysis planning. Nonetheless, to minimize infectious complications, patients should ideally undergo early creation of a functional AVF or timely placement of an AVG, to minimize or eliminate the time dialyzed through a catheter, if appropriate and given the patient's circumstances [32]. Further, coordination of care to ensure prompt removal of dialysis catheters after AVG/AVF maturation can decrease opportunities for infections when the catheter is no longer needed.

Evidence-Based Strategies for Preventing BSIs in Dialysis Facilities

In 2016, CDC provided the Core Interventions to BSI Prevention in Dialysis. The Core Interventions consist of nine interventions, largely focused on catheter care. They include: (1) BSI surveillance and feedback of data to clinical staff; (2) hand hygiene observations and feedback; (3) catheter/vascular access care observations and feedback; (4) development of staff infection prevention skills, demonstrated through competency assessments; (5) patient education and engagement in infection control processes; (6) efforts to decrease catheter prevalence; (7) use of alcohol-based chlorhexidine (>0.5%) as the first-line skin antiseptic for CVC exit site care; (8) catheter hub disinfection; and (9) polysporin triple ointment, or povidone-iodine ointment (or potential alternatives such as chlorhexidine-impregnated dressings) applied to catheter exit sites. Prior to publishing the Core Interventions, CDC conducted a demonstration project involving 17 dialysis facilities. This project showed a rapid reduction in BSI rates following the implementation of the Core Interventions [33]. The reduction in BSI rates was sustained for at least 4 years [34]. Further, a large cluster, randomized study involving approximately 400 facilities underscored the impact of CDC's Core Interventions on preventing BSI. The study implemented alcohol-based chlorhexidine for catheter exit-site care, and alcohol for disinfection of the catheter hub (i.e., scrub-the-hub) at the intervention facilities, which resulted in decreases in positive blood cultures and intravenous antibiotic starts [35]. CDC has also developed tools, protocols, and guidance to assist in the implementation of the interventions [36].

Catheter Devices

As previously discussed, one of the entry points of bacteria into the catheter and bloodstream is at the catheter hub. Accordingly, some catheter devices have been designed with the goal of reducing catheter contamination. A needlefree connector (Tego® needlefree hemodialysis connector), attached to the catheter hub, consists of a closed system with a silicone barrier to prevent bacteria from entering the catheter lumen. A quality improvement project in pediatric patients on hemodialysis showed a decrease in BSIs following the introduction of the Tego® connector [37]. Subsequently, a retrospective study comparing outcomes of patients on hemodialysis using the Tego® connector to those using standard catheter caps showed a decrease in IV antibiotic starts and IV antibiotic courses; however, there was not a statistically significant reduction in catheter-related BSIs [38]. In 2018, an open-label randomized control trial, compared the combination of Tego® and Curos (a cap impregnated with 70% isopropyl alcohol) to ClearGuard™HD. The ClearGuard™HD is a catheter cap that provides chlorhexidine to the catheter hub and contains a rod that releases chlorhexidine into the catheter lumen/lock solution. The trial, involving 40 dialysis facilities and over 600 patients, spanning a 13-month intervention period demonstrated that ClearGuard™HD was associated with a lower rate of BSI compared to the Tego and Curos group (0.28 versus 0.75 positive blood cultures per 1000 CVC-days, respectively; $P = 0.001$) [39].

While CDC's 2011 Guidelines for preventing intravascular catheter-related infections have a recommendation for using needleless system to access IV tubing, it does not contain a specific recommendation on the use of Tego or other needless connectors in the dialysis setting [40]. Further, there is no recommendation on the use of antiseptic-impregnated caps in any setting. At the time these guidelines were developed, there was little evidence in the literature to support their use and several of these products had not yet come to market. The Society for Healthcare Epidemiology of America (SHEA) guidance for acute hospitals recommends the use of an antiseptic-containing hub/connector cap/port protector to cover connectors as an additional approach for preventing central-line associated BSI (CLABSI) (i.e., when CLABSIs are not controlled after implementation of essential practices) but does not have a recommendation specific to the outpatient dialysis setting [41].

Antimicrobial Locks

An antimicrobial lock (AL) is a technique by which an antimicrobial solution is used to fill a catheter's lumen and then allowed to dwell for a period of time while the catheter is idle [42]. The antimicrobial agent is usually combined with an anticoagulant (heparin or citrate). Antimicrobial locks target the prevention of catheter contamination and biofilm formation within the catheter lumen. Antimicrobial locks can be classified as antibiotic locks and non-antibiotic locks. Gentamicin is the most studied antibiotic lock for preventing catheter-related bloodstream infections among hemodialysis patients. The studies on gentamicin locks are heterogeneous with varying concentrations of gentamicin locks combined with varying anticoagulants and anticoagulant doses. In a retrospective study assessing the effect of gentamicin lock (gentamicin 4 mg/mL and heparin) on catheter-related BSI over a 4-year period, gentamicin lock was associated with a decrease in BSI rates [43]. However, the gentamicin lock had to be discontinued due to an emergence of gentamicin resistance. A subsequent prospective study comparing a lower concentration of gentamicin in citrate lock (0.32 mg/mL in 4% citrate) with a heparin lock showed a lower rate of catheter-related BSI in the gentamicin lock group. Notably, gentamicin resistance was not found and there was a mortality benefit seen in the gentamicin group [44]. Non-antibiotic locks are of great interest because of the potential to avoid antibiotic resistance. Some non-antibiotic locks that have been evaluated and have shown promise in decreasing catheter-related BSI include taurolidine, methylene blue/parabens, ethanol, and citrate [45–48]. Some safety concerns have been raised regarding systemic absorption and associated toxicity and compromising catheter integrity [49]. For example, a fatal event occurred after infusing 46.7% of citrate into the catheter; likely secondary to calcium complexation leading to severe hypocalcemia and sudden death. Following this event in 2000, the FDA warned hemodialysis facilities against the use of 46.7% sodium citrate. In a meta-analysis including 30 randomized or quasi-randomized control trials comparing antimicrobial locks (i.e., antibiotic and non-antibiotic locks) to standard lock solutions in patients undergoing hemodialysis, antimicrobial locks reduced the incidence of catheter-related infections in both tunneled and non-tunneled catheters. However, the decrease in catheter-related infections was limited to tunneled catheters. The authors emphasized that their confidence in this evidence was low [50].

To date, there is no FDA-approved antimicrobial lock for preventing catheter-related BSIs in the United States, although some locks are approved in other countries. Hence, facilities that use antimicrobial locks and do not have a relationship with a pharmacy may have to prepare the locks within the facility, creating opportunities for contamination, and compounding and dosage errors. Training and quality audits should be performed regularly to ensure adherence to protocols to ensure patient safety. CDC and The *Kidney Disease Outcomes Quality Initiative* (KDOQI) do not recommend routinely using antimicrobial locks to prevent catheter-related BSI; they indicate specific populations and circumstances in which antimicrobial locks can be considered. CDC indicates that locks can be considered for patients with long-term catheters who have had multiple catheter-related BSI in spite of optimal adherence to maximal aseptic techniques, while KDOQI suggests that the selective use of specific prophylactic antimicrobial locks can be considered in patients in need of a long-term CVC who are at high risk of catheter-related BSI, especially in facilities with high rates catheter-related BSIs [32, 40].

Catheter Dressings

Catheter dressings prevent bacteria entry and colonization at the exit site. In the CDC's 2011 Guidelines for the Prevention of Intravascular Catheter-Related Infections, the recommended catheter dressing types were either a sterile gauze or a sterile transparent semi-permeable dressing to cover catheter sites [40]. For well-healed long-term cuffed and tunneled catheters (the predominant catheter used among patients on hemodialysis), a recommendation on the necessity of any catheter dressing was not given, as it was considered an unresolved issue [40]. The CDC's Core Interventions for preventing BSIs in outpatient dialysis facilities recommend the application of a triple antimicrobial ointment at the catheter exit site during each dressing change and suggest the use of chlorhexidine-impregnated dressings as an alternative to antimicrobial ointment [33]. Although the 2017 update to CDC's Guidelines for the Prevention of Intravascular Catheter-Related Infections included a recommendation for use of chlorhexidine-impregnated dressings to protect the insertion site of short-term, non-tunneled central venous catheters in patients aged 18 years and older, no recommendations were made for patients with long-term, tunneled catheters [51]. Studies examining the effect of chlorhexidine-impregnated dressings on reducing catheter-related bloodstream infections among hemodialysis patients are limited, and results are unclear [52–55]. Of note, in the demonstration project evaluating CDC's Core Interventions, several facilities used chlorhexidine-impregnated dressings (disks) and were able to show sustained reductions in BSIs [33].

Preventing Permanent Vascular Access (AVG/AVF) Infections

Contamination from skin flora is a source of permanent vascular access infections. During cannulation, bacteria from the skin can be introduced, leading to local and systemic infections. Washing the AVF/AVG site with water and soap, followed by prepping the site with appropriate antiseptic, and applying an aseptic technique during cannulation, can minimize this risk. Cannulation techniques can also contribute to the risk of access infections. Conventional cannulation (i.e., rope cannulation) is associated with a lower risk of infection compared to the buttonhole technique, a technique in which repeated cannulations occur at the same place so the scar tissue forms a tunnel [56]. Staff and patient trainings, regular audits, and annual competence evaluations can help to maintain good infection prevention standards [18, 56]. CDC's audit tools can be utilized to assess performances and promote good practices [13].

Strategies to Avoid Catheters and Promote Permanent Vascular Access

The best way to prevent a catheter-related infection is to avoid having a catheter, minimize the duration of catheter use, and ensure the timely removal of catheters when they are no longer needed. The AVF has been promoted as the optimal vascular access because of lower infectious risks, longer lifespan, and lower risk of thrombosis. In spite of national efforts to increase AVF uptake, the rates of catheter use at hemodialysis initiation have remained unchanged (~80%). Some studies have suggested that an AVF may not be the best access for all patient groups such as the elderly who may have limited life expectancy or poorer AVF patency outcomes [57, 58]. Consequently, there is a shift away from promoting AVF for all hemodialysis patients [31]. The most recent KDOQI guidelines recommend a patient-centered care and shared decision-making in vascular access selection, with the objective of getting the right access, in the right patient, at the right time, for the right reasons [31, 32].

Promoting permanent vascular access requires pre-dialysis CKD access planning, patient education, timely referral to vascular surgery, and coordination of care to ensure appropriate follow-up for monitoring for maturation and to allow for surgical revision, if necessary. When hemodialysis is initiated with a catheter, prompt placement of a permanent vascular access (when appropriate) can help limit the time the patient has a catheter. Coordination of care with radiology, vascular access surgeons, and nephrologists is integral to successful vascular access programs, but remains a challenge.

Antimicrobial Resistance

Multidrug-resistant organisms (MDROs) "defined as microorganisms, predominantly bacteria, that are resistant to 1 or more classes of antimicrobial agents," are a serious public health threat [59]. MDROs contribute to increased length of hospital stay, costs, and mortality. Hemodialysis patients are particularly vulnerable to infections and colonization with MDROs due to their frequent exposure to healthcare settings, surgical procedures, and the use of antibiotics. Not surprisingly, hemodialysis patients have been impacted by the epidemic of antimicrobial resistance. In the 1980s, one of the first cases of vancomycin-resistant enterococci (VRE) was from a renal unit in London, England [60]. VRE colonization is likely prevalent among hemodialysis patients. A meta-analysis of studies from 100 dialysis facilities across the world, involving 4800 patients (on hemodialysis and peritoneal dialysis) estimated an overall VRE colonization prevalence of 6% [61]. Another study assessing VRE colonization and VRE infections among hemodialysis patients at one dialysis facility found the prevalence of VRE rectal carriage to be 9% [62]. Hospitalization has been reported as risk factor for VRE [61]. Hospital acquisition of VRE was demonstrated in study that conducted serial VRE testing on hemodialysis patients admitted to a single hospital [63]. Among hemodialysis patients, receipt of vancomycin is another risk factor for VRE colonization, VRE infection, or VRE acquisition; thereby contributing to the overall burden of VRE [61, 63]. Vancomycin is widely used in dialysis facilities and is one of the most frequently used antibiotics among hemodialysis patients. From USRDS data spanning 1995–2005, vancomycin was the most commonly used IV antibiotic among hemodialysis patients [64]. In 2014, vancomycin accounted for 75% of intravenous antibiotic starts reported to NHSN [23]. Notably, among enterococci causing BSIs in hemodialysis patients, up to 11.4% have been reported to be resistant to vancomycin [23, 65–67].

Vancomycin resistance in *Staphylococcus aureus* has also been reported in dialysis patients. In 2002, the first patient found to be infected with a vancomycin-resistant *S. aureus* (VRSA) strain in the U.S. was an ESRD patient on hemodialysis [68]. From 2002 to date, a total of 16 cases of VRSA have been reported to CDC; the most recent VRSA case in an ESRD patient on chronic dialysis was reported in 2015 in a patient with a chronic wound [69–72]. Although person-to-person transmission of VRSA has not been demonstrated beyond the index patients, patients in healthcare settings including hemodialysis patients are vulnerable to acquiring MDROs [71]. CDC provides a guide to the investigation and control of VRSA including strategies for VRSA control in hemodialysis centers [73].

Methicillin-resistant *Staphylococcus aureus* (MRSA) was first isolated in the United States in 1968 [59]. Since then, MRSA prevalence has increased in healthcare settings. Most U.S. hemodialysis facilities are caring for patients colonized or infected with MRSA. From 1995 to 2002, the percentage of hemodialysis facilities reporting patients with MRSA infection or colonization increased from 40 to 76% [74, 75]. In 2014, MRSA accounted for 40% *of S. aureus* BSIs among hemodialysis patients in the United States [23]. Similar findings were reported in a United Kingdom study demonstrating MRSA accounted for 30% of *S. aureus* catheter-related infections among hemodialysis patients [76]. From 2009 to 2016, the incidence of invasive MRSA infections within the Emerging Infections Program catchment area among dialysis patients (including peritoneal and hemodialysis patients) has been decreasing steadily [77]. However, dialysis patients have more than 100-fold higher incidence of invasive MRSA infections than non-dialysis patients [77].

Clostridioides difficile has emerged as drug-resistant pathogen. *C. difficile*, a spore-forming, Gram-positive anaerobic bacillus, is a common cause of antibiotic-associated diarrhea. Patients with ESRD are at high risk of *C. difficile* infection (CDI) [78]. A meta-analysis showed a twofold higher mortality in patients with ESRD with CDI compared to those without CDI [79]. CDI contributes to hospitalizations and increased length of stay among patients with ESRD [80, 81]. An analysis of CMS ESRD data showed that among prevalent ESRD patients, the hospitalization rate for CDI in 2013 was 1.2 per 100 patient-years [80]. The UK Renal Registry reported a CDI incidence of 1.09 per 100 patient-years among hemodialysis patients in 2013–2014 [82]. A CDI outbreak investigation in a hemodialysis facility provided some understanding of potential risk factors for CDI in hemodialysis population [80]. Risk factors for CDI included high antibiotic exposure, use of β-lactam antibiotics, hospitalization within prior 30 days, and non-fistula dialysis access (i.e., AVG or CVC) [83]. In 2021, given the unique hemodialysis setting and the paucity of data on *C. difficile* transmission in the outpatient dialysis setting, the American Society of Nephrology's Nephrologists Transforming Dialysis Safety committee provided strategies to prevent and control *C. Difficile* transmission in outpatient hemodialysis (Table 4.2). The committee adapted the 2017 clinical practice guidelines for CDI prevention from the Infectious Diseases Society of America (IDSA) and the Society of Healthcare Epidemiology of American (SHEA) to the hemodialysis setting [84].

In order to prevent transmission of MDROs in the outpatient hemodialysis setting, one must understand the transmission kinetics involved with each organism. While Contact Precautions are used in the acute care setting for certain MDROs, including MRSA and VRE, [17] CDC has not recommended the routine use of contact precautions in outpatient hemodialysis centers for patients infected or colonized with these MDROs. Transmission of pathogenic bacteria is well documented in hospitals, and at least one study has suggested that the majority of transmission and acquisition of resistant pathogens among dialysis patients occur when these patients are admitted to the acute care setting [63]. However, other studies have demonstrated MDRO spread in dialysis centers [83, 85]. Some potential reasons why spread is less common in dialysis centers enhanced environmental cleaning and

Table 4.2 Summary of suggestions for the prevention of *Clostridioides difficile* spread within outpatient dialysis and hemodialysis facilities provided by Nephrologists Transforming Dialysis Safety Committee

Questions	Suggestions
1. What IPC resources/activities should outpatient hemodialysis facilities have in place for the prevention of CDI transmission and care of patients with CDI?	• Develop and maintain a robust IPC program that is integrated within the QAPI program • Assure at least one individual with training in IPC is regularly available to the facility • Have a written policy detailing IPC precautions specifically designed to prevent the transmission of *C. difficile* • Provide education and training to all HCP on the basic principles and practices for preventing the spread of CDI • Provide CDI education to patients • Conduct regular surveillance for CDI, calculate facility rates, and share results with front-line clinical staff • Encourage judicious use of antimicrobials through implementation of antimicrobial stewardship activities • Ensure open communication with other health care facilities • Contact local or state health department if an outbreak or cluster is detected or if transmission is identified within the facility
2. What are the preferred hand hygiene measures for HCP when caring for a patient with suspected or confirmed CDI?	• Wear gloves when caring for patients with CDI to reduce hand contamination • Perform hand hygiene before donning gloves and after removing gloves • Soap and water are preferred; however, use of an alcohol-based hand rub is acceptable unless there is an outbreak or concern for horizontal transmission within the facility • Perform handwashing with soap and water if there has been direct contact with feces or an area where fecal contamination is likely • Encourage patients to perform hand hygiene and increase personal hygiene measures before their dialysis session • Audit HCP hand hygiene compliance and provide feedback
3. What PPE should be worn when caring for a patient with suspected or confirmed CDI?	• Wear gloves when caring for CDI patients and remove and immediately discard gloves when finished • Wear a new gown over usual clothing during high-contact patient care activities • Use disposable face shields for each interaction that warrants face protection and immediately discard after each use • Remove PPE slowly and deliberately in a sequence that prevents self-contamination
4. What is the preferred placement for dialysis treatment for patients with CDI?	• Assess patients for signs and symptoms of CDI before their entry to the treatment area • Provide dialysis during sessions with the fewest number of other patients or minimal number of adjacent stations as possible • Consider using isolation room if there are no hepatitis B-infected patients being cared for in the facility, and the room has been terminally cleaned • The dialysis station or isolation room should be thoroughly cleaned with *C. difficile*-active disinfectants after dialysis of patients with CDI

(continued)

Table 4.2 (continued)

Questions	Suggestions
5. What bathroom facilities should be provided to dialysis patients with CDI?	• Bathroom facilities should be thoroughly cleaned with *C. difficile*-approved disinfectants after use by a patient with CDI • Assess the patient before entering the treatment floor to determine if he/she is having active diarrhea or incontinence • Limit use of bedpans and bedside commodes in the treatment floor • Roll-out screens, if used for toileting privacy, should be nonporous and immediately cleaned and disinfected with *C. difficile*-approved disinfectants after use • Change and discard all PPE and perform hand hygiene with soap and water, immediately after assisting the patient with toileting activities
6. What is the appropriate length of time to maintain precautions?	• CDI-specific precautions should be continued for at least 48 h after the diarrhea has ceased • If signs and symptoms of CDI recur after precautions have been discontinued, CDI-specific precautions should be resumed • CDI-specific precautions beyond 48 h should be considered if CDI rates remain high despite implementation of CDI IPC measures
7. What are the optimal measures for environmental disinfection?	• Thoroughly clean and disinfect the station after the patient with CDI completes his/her dialysis treatment and exits the station • Use disinfectants from the EPA's registered antimicrobial products effective against the spores of *C. difficile* (list K) • Limit multiuse items and dedicate patient care items that are typically multiuse to the care of the patient with CDI • Audit staff practices to ensure effective environmental disinfection is occurring and provide feedback

CDI Clostridioides difficile infection, *EPA* Environmental Protection Agency, *HCP* health care personnel, *IPC* infection prevention and control, *PPE* personal protective equipment, *QAPI* Quality Assessment and Performance Improvement

*Adapted from D'Agata EMC, Apata IW, Booth S, et al. Suggestions for the prevention of Clostridioides difficile spread within outpatient hemodialysis facilities. *Kidney Int.* May 2021;99(5):1045–1053. doi:10.1016/j.kint.2021.02.028

disinfection that occurs frequently throughout the day between patients and the amount of time an individual patient spends at the dialysis center (compared to the acute care setting). CDC recommends additional precautions be used during treatment of patients who might be at higher risk for transmitting pathogenic bacteria (i.e., those with an infected skin wound with drainage that is not contained by dressings, fecal incontinence, or uncontrolled diarrhea). These additional precautions include: (1) HCP treating the patient should wear a separate gown over their usual clothing and remove the gown when finished caring for the patient and (2) dialyzing the patient at a station away from the main flow of traffic and with as few adjacent stations as possible (e.g., at the end or corner of the unit) [17]. More work is needed to understand the transmission of MDROs including targeted MDRO (i.e., those with novel or pan-resistance patterns such as vancomycin-resistant *Staphylococcus aureus* or carbapenem-resistant Enterobacteriaceae) in dialysis settings and the effectiveness of interventions to reduce transmission [73].

As more is learned about the spread of targeted MDROs among dialysis patients and as other emerging pathogens of concern are identified, recommendations may change. Although most MDROs are bacteria, there are also emerging fungal pathogens, including *Candida auris*, that are resistant to multiple antifungals [86]. CDC has released on its website recommendations for infection control to prevent transmission of *C. auris*, including dialysis-specific recommendations [86, 87]. CDC has released on its website recommendations for infection control to prevent transmission of *C. auris*, including dialysis-specific recommendations [87]. Dialysis centers should consider how they will minimize exposure to other patients (i.e., dialyzing at a station with as few adjacent stations as possible, dialyzing patient on the last shift of the day) when dialyzing patients with targeted MDROs. While challenges may exist in implementing such practices, it is critical that dialysis centers become adept at incorporating these procedures as the number of patients identified with these targeted MDROs is likely to increase in the future. If questions exist about how to safely dialyze patients with certain MDROs in the outpatient setting, for dialysis facility staff or administrators should contact local or state health departments for assistance.

Antimicrobial Stewardship

Antibiotic resistance is one of the unintended consequences of antibiotic use; other unintended consequences are adverse drug events such as allergic reactions and nephrotoxicity. Antibiotic stewardship, defined as "the effort to measure and improve how antibiotics are prescribed by clinicians and used by patients, focuses on improving treatment outcomes in patients and minimizing inappropriate antibiotic prescribing" [88]. Given the burden of infections and significant morbidity and mortality from these infections, antibiotic use in the hemodialysis population is high. A national study in 1998 showed that approximately 30% of hemodialysis patients received at least 1 dose of antibiotics in a given year [64]. Vancomycin, cefazolin, and third and fourth-generation cephalosporins are some antibiotics commonly used in the hemodialysis setting [64, 89]. In a study involving two hemodialysis facility, as many as 30% of IV antibiotics were found to be inappropriate (i.e., unnecessary or not indicated) [89]. Reasons for those inappropriate uses and possible strategies for improving antibiotic prescribing in dialysis facilities have been proposed [90]. More data are needed to understand the relationship between antibiotic prescribing patterns in dialysis centers and antibiotic resistance to better target potential stewardship activities.

In 2020, CDC and the American Society of Nephrology (ASN) developed a white paper describing what is known regarding antibiotic use and opportunities for optimizing antibiotic prescribing in outpatient hemodialysis facilities [91]. CDC developed the Core Elements of Antibiotic Stewardship to provide facilities and providers a set of key principles to guide efforts to improve antibiotic use and advance patient safety and outcomes [88]. Since there are no Core Elements for antibiotic stewardship specific to outpatient hemodialysis facilities (due to limited research and evidence for antibiotic stewardship in this setting), a joint effort aimed to offer strategies that could be applied to improve antibiotic prescribing in dialysis settings. Key strategies outlined in the white paper include standardization of blood culture collection, enhanced communication across care transitions (e.g., communicating blood culture results and antibiotic course and plan from hospital to outpatient dialysis facility), and appropriate de-escalation of antibiotics (Fig. 4.1). The white paper also outlines population- and setting-specific considerations and research gaps.

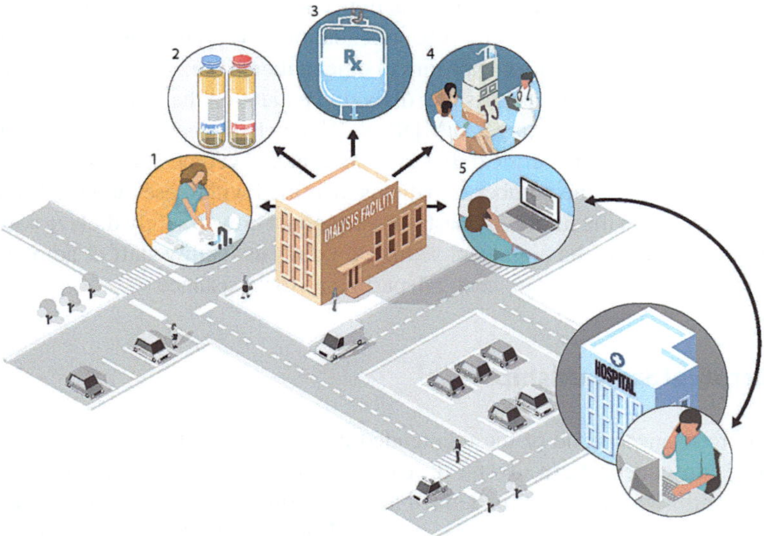

Suggested Strategy	Description	Examples
1. **Infection prevention and sepsis prevention efforts**	Engage all staff and patients in preventing infections such as bloodstream infection and vascular access infection.	• Conduct routine competency assessments for all dialysis staff involved in catheter care. • Implement influenza vaccine campaign. • Involve patients in hand hygiene observations
2. **Blood culture practices**	Implement standardized practices to improve blood culture collection.	• Train staff on how blood culture should be obtained (e.g. sites of collection, blood volume). • Evaluate adherence to blood culture collection prior to antibiotic initiation.
3. **Treatment of methicillin-susceptible Staphylococcus aureus (MSSA) infections**	Treat MSSA infections with ß-lactams instead of vancomycin for better treatment outcomes.	• Incorporate automated alert in electronic medical record to prompt providers to review appropriateness of antibiotic therapy. • Develop a process to receive and notify providers of culture results.
4. **Communication with prescribing providers**	Implement practices to improve communication between onsite nurses and prescribing physicians or physician extenders.	• Develop a structed method of communicating critical information such as SBAR (Situation, Background, Assessment and Recommendation).
5. **Communication across care transitions**	Implement practices to improve communication across transitions of care between the outpatient dialysis facility and other healthcare settings.	• Work with local hospitals to establish data sharing agreements for bidirectional communication. • Implement standard transfer form/sign out between dialysis facility and nursing home.

Fig. 4.1 Suggested strategies for improving antibiotic use in outpatient hemodialysis facilities. [Reprinted from Apata IW, Kabbani S, Neu AM, et al. Opportunities to Improve Antibiotic Prescribing in Outpatient Hemodialysis Facilities. Am J Kidney Dis. 2020 Oct 9 (205)]

Viral Bloodborne Infections

Hepatitis B

HBV is transmitted by percutaneous (i.e., puncture through the skin) or mucosal exposure to infectious blood, semen, or other body fluids. The virus is relatively stable in the environment and can remain infectious on environmental surfaces for at least 7 days [92]. Improper cleaning and disinfection of blood-contaminated surfaces can lead to HBV transmission via dialysis HCP. HBV can be present on environmental surfaces in the absence of visible blood and still cause infection. It has been detected in dialysis facilities on hemostats, gloved hands, dialysis machine control panels, and door knobs [92].

Epidemiology

In the early 1970s, hemodialysis facilities were a reservoir of HBV, and infections were endemic, and outbreaks were common. From 1976 through 1983, a dramatic decline in hepatitis B incidence and prevalence among hemodialysis patients was seen. This decline coincided with the publication of control measures for hepatitis B in the hemodialysis setting in 1977, followed by the widespread implementation of these recommendations in the 1980s [93]. Similar trends were seen in the HBV incidence and prevalence among HCP [94, 95]. With the advent of the hepatitis B vaccine in 1982, which was recommended for all susceptible patients and HCP in hemodialysis further declines were seen in incidence and prevalence among patients on chronic hemodialysis. In 2002, the incidence of HBV infection among hemodialysis patients was 0.12% and the HBV infection prevalence was 1% [75]. Data from 2002 also showed that newly acquired HBV infections were reported by 2.8% of U.S. hemodialysis facilities and 27.3% of facilities reported one or more patients with chronic HBV infection [75]. In addition to widespread adoption of HBV-specific infection control measures and HBV vaccine uptake, improved blood donor screening (safer blood) and introduction of erythrocyte stimulating agents (leading to decreased need for blood transfusion) may have contributed to declines in HBV incidence and prevalence in the dialysis population.

Risk factors for acquiring HBV infection include injection drug use, sexual and household exposure to HBV-infected contacts, exposure to multiple sexual partners, male-to-male sexual contact (MMSC), and perinatal exposure [96]. Some of the reported independent risk factors for acquiring HBV infection among patients on chronic hemodialysis have been the presence of at least one HBV-infected patient in the hemodialysis facility who was not isolated, and a facility vaccination rate <50% among patients [97]. All patients with active HBV infection (HBsAg positive) should be educated about risk factors of HBV transmission; their sexual partners and household contacts should be informed and vaccinated [98, 99]. All HBV-infected patients should be evaluated for HBV treatment.

Over the past 20 years, reports of HBV transmission in U.S. hemodialysis facilities have become rare. A single case of dialysis-associated HBV transmission was reported in the U.S. more recently, in the setting of HBV reactivation in a patient with HIV infection who had previous resolved HBV infection and had received immunosuppressive therapy for kidney transplantation [100]. The patient was not dialyzed under HBV isolation, given his known HBsAg negative status. The epidemiological investigation revealed that the source patient and index patient (a vaccine non-responder) had shared a dialysis station several times. It also identified several infection control breaches, including preparation of injectable medications on a mobile cart near dialysis stations, failure to thoroughly disinfect dialysis stations, and movement of patient-care materials between stations [100]. An important finding of the investigation was the failure of the dialysis facility to recognize a discordant HBV serology result for the source patient, that signaled possible HBV reactivation. It underscores the need for dialysis clinicians to know how to interpret HBV serology or seek assistance when necessary. In recent years, CDC has received other reports of atypical hepatitis B serology results among dialysis patients that may have represented reactivation of HBV infection or HBV mutant strains; however, no cases of dialysis-related transmission related to these instances were identified [101, 102].

Screening and Diagnostic Tests

HBV serology including HBV antigens [i.e., hepatitis B surface antigen (HBsAg), hepatitis B core antigen (HBcAg), and hepatitis B e antigen (HBeAg)] and HBV antibodies [i.e., antibody to HBsAg (anti-HBs), antibody to hepatitis B core antigen (anti-HBc), and antibody to HBeAg (anti-HBe)] can be used to distinguish acute HBV infection, chronic HBV infection, resolved HBV infection, or vaccine immunity (Table 4.3). There are commercially available assays for these serological markers [103]. One or more of these serologic markers are present during different

Table 4.3 Interpretation of serological test results for hepatitis B virus infection

Serologic markers				
HBsAg[a]	Total anti-HBc[b]	IgM[c] anti-HBc	Anti-HBs[d]	Interpretation
–	–	–	–	Susceptible, never infected
+	–	–	–	Acute infection, early incubation[e]
+	+	+	–	Acute infection
–	+	+	–	Acute resolving infection
–	+	–	+	Past infection, recovered and immune
+	+	–	–	Chronic infection
–	+	–	–	False positive (i.e., susceptible), past infection, or low-level chronic infection
–	–	–	+	Immune if titer ≥10 mIU/mL (or the lab-specific level that represents immunity)

[a]Hepatitis B surface antigen
[b]Antibody to hepatitis B core antigen
[c]Immunoglobulin M
[d]Antibody to hepatitis B surface antigen
[e]Transient HBsAg positivity might be detected in some patients following vaccination

phases of HBV infection and can help distinguish between acute or chronic infection [103] (Table 4.3). HBV DNA quantitative and qualitative tests can also detect HBV infections and can be used to evaluate when HBV reactivation or infection with an HBV mutant strain is suspected [104, 105]. HBsAg mutant strains may evade some commercial assays [101, 102].

The presence of HBsAg usually correlates with viremia (positive HBV DNA) and is indicative of ongoing HBV infection and potential infectiousness. In newly infected individuals, HBsAg is present in serum on average 30 days (range 6–60 days) after exposure to HBV and persists for variable periods. Anti-HBc develops in all HBV infections and persists for life. Acute or recently acquired infection can be distinguished by presence of the immunoglobulin M (IgM) class of anti-HBc, which persists for approximately 6 months. In individuals who recover from HBV infection, HBsAg and HBV DNA are usually eliminated from the blood and anti-HBs appear. After recovery from natural infection, most individuals will be positive for both total anti-HBc and anti-HBs, whereas only anti-HBs develop in individuals who are successfully vaccinated. Most individuals who do not recover and remain chronically infected remain HBsAg, total anti-HBc, and HBV DNA positive. HBeAg can be detected in acute or chronic HBV infection and usually correlates with viral replication and high-level viremia (i.e., high infectivity) while anti-HBe correlates with loss of replicating virus and lower levels of virus.

In some individuals, the only HBV serologic marker detected is total anti-HBc (i.e., isolated anti-HBc). This pattern can occur after HBV infection among individuals who have recovered but whose anti-HBs have waned; or among individuals who have low-level chronic HBV infection and failed to develop anti-HBs. It may also represent a false positive total anti-HBc result or someone in the early convalescent period after natural infection before the appearance of anti-HBs. HBV DNA has been detected in <10% of individuals with isolated anti-HBc, and these individuals are unlikely to be infectious to others except under unusual circumstances involving direct percutaneous exposures to large quantities of blood (e.g., transfusion) or organ transplantation [106–111]. However, the rare individual with high titers of HBV DNA and isolated anti-HBc is likely infectious, even if HBsAg negative and should be dialyzed in isolation while the diagnostic workup proceeds with expert consultation [101]. In most persons with isolated anti-HBc in the general population, the result appears to be false positive. Data from several studies have demonstrated that a primary anti-HBs response develops in most of these individuals after a three-dose series of hepatitis B vaccine [112, 113]. No data exist on response to vaccination among hemodialysis patients with this serologic pattern. Testing and follow-up recommendations for hemodialysis patients with isolated anti-HBc are available [17]. The suggested approach includes retesting the patient to confirm the total anti-HBc result, and if total anti-HBc remains positive and IgM anti-HBc remains negative, the patient may undergo vaccination and post-vaccination testing for anti-HBs. HBV DNA testing can also be considered early in this situation, to determine if the patient is susceptible and would benefit from vaccine or has "low-level" chronic infection.

Table 4.4 Schedule for routine testing for hepatitis B virus (HBV) and hepatitis C virus (HCV)

Patient status	On admission[a]	Monthly	Semi-annual	Annual
All patients	HBsAg[b], anti-HBc (total), anti-HBs, anti-HCV, ALT			
HBV susceptible		HBsAg[b]		
Anti-HBs positive (≥10 mIU/mL), anti-HBc negative				Anti-HBs
Anti-HBs and total anti-Hbc positive[c]				
Anti-HCV negative		ALT	Anti-HCV	

HBsAg hepatitis B surface antigen, *anti-HBs* antibody to HBsAg, *anti-HBc* antibody to hepatitis B core antigen, *ALT* alanine aminotransferase, *anti-HCV* antibody to hepatitis C virus
[a]Results of HBV testing should be known before patient begins dialysis
[b]Test for HBsAg with an assay that can detect HBsAg mutants
[c]No ongoing HBV infection monitoring is recommended for patients with evidence of past, resolved infection. Screening for reappearance of HBsAg at regular intervals can be considered

Recommendations for routine testing for HBV in maintenance hemodialysis patients are described in Table 4.4. Routine testing for HBV depends on the patient's HBV status such as HBV susceptible and HBV vaccine immune. Interpreting and responding to HBV serology appropriately in the dialysis clinic have implications for HBV infection control measures. A false positive HBV result may result in placing a patient without HBV infection at risk of acquiring HBV, if placed in HBV isolation. On the other hand, failing to place a patient with HBV infection in isolation can put HBV-susceptible patients at risk of acquiring HBV infection. Because of the potentially serious consequences of missing an individual with HBV infection in a dialysis center, dialysis providers should routinely use HBsAg assays that are capable of detecting common HBV mutant strains [101, 102]. All HBsAg-positive patients are potentially infectious. Patients' HBsAg status should be determined upon admission to (or first treatment within) a dialysis facility, and HBsAg-positive patients should be placed on isolation precautions.

Prevention of HBV Transmission

Most HBV outbreaks among hemodialysis patients have been caused by cross-contamination to patients via (1) environmental surfaces, supplies (e.g., hemostats, clamps), or equipment that was not routinely cleaned and disinfected after each use; (2) multiple-dose vials or intravenous solutions that were not used exclusively for one patient; (3) medications for injections that were prepared adjacent to areas where blood samples were handled; and (4) HCP who simultaneously provided care for both infected (HBsAg-positive) patients and susceptible patients [97, 114–121]. Once the factors that promote HBV transmission among hemodialysis patients were identified, recommendations for control were published [93].

The following recommendations can be applied to prevent transmission of HBV in hemodialysis facilities (Tables 4.1 and 4.4): (1) serologic screening of all patients for HBV infection at admission; (2) monthly testing of all susceptible patients for

HBsAg; (3) HBV vaccination of susceptible patients [and HCP without documented immunity per Advisory Committee on Immunization Practices (ACIP) recommendations]; [122] (4) isolation of all HBsAg-positive patients in a separate room; (5) assignment of HCP to HBsAg-positive patients and not to HBV-susceptible patients during the same or overlapping shift; (6) assignment of dedicated dialysis equipment and supplies to HBsAg-positive patients; (7) cleaning and disinfection of non-disposable items (e.g., hemostats, clamps) before use on another patient; (8) glove use whenever patient or hemodialysis equipment is touched and glove changes and hand hygiene between each patient (and station); and (9) routine cleaning and disinfection of equipment and environmental surfaces [93, 123]. Patients who are not documented vaccine responders should not be cared for by HCPs who are also caring for HBV-infected patients.

Hepatitis C

Hepatitis C virus (HCV) is a bloodborne virus with transmission occurring primarily through direct percutaneous exposure to blood such as injection drug use, unsafe injection practices, and unscreened blood products. HCV is moderately stable in the environment, and the infectious virus can persist on surfaces when exposed to room temperature for at least 16 h [124]. Longer persistence of up to several weeks has been reported [125]. No vaccine is available to prevent HCV infection. HCV transmission continues to occur among hemodialysis patients due to lapses in infection control, in contrast to vaccine-preventable HBV, which is more efficiently transmitted but now rarely acquired in the US dialysis setting.

Epidemiology

Hepatitis C virus (HCV) was first identified in 1989. According to the World Health Organization, in 2019 an estimated 58 million people in the world have chronic HCV infection [126]. Chronic HCV infection can lead to cirrhosis, hepatocellular carcinoma, and other extrahepatic effects such as mixed cryoglobulinemia and membranoproliferative kidney disease resulting in chronic kidney disease with the potential for progression to ESRD [126, 127]. In the United States, improved screening of blood donors led to decrease in post-transfusion HCV infections even before the discovery of HCV. The introduction of improved HCV testing of blood products including anti-HCV (introduced in 1990) and nucleic acid testing (NAT) (introduced in 1999) led to further reductions in transfusion-transmitted HCV; the current estimated risk is <1 in a million per unit transfused [128]. With improved blood donor screening, injection drug use is the most important risk factor for HCV acquisition in the US [96, 129].

Prevalence rates of HCV in dialysis patients are higher than in patients without kidney disease. HCV infection is reported to be an independent risk factor for mortality in the hemodialysis population and portends increased morbidity and lower quality of life [130]. Efforts have been made to determine HCV prevalence among patients on dialysis. For the period spanning 1997–2001, the Dialysis Outcomes and Practice Patterns Study (DOPPS) reported a mean HCV facility prevalence of

13.5% (range 2.6–22.9%) among 308 hemodialysis facilities across seven countries including the United States; the mean HCV prevalence in the US was 14% (range 13.6–14.5%). Black race, male gender, presence of diabetes mellitus, HBV infection, prior renal transplant, history of GI bleed, drug and alcohol abuse were associated with higher HCV prevalence [131]. Subsequent data from DOPPS showed that HCV prevalence among dialysis patients decreased in the United States from 11.5% (years 1996–2001) to 6.9% (years 2012–2015) [132]. HCV prevalence among US Black patients on hemodialysis remained higher than in non-Black patients (spanning DOPPs period from 1997 to 2015). The DOPPS study also examined trends in HCV incidence (i.e., seroconversion among patients with initial HCV-negative serology); HCV incidence in the United States decreased from 3.5 per 100 patient years to less than 1 per 100 patient years from 1997 to 2015. Patient characteristics associated with HCV seroconversion were dialysis vintage (i.e., number of years on dialysis) of greater than 10 years, HBV infection, and HIV infection. Facility HCV prevalence of greater than 20% was associated with a higher HCV incidence [132].

Elimination of post-transfusion HCV infections through improved screening of the blood supply, as well as the introduction of erythrocyte stimulating agents (like epoetin alpha) that reduced the need for transfusion likely played a role in the decrease in HCV incidence rates among dialysis patients. Nonetheless, HCV seroconversions continue to occur in hemodialysis patients, and the evidence supports nosocomial acquisition as a contributing factor.

Screening and Diagnostic Tests

Antibodies to HCV (anti-HCV) can be detected as early as 10 weeks post-exposure using FDA-approved third-generation testing platforms, while HCV RNA can be detected as early as 1-week post-exposure using FDA-approved nucleic acid tests (NAT). Increases in alanine aminotransferase (ALT) can occur before the anti-HCV becomes positive. A positive anti-HCV antibody test represents either current or resolved past infection. A positive HCV RNA test signifies the presence of active HCV infection and HCV viremia. Screening for HCV should start with an anti-HCV test. All patients who test positive for anti-HCV should have HCV RNA testing done [133].

CDC recommends routine HCV screening for patients on (chronic) hemodialysis with anti-HCV testing on admission to the outpatient facility (Table 4.4). For patients with a negative anti-HCV test on admission, CDC recommends: (1) anti-HCV testing every 6 months and (2) monthly alanine aminotransferase. For patients with a positive anti-HCV test, CDC recommends further testing for HCV RNA with NAT testing (Table 4.4, Fig. 4.2). Kidney Disease: Improving Global Outcomes (KDIGO) also recommends routine HCV screening upon admission to an outpatient dialysis facility [134]. However, they recommend that screening should be done by NAT testing or by immunoassay followed by NAT, if immunoassay is positive. KDIGO also recommends this testing for follow-up screening in HCV-susceptible patients (or HCV-negative patients). The frequency of follow-up screening (every 6 months) and recommendations for monthly ALT testing is consistent with CDC's recommendations. Currently, CMS does not require or reimburse HCV screening

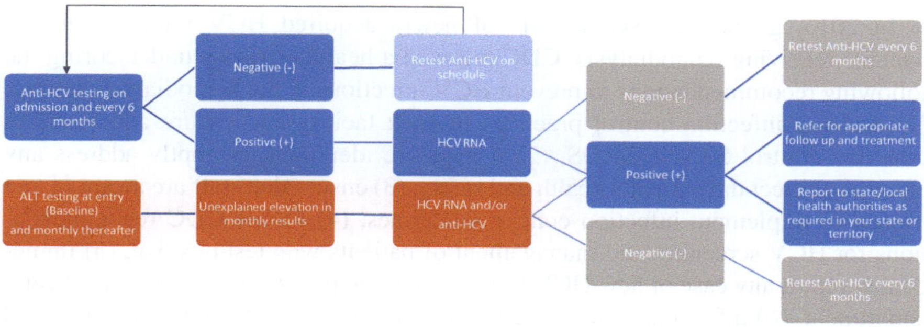

Fig. 4.2 Hepatitis C screening algorithm for outpatient hemodialysis facilities. If the anti-HCV is positive, but the HCV RNA test is negative (e.g., after treatment with a sustained virologic response) subsequent anti-HCV screening tests are replaced with HCV RNA tests. A change in HCV infection status (i.e., new infection or seroconversion) should be reported to the state or local health department. *ALT* alanine aminotransferase, *anti-HCV* antibody to hepatitis C virus, *HCV-RNA* hepatitis C virus ribonucleic acid. (Reprinted from Nephrologists Transforming Dialysis Safety)

for patients treated in hemodialysis facilities, possibly causing a barrier in identifying and reporting all new HCV cases in U.S. facilities. For patients with resolved HCV infections (anti-HCV positive and negative HCV RNA) or patients who have successfully been treated for HCV, KDIGO recommends that NAT testing to be conducted every 6 months to assess for reinfection [134].

Prevention of HCV Transmission

From 2008 to 2019, 22 HCV outbreaks involving a combined total of 104 new HCV infections, in the outpatient hemodialysis setting in the US were reported to CDC [6]. The epidemiology investigations identified multiple plausible mechanisms for transmission, including breaches in infection control practices including improper hand hygiene and glove changing practices (e.g., failing to change gloves and perform hand hygiene between patients), inadequate cleaning and disinfection of environmental surfaces and equipment between patients (e.g., dialysis station, dialysis chair, clamps, and priming bucket), and poor medication preparation procedures (e.g., medication preparation close to the treatment area, and the use of single-dose vials for more than 1 patient). Similar findings were reported in an epidemiological study aimed at identifying patient-care practices associated with HCV prevalence in outpatient dialysis facilities [2]. Specifically, reusing priming receptacles without disinfection, handling blood specimens adjacent to medications and clean supplies, and using mobile carts to deliver injectable medications were patient-care practices associated with a higher prevalence of HCV infection [135]. Other reported risk factors associated with HCV infection included receiving dialysis at a station in close proximity to an HCV-infected patient, receiving dialysis treatment using the same station/machine (on consecutive shifts) to an HCV-infected patient, and receiving care from a dialysis staff who also cared for an HCV-infected patient [2, 135].

In 2016, given increased reports of newly acquired HCV infection among patients receiving hemodialysis, CDC released a health advisory underscoring the following recommendations to prevent HCV infections in the hemodialysis setting: (1) evaluate infection control practices in each facility and ensure adherence to infection control STANDARDS, (2) if gaps are identified, promptly address any issues to protect the patient's health and safety, (3) ensure that staff are aware of and trained to implement infection control guidelines, (4) follow CDC recommendations for HCV screening and management of patients who test positive, (5) immediately report any case of new HCV infection among patients to state or local health department, (6) inform patients if HCV transmission is suspected to have occurred within the facility and explain steps being taken to address the problem [136].

In the U.S., the management of HCV-positive patients in the outpatient dialysis setting differs from HBV-positive patients. CDC and KDIGO do not recommend isolation or separation of HCV-positive patients from HCV-negative patients, nor do they recommend using a dedicated dialysis machine for HCV-positive patients. Some countries (or some facilities outside the United States) may separate HCV-positive patients from HCV-negative patients. The DOPPS study involving seven countries revealed 11.4% of facilities reported using isolation stations for dialyzing HCV-positive patients, although delineation was not made regarding if the isolation stations were in a separate room. Further, isolation of HCV-positive patients in a facility was not associated with a lower risk of HCV seroconversion [131].

Treatment and cure of patients with HCV is a potential strategy for prevention in the dialysis facility, as HCV prevalence is a risk factor for transmission. All patients who are HCV-positive should be referred for evaluation and treatment [137–141]. Treatment for hepatitis C is associated with improved survival among patients on dialysis. In recent years, advances have been made in HCV treatment with the advent of direct-acting antivirals (DAA). Effective and safe treatment options are available for patients with advanced kidney disease, including ESRD [142]. Elimination of hepatitis C from dialysis units through diagnosis and treatment of HCV infection is both feasible and desirable [137].

Managing New HCV Infection

HCV seroconversion (i.e., new HCV infection) in a patient on hemodialysis may be detected on routine HCV screening or during HCV testing for evaluation of acute hepatitis. When a new HCV infection is identified (i.e., HCV seroconversion), the patient's laboratory data and medical records should be reviewed to ensure that the patient had previously tested anti-HCV negative and had seroconverted to anti-HCV positive. A newly identified HCV seroconversion should prompt a thorough investigation and notification to the local public health department. The hepatitis C screening algorithm can be used as an aid for the initial laboratory investigation of new HCV seroconversion (Fig. 4.2) [143]. In addition, a newly identified HCV seroconversion investigation should include an assessment of the patient's risk factors for HCV not limited to dialysis healthcare but also including considerations such as other healthcare exposures, IV drug use, and potential patient interactions outside the facility. Auditing and observations of staff/facility infection control procedures,

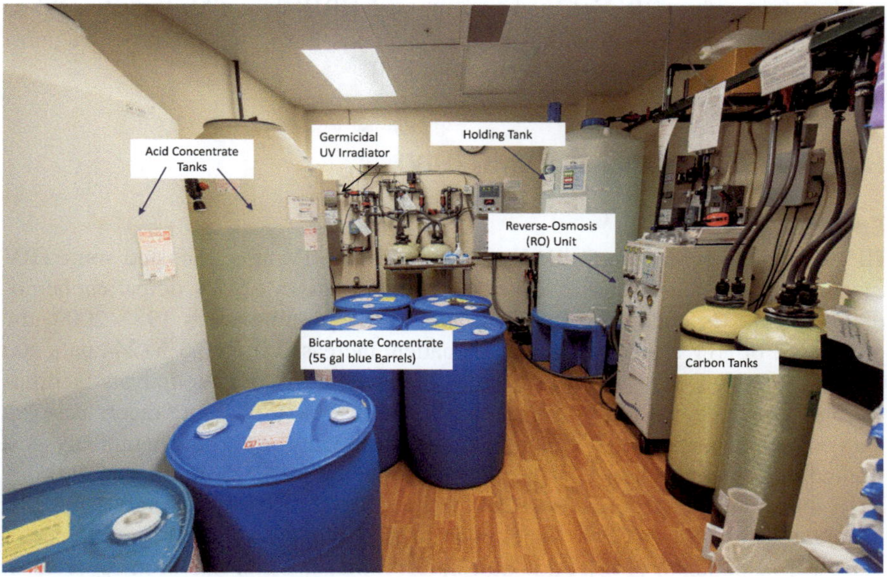

Fig. 4.3 Water room in outpatient dialysis facility: selected components of water system, acid tanks, and bicarbonate tanks

developing and implementing solutions to mitigate gaps identified, reviewing of HCV tests in all patients in the facility to identify if there are new cases and likely retesting of all patients in the facility for HCV. The local health department can assist and support the investigation, including coordinating molecular testing as available from local, state, or federal public health laboratories to determine the genetic sequence of new cases with previously infected cases to determine the probability of HCV transmission occurring in the dialysis facility (Fig. 4.3).

Hepatitis D

Hepatitis D, also known as "delta hepatitis," is caused by the hepatitis delta virus (HDV). HDV causes infections only in persons with active HBV infection. The prevalence of HDV infection in is very low in the United States [144]. HDV prevalence was found to be higher among intravenous drug users and persons with high risk sexual behaviors [145]. There is little data regarding the prevalence of HDV infection among chronic hemodialysis patients.

In the U.S., there has been only one report of HDV transmission among hemodialysis patients [15]. This transmission event occurred in the 1980s and transmission occurred from patient chronically infected with HBV and HDV (with a risk factor of IV drug use) to a HBsAg-positive patient following a massive bleeding incident resulting in environmental contamination. Both patients shared the same dialysis station. Therefore, in hemodialysis settings, HDV-infected patients should be isolated from other HBV-infected patients and HBV-susceptible patients. While there is no vaccine to prevent hepatitis D, hepatitis B vaccine can protect against hepatitis B and future hepatitis D infections [15].

Human Immunodeficiency Virus (HIV)

Epidemiology

HIV infections contribute to the burden of ESRD; HIV infections and some HIV medications can cause chronic kidney disease. In a survey of U.S. outpatient hemodialysis facilities conducted by CDC and CMS spanning years 1985–2002, the prevalence of HIV among hemodialysis patient increased from 0.3% (244 patients) to 1.5% (4019). During the same period, the percentage of hemodialysis facilities caring for patients with HIV increased from 11 to 39% [75]. More recent national data on the prevalence of HIV infections among patients on chronic hemodialysis is limited due to changes in HIV status data collected by CMS starting in 2005. A study analyzing data from 2004 to 2014 from one of the two largest dialysis providers in the United States (2900 facilities from 47 states) found an HIV prevalence of 1.3% (5348 patients) [146]. Although no HIV transmission has been reported in hemodialysis facilities in the United States, several countries have reported HIV transmission in hemodialysis facilities [147–150].

Screening

CDC does not recommend routine testing for the purpose of infection control in outpatient hemodialysis facilities [17]. However, CDC recommends HIV screening for anyone aged 13–64 years, and repeat screening is recommended at least annually for those at high risk for HIV, including injection drug users and their sexual partners, persons who exchange sex for money or drugs, sex partners of HIV-infected persons, MSMs (men who have sex with men), or heterosexual persons who themselves or whose sex partners have had more than one sex partner since their most recent HIV test [151].

Prevention of HIV Transmission

Although HIV transmission associated with dialysis is rare, reports of HIV transmission in this setting highlight the importance of adhering to recommended infection control practices. HIV transmission in outpatient dialysis facilities have been linked to breaches in infection control practices, including the use of multidose heparin vial, inadequate disinfection of hemodialysis equipment, dialysis staff using blood-contaminated gloves during vascular access manipulation for multiple patients, [148] vascular access needle reuse and inadequate needle disinfection, [150] and shared syringes between patients (using the same syringe to flush the bloodline of multiple patients) [147, 148]. Adherence to recommended infection control procedures and practices is considered adequate to prevent HIV transmission in the hemodialysis setting. Consequently, there are no HIV specific infection control recommendations, and isolation of HIV-infected patients from other patients is not recommended.

Infection Prevention—Water Systems

Potential for Microbial Contamination

Hemodialysis systems are complex and contain a variety of fluid pathways that transport water, dialysate, dialysate effluent, and blood. Many microbiologic parameters were not accounted for in the design of hemodialysis machines and their respective water supply systems. Consequently, there are situations where certain types of organisms (most commonly Gram-negative water bacteria) can persist and actively multiply in the aqueous environments associated with hemodialysis equipment. This can result in massive numbers of Gram-negative bacteria, which can directly or indirectly lead to septicemia or endotoxemia [152–163]. These bacteria can adhere to surfaces and form biofilms, which are virtually impossible to eradicate [10, 154, 164, 165]. Control strategies are not designed to eradicate bacteria but instead to reduce their concentration to relatively low levels and prevent their regrowth.

Water Treatment

Water used to make dialysate is typically obtained from the municipal water system and must be treated to remove chemical and microbial contaminants. The Association for the Advancement of Medical Instrumentation (AAMI) has published guidelines and recommended practices for the chemical and microbial quality of water used to prepare dialysate and reprocess hemodialyzers (Table 4.5) [166–168]. Maximum contaminant levels are an indication that the fluid quality of a dialysis system is approaching levels that may cause adverse health effects in patients and may need to be taken offline so appropriate measures can be immediately taken to correct the contamination. Action levels or limits are the concentrations at which additional steps should be taken to prevent the maximum contaminant levels from occurring. CMS has incorporated into their ESRD facility conditions for coverage infection prevention requirements based on AAMI guidelines and recommended practices detailing the minimum regulatory requirements that dialysis facilities need to follow, including water quality standards [169].

The components in a typical water system will vary based on a chemical analysis of the source water but most include (1) pre-filters, (2) a water softener, (3) carbon adsorption tanks (at least two in series), (4) a particulate filter (to protect the reverse osmosis membrane), and (5) a reverse osmosis (RO) unit (Fig. 4.3). As the incoming municipal water passes through the system components, it becomes more chemically pure, but the level of microbial contamination increases as some components of the water treatment system may allow for amplification of bacteria (e.g., filters particularly if they are not adequately disinfected or changed at the appropriate frequency).

Table 4.5 CMS and AAMI requirements for dialysis fluids

Types of fluid	Microbial bioburden[a] Maximum contaminant level	Microbial bioburden[a] Action level	Endotoxin Maximum contaminant level	Endotoxin Action level
Dialysis fluid quality standards adopted by reference in CMS conditions for coverage				
Water for all purposes	200 CFU/mL	50 CFU/mL	2 EU/mL	1 EU/mL
Conventional dialysate	200 CFU/mL	50 CFU/mL	2 EU/mL	1 EU/mL
AAMI 23500 Dialysis Fluid Quality Standards				
Water for all purposes	100 CFU/mL	50 CFU/mL	0.25 EU/mL	0.125 EU/mL
Conventional dialysate	100 CFU/mL	50 CFU/mL	0.5 EU/mL	0.25 EU/mL
Ultrapure dialysate[b]	1 CFU/10 mL	–	0.03 EU/mL	–
Dialysate for infusion	This online process shall be validated by the manufacturer to produce fluid that is sterile and nonpyrogenic			

Minimum regulatory requirements as per CMS 2008 Conditions for Coverage based on AAMI RD52

[a]Compliance with a maximum bacterial level of 10^{-6} CFU/mL cannot be demonstrated by culturing, but by processes developed by the machine manufacturers

[b]Culture and endotoxin assays are not required if machine is fitted with an appropriate capacity bacterial and endotoxin retentive filter validated by the manufacture and used according to the instructions for use (IFUs)

RO is an effective water treatment modality that is used in almost 100% of U.S. hemodialysis facilities. RO removes a variety of substances including microorganisms and endotoxin from supply water based primarily on particle size and adsorption to the membrane. RO units must be routinely disinfected as they can become colonized with bacteria in several ways. For example, low numbers of organisms may penetrate the membrane or by other means (i.e., leaks around seals) and colonize downstream portions of the water distribution system such as the RO.

Dialysis Fluids (Dialysate)

Dialysate is most commonly produced using a three-stream proportioning system, where acid and base concentrates are mixed with AAMI grade water in specific ratios that allow for individualized dialysate prescription [170]. In a proportioning system, the dialysis machine mixes the acid concentrate, the base concentrate (most commonly bicarbonate), and AAMI grade water in situ, so a dialysate storage tank is not needed.

Bicarbonate concentrate provides an excellent medium for bacterial growth. Depending on the delivery method, specific procedures are needed to ensure clean, safe bicarbonate is delivered to all patients [171]. Mixing and delivery systems for bicarbonate include (1) jugs that are physically carried to the hemodialysis station,

(2) large mechanical mixing tanks, and (3) prefilled cartridges or bags that connect directly to the hemodialysis machine. Large mixing tanks are most commonly used in outpatient hemodialysis facilities as they allow for the production of dialysate for a large number of patients at the same time. A large tank is prefilled with AAMI grade water, and then bicarbonate powder or liquid is added to create the base concentrate. The concentrate is delivered to dialysis machines (in series) through a distribution loop. The bicarbonate storage tank (or jugs) and delivery loop must be adequately cleaned, disinfected, and rinsed on a routine basis.

Distribution Systems

The water distribution system functions to distribute dialysis fluids (dialysis water and concentrates) from a central point to an individual or multiple dialysis machines. Product water (water treated by reverse osmosis or deionization) passes through the water distribution system to individual dialysis machines, where it is combined with dialysate concentrates and to a reprocessing area if a facility reprocesses hemodialyzers. It may also be combined with acid and base concentrates at a central location where the resulting dialysate is supplied to the individual machines. Medically inert, the biocompatible pipe is then used to distribute water or dialysis fluids to the dialysis machines. Distribution systems should be loop-based system and have no dead-end pipes. Outlets to dialysis machines should have a relatively short path with minimal dead space. Voids, dead ends, and large surface areas serve as sites for microbial colonization. Large diameter pipes decrease fluid velocity and increase the wetted surface area available for microbial colonization. In addition, long pipe runs also increase the available surface area for colonization. Bacteria in fluids remaining in pipes overnight can rapidly multiply and colonize wetted surfaces of the distribution system. Biofilm, which are difficult to remove and protect the bacteria and other organisms from disinfection, can form [172]. Inadequate disinfection of the water distribution system has been implicated in past outbreaks [156, 157, 172–177].

Machines

In the 1970s, most dialysis machines were of the recirculating variety; their design contributed to relatively high levels of Gram-negative bacterial contamination in dialysis fluid. At present, virtually all dialysis machines in the United States are single-pass machines (i.e., the dialysate flows through the machine once). Single-pass machines tend to respond to adequate cleaning and disinfection procedures and, in general, have lower levels of bacterial contamination than do recirculating machines. Levels of contamination in single-pass machines depend primarily on the microbiologic quality of the incoming water and the method of machine disinfection [154, 178]. Earlier dialysis machines had a port (waste-handling option) that allowed disposal of the extracorporeal circuit priming fluids. If one-way check valves in the waste-handling option are not maintained, checked for competency, or disinfected as recommended, they allow backflow from the effluent dialysate path into and contamination of the port and the attached bloodline. This led to outbreaks of infections among HD patients [174, 176, 179]. Currently, the waste-handling option is used less frequently.

Waste

Waste (or effluent) leaves the dialysis machine via a waste line and empties into the sanitary sewer system. The waste line connects to a drain in a wall box. Wall boxes are recessed areas in the walls at each dialysis station that contain connections to allow dialysis machines to attach to the water supply, acid and base concentrates, and waste drain (Fig. 4.4). Dialysis effluent is rich in nutrients and protein and provides an environment conducive to the growth of microorganisms leading to the formation of biofilms and proliferation of microorganisms in effluent drains. During a large outbreak of Gram-negative organisms including *Serratia marcescens*, dialysis wall boxes were identified as a source of infections [11]. Soon after, a second cluster of BSIs related to wall boxes was reported from a different state [180]. CDC has developed a set of recommended strategies to decrease the risk of patient infections related to wall boxes [181]. Routine cleaning and disinfection of wall boxes are likely not happening in most dialysis centers.

Monitoring Water and Dialysis Fluids

Dialysate samples should be collected during or at the end of the dialysis treatment from a source close to where the dialysis fluid either enters or leaves the dialyzer. Dialysate samples should be collected at least monthly from a representative number of dialysis machines. At least two machines should be sampled during each sampling period and sampling should be rotated to ensure that all machines are tested at least once per year.

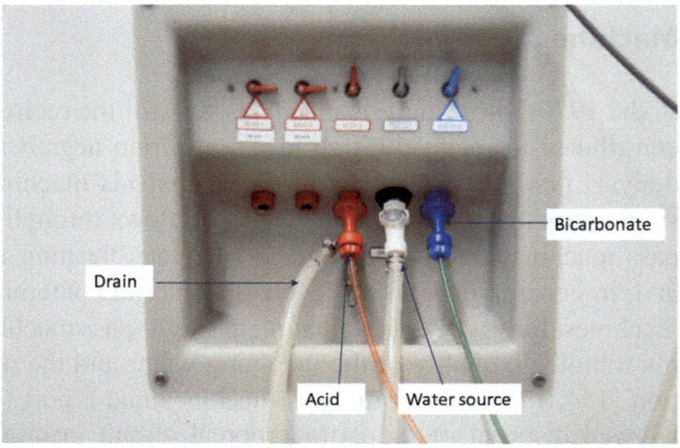

Fig. 4.4 Wall box at dialysis station

Water samples for routine testing should be collected from a source as close as possible to where water enters the dialysate proportioning unit. In most cases, this is the tap (not from the hose connecting the tap to the dialysis machine) at the dialysis station. Water samples should be collected at least monthly from several locations within the dialysis unit. Samples should also be collected using a similar approach after any modifications or maintenance have been made to the water treatment system or water distribution system.

Samples of water and dialysate should also be collected when a pyrogenic reaction is suspected. If centers reprocess hemodialyzers for reuse, water used to prepare disinfectant and rinse dialyzers should also be assayed monthly. Methods for microbiological and endotoxin testing are available elsewhere [167, 182, 183]. In an outbreak investigation, the assay methods may need to be both qualitative and quantitative; detection of nontuberculous mycobacteria and in some cases fungi in water or dialysate may be desirable. In such instances, laboratories should be notified of special testing requests outside of routine water testing, e.g., if the facilities would like to look for specific pathogens.

Disinfecting System and Machines

Disinfection of the water or dialysate distribution system should be performed on a regular basis so that the microbial quality of the fluids is within the acceptable standards range. The frequency of disinfection should be validated by each facility and should be performed at least monthly and following any changes or modifications to the system [178, 184]. AAMI standards and recommended practices are community consensus standards and do not specify a schedule for disinfection other than to suggest that routine disinfection be conducted. In many instances, microbiologic monitoring can be used to determine the frequency of disinfection of the distribution system [178, 185]. In some circumstances, repeat disinfection of the system cannot adequately control microbial growth due to established biofilms and replacement of the system is the only option.

If used, storage tanks should be routinely cleaned, disinfected, and drained. In order to remove biofilm, use of strong oxidizers may aid in stripping biofilm from surfaces, however physical scrubbing of the inner surfaces of the tank may be necessary. Routine disinfection of isolated components of the dialysis system frequently produces inadequate results. Consequently, the total dialysis system (water treatment system, distribution system, and dialysis machine) should be included in the disinfection procedure.

Disinfection of dialysis systems usually employs sodium hypochlorite solutions, hydrogen peroxide solutions, commercially available peracetic acid disinfectants, ozone, and in some systems, hot-water pasteurization. Sodium hypochlorite solutions are convenient and effective in most parts of the dialysis system when used at the manufacturer's recommended concentrations. The test for residual available chlorine to confirm adequate rinsing is simple and sensitive. However, because chlorine is corrosive, it is usually rinsed from the system after a relatively short dwell time of 20–30 min. The rinse water invariably contains organisms that can multiply to significant levels, if the system is permitted to stand overnight [184]. Therefore, disinfection with chlorine-based disinfectants are best used before the start of the first patient treatment session rather than at the end of the day. However, for models of machines that most dialysis facilities are currently using, options for disinfection include heat at the end of the day and use of other disinfectants with longer contact time that also require overnight dwell. There is no need to disinfect the fluid pathway between patients.

Aqueous formaldehyde, peroxyacetic acid, hydrogen peroxide, or glutaraldehyde solutions can produce good disinfection results [165, 186, 187]. These products are not as corrosive as hypochlorite solutions and can be allowed to dwell in the system for long periods of time when the system is not in operation. Some dialysis systems (water treatment, distribution systems, and some hemodialysis machines) utilize hot-water disinfection (pasteurization) for the control of microbial contamination. In this type of system, water is heated to >80 °C (176 °F) and is passed through the water distribution system and hemodialysis machine, or just the hemodialysis machine at the end of the day. These systems are excellent for controlling microbial contamination. However, it should be noted that heat disinfection of the hemodialysis machine would not control microbial contamination of the intake lines, waste lines, and effluent drains. Additional processes may be needed to disinfect intake lines, waste lines, drains, and wall boxes.

Respiratory Infections

Hemodialysis patients are at high risk for acquiring and suffering morbidity and mortality related to respiratory infections, both bacterial and viral [188, 189]. One study found pneumonia was the third most common cause of infection (after vascular access and lower extremity skin and soft tissue infections) and accounted for 13% of all infections [190]. Per the ACIP, chronic renal failure is considered a medical condition that increases the risk of pneumococcal disease [191, 192]. Accordingly, patients on dialysis should receive pneumococcal vaccine according to the recommended dosing schedule [191, 192].

Patients with chronic kidney diseases, including hemodialysis patients, are at high risk for developing complications of seasonal influenza [193]. Influenza vaccination is associated with lower risk of hospitalization and death in patients with ESRD [194]. Vaccination for HCP has been shown to decrease absenteeism and healthcare-facility acquired influenza [195–197]. Influenza outbreaks in hemodialysis facilities have not been commonly described in the literature; however, an influenza (H1N1) outbreak in a dialysis facility in Brazil highlights the potential for an outbreak among patients and staff [198]. Annual vaccination is recommended for both dialysis patients and HCP [193]. However, coverage among both patients on dialysis and HCP is suboptimal. According to United States Renal Data System

(USRDS) data in 2020, 77% of patients on dialysis received the influenza vaccine [199]. Only 73% of HCP in dialysis facilities received influenza vaccination in 2011–2012 season [200].

Patients with ESRD are at higher risk of developing tuberculosis (TB) than the general population [201]. For this reason, as well as implications for infection control within a healthcare setting, CDC recommends that all dialysis patients be tested at least once upon admission for *M. tuberculosis* infection using a TB blood test (Interferon-Gamma Release Assay [IGRA]); a tuberculin skin test (TST) is an acceptable alternative [202–204]. Annual retesting is indicated if ongoing exposure to *M. tuberculosis* is probable. Patients with a positive test should be evaluated to rule out TB disease; patients with a positive test for whom TB disease is ruled out have latent TB infection. Patients with either latent TB infection or TB disease should be treated accordingly. In the setting of TB symptoms or recent exposure to an infectious TB case, a negative TST or IGRA does not rule out TB disease and a full diagnostic evaluation should be conducted. TB transmission in U.S. dialysis facilities is uncommon [205]. The most recent published instance of transmission in a U.S. dialysis facility occurred in 2003 when an infected HCP transmitted the bacteria to patients and other HCP [206]. Suspected or confirmed TB exposure, as well as any suspect TB disease case, occurring within a dialysis facility should be reported to the appropriate state or local public health authority. Some jurisdictions also require reporting of cases of latent TB infection; dialysis facility management should maintain familiarity with their local disease reporting requirements.

The COVID-19 pandemic illustrated the vulnerability of this patient population; ESRD patients on dialysis with SARS-CoV-2 infections suffered from high morbidity and mortality [207–209]. Patients on hemodialysis must present multiple times a week and receive treatments in close proximity to others which may increase their risk of acquiring SARS-CoV-2 infections, particularly when community levels are high. While there were some reports of transmission in dialysis facilities in the literature, [210] the lack of widespread outbreaks, as was seen in other settings, illustrates that adherence to recommended infection prevention practices can decrease the risk of transmission in this setting [211–215]. Furthermore, COVID-19 vaccinations have been shown to be efficacious in this population and vaccination of both patients and HCP is recommended [216–218]. Future research is needed to better define vaccine effectiveness and schedules in this population.

The COVID-19 pandemic reinforced the importance of facilities having processes in place to prevent the transmission of respiratory infections, including systems to detect patients with respiratory symptoms upon presentation to the facilities and implement interventions to decrease transmission (e.g., adequate spacing between patients during treatment, optimizing building ventilation). Facilities should educate patients about respiratory hygiene and cough etiquette and provide necessary supplies such as tissues, masks, and hand hygiene materials. Facilities should also have policies that encourage dialysis HCP not to work while sick with a respiratory infection [219].

Conclusion and Future Direction

Infections among patients on chronic hemodialysis can have devastating consequences and a deleterious impact on the quality of life in a patient population with a high burden of comorbidities, already facing the burden of three dialysis sessions a week. The case presentation provided in this chapter highlights a complication of VAIs, (i.e., embolic stroke) and underscores the importance of infection prevention efforts. Studies have shown how infection prevention efforts in the outpatient hemodialysis setting can lead to sustainable reduction in infection rates (such as BSIs) on a facility and national level. Preventing transmission of pathogens and reducing HAIs among patients on chronic hemodialysis patients requires implementation of a comprehensive infection control program that can support consistent adherence to infection control recommendations (Table 4.1) among HCP. The components of such a program include routine implementation of infection prevention practices specifically designed for the hemodialysis setting: (1) Each dialysis facility should have at least one HCP with infection prevention knowledge and experience in addition to being able to access personnel with advanced expertise; (2) infection prevention training and education should be provided to both HCP and patients; (3) regular auditing of infection prevention practices (audit and assessment tools are available at https://www.cdc.gov/dialysis/prevention-tools/index.html); [13] (4) development of a safety culture, engaged leadership, and involvement of frontline HCP in infection prevention efforts; (5) routine serologic testing and immunization of patients and HCP; (6) infection surveillance and use of the data for continuous quality improvement; and (7) systems in place for public health reporting. A review of those essential components of an infection prevention program is available elsewhere [220]. CDC has also published recommendations describing these components in detail [17].

Innovation and research are needed to continue to advance patient safety in infection prevention and control in hemodialysis. This may include improving facility design/layout to facilitate HCP adherence to best practices and implementation of infection control recommendations. Additional interventions are needed to further reduce VAI rates. HBV infection prevention strategies among hemodialysis patients have been well-established; however, some questions remain. More work is needed to determine the ideal hepatitis B vaccine dosage regimen for pre-dialysis and dialysis pediatric patients and for pre-dialysis adult patients, as well as the optimal timing for follow-up testing and administration of booster doses among vaccine responders. Further, recent reports of patients with mutant HBV, patients with reverse seroconversion, and patients with atypical HBV serology highlight the need for more research to evaluate their significance in the dialysis population. Further work is also needed to clarify the specific factors responsible for transmission of HCV among hemodialysis patients and to evaluate the effect of current prevention recommendations. The Department of Health and Human Services has developed a plan to eliminate hepatitis C in the United States by 2030; treatment of dialysis patients with hepatitis C is a key component of that strategy and is strongly recommended due to the survival advantage conferred by treatment of hepatitis C [221].

Other important questions about the role hemodialysis centers play in the spread of MDROs and the effectiveness of interventions designed to prevent MDRO transmission require further investigation. A better understanding of the relationship between facility design, staffing, and infection risks could help expand prevention strategies in this highly vulnerable population. Finally, in the near future, home dialysis and dialysis in nursing homes may become more common. It will be important to ensure uptake of standard infection prevention practices in these settings and be vigilant for the development issues that contribute to infection risk that would necessitate specific infection control guidance in this setting.

Acknowledgments The authors extend their gratitude to Danae Bixler, Stephanie Booth, Anne Moorman and Rebekah Stewart for providing their knowledge and expertise to this chapter.

References

1. National Institute of Diabetes and Digestive and Kidney Diseases. United States Renal Data System, 2021 USRDS annual data report: epidemiology of kidney disease in the United States. Bethesda: National Institutes of Health; 2021.
2. Nguyen DB, Bixler D, Patel PR. Transmission of hepatitis C virus in the dialysis setting and strategies for its prevention. Semin Dial. 2019;32(2):127–34.
3. Centers for Disease Control and Prevention. Dialysis-related outbreaks: current. 2022. https://www.cdc.gov/dialysis/reports-news/outbreaks.html. Accessed 10 Nov 2022.
4. Syed-Ahmed M, Narayanan M. Immune dysfunction and risk of infection in chronic kidney disease. Adv Chronic Kidney Dis. 2019;26(1):8–15.
5. Vanholder R, Ringoir S. Polymorphonuclear cell function and infection in dialysis. Kidney Int Suppl. 1992;38:S91–5.
6. Prevention, C.f.D.C.a. Healthcare-Associated Hepatitis B and C Outbreaks (≥2 cases) reported to the CDC 2008–2018. https://www.cdc.gov/hepatitis/outbreaks/healthcarehepoutbreaktable.htm. Accessed 31 Dec 2019.
7. Patel PR, Brinsley-Rainisch K. The making dialysis safer for patients coalition: a new partnership to prevent hemodialysis-related infections. Clin J Am Soc Nephrol. 2017;13(1):175–81.
8. Patel PR, Tanz LJ, Hamilton E, Swanzy K, et al. Assessment of provision of COVID-19 vaccination in dialysis clinics and patient vaccination coverage. JAMA Intern Med. 2022;182(6):676–8.
9. Silberzweig J, Bhat JG, Dittrich MO, Durvasula R, et al. Collaboration between dialysis providers. J Am Soc Nephrol. 2022;33(8):1440–4.
10. Favero MS, Carson LA, Bond WW, Petersen NJ. *Pseudomonas aeruginosa*: growth in distilled water from hospitals. Science. 1971;173(999):836–8.
11. Novosad SA, Lake J, Nguyen D, Soda E, et al. Multicenter outbreak of Gram-negative bloodstream infections in hemodialysis patients. Am J Kidney Dis. 2019;74(5):610–9.
12. Centers for Disease Control and Prevention. Core Interventions. https://www.cdc.gov/dialysis/prevention-tools/core-interventions.html. Accessed 5 Nov 2020
13. Centers for Disease Control and Prevention. Audit tools and checklists. https://www.cdc.gov/dialysis/prevention-tools/audit-tools.html. Accessed 31 Dec 2019.
14. Sehulster L, Chinn RY. Guidelines for environmental infection control in health-care facilities. Recommendations of CDC and the Healthcare Infection Control Practices Advisory Committee (HICPAC). MMWR Recomm Rep. 2003;52(RR-10):1–42.
15. Lettau LA, Alfred HJ, Glew RH, Fields HA, et al. Nosocomial transmission of delta hepatitis. Ann Intern Med. 1986;104(5):631–5.

16. Grohskopf LA, Roth VR, Feikin DR, Arduino MJ, et al. *Serratia liquefaciens* bloodstream infections from contamination of epoetin alfa at a hemodialysis center. N Engl J Med. 2001;344(20):1491–7.
17. Centers for Disease Control and Prevention. Recommendations for preventing transmission of infections among chronic hemodialysis patients. MMWR Recomm Rep. 2001;50(RR-5):1–43.
18. Kumbar L, Yee J. Current concepts in hemodialysis vascular access infections. Adv Chronic Kidney Dis. 2019;26(1):16–22.
19. Oyong K, Marquez P, Terashita D, English L, et al. Outbreak of bloodstream infections associated with multiuse dialyzers containing O-rings. Infect Control Hosp Epidemiol. 2014;35(1):89–91.
20. Centers for Disease Control and Prevention. Tracking infections in outpatient dialysis facilities. https://www.cdc.gov/nhsn/dialysis/index.html. Accessed 31 Dec 2019.
21. Services, C.f.M.M. ESRD Quality Incentive Program. https://www.cms.gov/Medicare/Quality-Initiatives-Patient-Assessment-Instruments/ESRDQIP/index. Accessed 31 Dec 2019.
22. Centers for Disease Control and Prevention. Dialysis event surveillance protocol. https://www.cdc.gov/nhsn/PDFs/pscManual/8pscDialysisEventcurrent.pdf. Accessed 31 Dec 2019.
23. Nguyen DB, Shugart A, Lines C, Shah AB, et al. National Healthcare Safety Network (NHSN) dialysis event surveillance report for 2014. Clin J Am Soc Nephrol. 2017;12(7):1139–46.
24. Klevens RM, Edwards JR, Andrus ML, Peterson KD, et al. Dialysis surveillance report: National Healthcare Safety Network (NHSN)-data summary for 2006. Semin Dial. 2008;21(1):24–8.
25. Klevens RM, Tokars JI, Andrus M. Electronic reporting of infections associated with hemodialysis. Nephrol News Issues. 2005;19(7):37–8.
26. Centers for Disease Control and Prevention. Surveillance summary of Bloodstream Infections (BSI) in outpatient hemodialysis facilities. National Healthcare Safety Network, 2014–2019. https://www.cdc.gov/dialysis/published-studies/index.html.
27. Lok CE, Sontrop JM, Tomlinson G, Rajan D, et al. Cumulative patency of contemporary fistulas versus grafts (2000–2010). Clin J Am Soc Nephrol. 2013;8(5):810–8.
28. Lee T. Fistula first initiative: historical impact on vascular access practice patterns and influence on future vascular access care. Cardiovasc Eng Technol. 2017;8(3):244–54.
29. Allon M, Dinwiddie L, Lacson E Jr, Latos DL, et al. Medicare reimbursement policies and hemodialysis vascular access outcomes: a need for change. J Am Soc Nephrol. 2011;22(3):426–30.
30. Brown RS. Barriers to optimal vascular access for hemodialysis. Semin Dial. 2020;33(6):457–63.
31. Murea M, Grey CR, Lok CE. Shared decision-making in hemodialysis vascular access practice. Kidney Int. 2021;100(4):799–808.
32. Lok CE, Huber TS, Lee T, Shenoy S, et al. KDOQI clinical practice guideline for vascular access: 2019 update. Am J Kidney Dis. 2020;75(4 Suppl 2):S1–S164.
33. Patel PR, Yi SH, Booth S, Bren V, et al. Bloodstream infection rates in outpatient hemodialysis facilities participating in a collaborative prevention effort: a quality improvement report. Am J Kidney Dis. 2013;62(2):322–30.
34. Yi SH, Kallen AJ, Hess S, Bren VR, et al. Sustained infection reduction in outpatient hemodialysis centers participating in a collaborative bloodstream infection prevention effort. Infect Control Hosp Epidemiol. 2016;37(7):863–6.
35. Rosenblum A, Wang W, Ball LK, Latham C, et al. Hemodialysis catheter care strategies: a cluster-randomized quality improvement initiative. Am J Kidney Dis. 2014;63(2):259–67.
36. Centers for Disease Control and Prevention. Infection prevention tools. https://www.cdc.gov/dialysis/prevention-tools/index.html. Accessed 31 Dec 2019.
37. McAfee N, Seidel K, Watkins S, Flynn JT. A continuous quality improvement project to decrease hemodialysis catheter infections in pediatric patients: use of a closed luer-lock access cap. Nephrol Nurs J. 2010;37(5):541–4.

38. Brunelli SM, Njord L, Hunt AE, Sibbel SP. Use of the Tego needlefree connector is associated with reduced incidence of catheter-related bloodstream infections in hemodialysis patients. Int J Nephrol Renovasc Dis. 2014;7:131–9.
39. Brunelli SM, Van Wyck DB, Njord L, Ziebol RJ, et al. Cluster-randomized trial of devices to prevent catheter-related bloodstream infection. J Am Soc Nephrol. 2018;29(4):1336–43.
40. O'Grady NP, Alexander M, Burns LA, Dellinger EP, et al. Guidelines for the prevention of intravascular catheter-related infections. Clin Infect Dis. 2011;52(9):e162–93.
41. Buetti N, Marschall J, Drees M, Fakih MG, et al. Strategies to prevent central line-associated bloodstream infections in acute-care hospitals: 2022 update. Infect Control Hosp Epidemiol. 2022;43(5):553–69.
42. Fernandez-Hidalgo N, Almirante B. Antibiotic-lock therapy: a clinical viewpoint. Expert Rev Anti-Infect Ther. 2014;12(1):117–29.
43. Landry DL, Braden GL, Gobeille SL, Haessler SD, et al. Emergence of gentamicin-resistant bacteremia in hemodialysis patients receiving gentamicin lock catheter prophylaxis. Clin J Am Soc Nephrol. 2010;5(10):1799–804.
44. Moore CL, Besarab A, Ajluni M, Soi V, et al. Comparative effectiveness of two catheter locking solutions to reduce catheter-related bloodstream infection in hemodialysis patients. Clin J Am Soc Nephrol. 2014;9(7):1232–9.
45. Maki DG, Ash SR, Winger RK, Lavin P. A novel antimicrobial and antithrombotic lock solution for hemodialysis catheters: a multi-center, controlled, randomized trial. Crit Care Med. 2011;39(4):613–20.
46. Zhao T, Liu H, Han J. Ethanol lock is effective on reducing the incidence of tunneled catheter-related bloodstream infections in hemodialysis patients: a systematic review and meta-analysis. Int Urol Nephrol. 2018;50(9):1643–52.
47. Murray EC, Deighan C, Geddes C, Thomson PC. Taurolidine-citrate-heparin catheter lock solution reduces *Staphylococcal* bacteraemia rates in haemodialysis patients. QJM. 2014;107(12):995–1000.
48. Winnicki W, Herkner H, Lorenz M, Handisurya A, et al. Taurolidine-based catheter lock regimen significantly reduces overall costs, infection, and dysfunction rates of tunneled hemodialysis catheters. Kidney Int. 2018;93(3):753–60.
49. Mermel LA, Alang N. Adverse effects associated with ethanol catheter lock solutions: a systematic review. J Antimicrob Chemother. 2014;69(10):2611–9.
50. Arechabala MC, Catoni MI, Claro JC, Rojas NP, et al. Antimicrobial lock solutions for preventing catheter-related infections in haemodialysis. Cochrane Database Syst Rev. 2018;4:Cd010597.
51. Centers for Disease Control and Prevention. Updated recommendations on the use of chlorhexidine-impregnated dressings for prevention of intravascular catheter-related infections. 2017. https://www.cdc.gov/infectioncontrol/guidelines/bsi/c-i-dressings/recommendations.html. Accessed 31 Dec 2019.
52. Apata IW, Hanfelt J, Bailey JL, Niyyar VD. Chlorhexidine-impregnated transparent dressings decrease catheter-related infections in hemodialysis patients: a quality improvement project. J Vasc Access. 2017;18(2):103–8.
53. Camins BC, Richmond AM, Dyer KL, Zimmerman HN, et al. A crossover intervention trial evaluating the efficacy of a chlorhexidine-impregnated sponge in reducing catheter-related bloodstream infections among patients undergoing hemodialysis. Infect Control Hosp Epidemiol. 2010;31(11):1118–23.
54. Onder AM, Chandar J, Coakley S, Francoeur D, et al. Controlling exit site infections: does it decrease the incidence of catheter-related bacteremia in children on chronic hemodialysis? Hemodial Int. 2009;13(1):11–8.
55. Righetti M, Palmieri N, Bracchi O, Prencipe M, et al. Tegaderm CHG dressing significantly improves catheter-related infection rate in hemodialysis patients. J Vasc Access. 2016;17(5):417–22.

56. Lyman M, Nguyen DB, Shugart A, Gruhler H, et al. Risk of vascular access infection associated with buttonhole cannulation of fistulas: data from the National Healthcare Safety Network. Am J Kidney Dis. 2020;76(1):82–9.
57. DeSilva RN, Patibandla BK, Vin Y, Narra A, et al. Fistula first is not always the best strategy for the elderly. J Am Soc Nephrol. 2013;24(8):1297–304.
58. Woo K, Goldman DP, Romley JA. Early failure of dialysis access among the elderly in the era of fistula first. Clin J Am Soc Nephrol. 2015;10(10):1791–8.
59. Siegel JD, Rhinehart E, Jackson M, Chiarello L, et al. Management of multidrug-resistant organisms in health care settings, 2006. Am J Infect Control. 2007;35(10 Suppl 2):S165–93.
60. Uttley AH, George RC, Naidoo J, Woodford N, et al. High-level vancomycin-resistant enterococci causing hospital infections. Epidemiol Infect. 1989;103(1):173–81.
61. Zacharioudakis IM, Zervou FN, Ziakas PD, Rice LB, et al. Vancomycin-resistant enterococci colonization among dialysis patients: a meta-analysis of prevalence, risk factors, and significance. Am J Kidney Dis. 2015;65(1):88–97.
62. Fishbane S, Cunha BA, Mittal SK, Ruggian J, et al. Vancomycin-resistant enterococci in hemodialysis patients is related to intravenous vancomycin use. Infect Control Hosp Epidemiol. 1999;20(7):461–2.
63. D'Agata EM, Green WK, Schulman G, Li H, et al. Vancomycin-resistant enterococci among chronic hemodialysis patients: a prospective study of acquisition. Clin Infect Dis. 2001;32(1):23–9.
64. St. Peter WL, S.C. Outpatient IV antibiotic use in the U.S. hemodialysis population, 1995–2007.
65. Dopirak M, Hill C, Oleksiw M, Dumigan D, et al. Surveillance of hemodialysis-associated primary bloodstream infections: the experience of ten hospital-based centers. Infect Control Hosp Epidemiol. 2002;23(12):721–4.
66. Taylor G, Gravel D, Johnston L, Embil J, et al. Prospective surveillance for primary bloodstream infections occurring in Canadian hemodialysis units. Infect Control Hosp Epidemiol. 2002;23(12):716–20.
67. Tokars JI, Miller ER, Stein G. New national surveillance system for hemodialysis-associated infections: initial results. Am J Infect Control. 2002;30(5):288–95.
68. Chang S, Sievert DM, Hageman JC, Boulton ML, et al. Infection with vancomycin-resistant *Staphylococcus aureus* containing the vanA resistance gene. N Engl J Med. 2003;348(14):1342–7.
69. Finks J, Wells E, Dycke T, Husain N, et al. Vancomycin-resistant *Staphylococcus aureus*, Michigan, USA, 2007. Emerg Infect Dis. 2009;15(6):943–5.
70. Sievert DM, Rudrik JT, Patel JB, McDonald LC, et al. Vancomycin-resistant *Staphylococcus aureus* in the United States, 2002–2006. Clin Infect Dis. 2008;46(5):668–74.
71. Walters MS, Eggers P, Albrecht V, Travis T, et al. Vancomycin-resistant *Staphylococcus aureus*—Delaware, 2015. MMWR Morb Mortal Wkly Rep. 2015;64(37):1056.
72. Centers for Disease Control and Prevention. CDC Reminds Clinical Laboratories and Healthcare Infection Preventionists of their Role in the Search and Containment of Vancomycin-Resistant *Staphylococcus aureus* (VRSA). 2022. https://www.cdc.gov/hai/settings/lab/vrsa_lab_search_containment.html#:~:text=The%20Centers%20for%20Disease%20Control%20and%20Prevention%20%28CDC%29,case%20identified%20in%20the%20United%20States%20in%202021. Accessed 22 Dec 2022.
73. Walters M, Lonsway D, Rasheed K, Albrecht V, et al. Investigation and control of vancomycin-resistant *Staphylococcus aureus*: a guide for health departments and infection control personnel. CDC; 2015. https://www.cdc.gov/hai/pdfs/vrsa-investigation-guide-05_12_2015.pdf
74. Tokars JI, Miller E, Alter MJ, Arduino MJ. National surveillance of dialysis-associated diseases in the United States, 1995. Altanta: US Department of Health and Human Services; 1998.
75. Finelli L, Miller JT, Tokars JI, Alter MJ, et al. National surveillance of dialysis-associated diseases in the United States, 2002. Semin Dial. 2005;18(1):52–61.
76. Fluck R, Rao R, van Schalkwyk D, Ansell D, et al. The UK Vascular Access Survey—follow-up data and repeat survey (chapter 5). Nephrol Dial Transplant. 2007;22(Suppl 7):751–7.

77. Prevention, C.f.D.C.a. Healthcare-Associated Infections-Community Interface (HAIC): Emerging Infections Program (EIP) Network Report Invasive *Staphylococcus aureus*. 2016. https://www.cdc.gov/hai/eip/pdf/2016-MRSA-Report-508.pdf. Accessed 31 Dec 2019.
78. Phatharacharukul P, Thongprayoon C, Cheungpasitporn W, Edmonds PJ, et al. The risks of incident and recurrent *Clostridium difficile*-associated diarrhea in chronic kidney disease and end-stage kidney disease patients: a systematic review and meta-analysis. Dig Dis Sci. 2015;60(10):2913–22.
79. Thongprayoon C, Cheungpasitporn W, Phatharacharukul P, Mahaparn P, et al. High mortality risk in chronic kidney disease and end stage kidney disease patients with *Clostridium difficile* infection: a systematic review and meta-analysis. J Nat Sci. 2015;1(4):e85.
80. Wetmore JB, Li S, Molony JT, Guo H, et al. Insights from the 2016 peer kidney care initiative report: still a ways to go to improve care for dialysis patients. Am J Kidney Dis. 2018;71(1):123–32.
81. Keddis MT, Khanna S, Noheria A, Baddour LM, et al. *Clostridium difficile* infection in patients with chronic kidney disease. Mayo Clin Proc. 2012;87(11):1046–53.
82. Evans R, Caskey F, Fluck R, Crowley L, et al. UK Renal Registry 18th annual Report: chapter 12 epidemiology of reported infections amongst patients receiving dialysis for established renal failure in England 2013 to 2014: a Joint Report from Public Health England and the UK Renal Registry. Nephron. 2016;132(Suppl 1):279–88.
83. See I, Bagchi S, Booth S, Scholz D, et al. Outbreak of *Clostridium difficile* infections at an outpatient hemodialysis facility-Michigan, 2012–2013. Infect Control Hosp Epidemiol. 2015;36(8):972–4.
84. D'Agata EMC, Apata IW, Booth S, Boyce JM, et al. Suggestions for the prevention of *Clostridioides difficile* spread within outpatient hemodialysis facilities. Kidney Int. 2021;99(5):1045–53.
85. Pop-Vicas A, Strom J, Stanley K, D'Agata EM. Multidrug-resistant Gram-negative bacteria among patients who require chronic hemodialysis. Clin J Am Soc Nephrol. 2008;3(3):752–8.
86. Vallabhaneni S, Kallen A, Tsay S, Chow N, et al. Investigation of the first seven reported cases of *Candida auris*, a globally emerging invasive, multidrug-resistant fungus-United States, May 2013–August 2016. MMWR Morb Mortal Wkly Rep. 2016;65(44):1234–7.
87. Centers for Disease Control and Prevention. Infection prevention and control for *Candida auris*. https://www.cdc.gov/fungal/candida-auris/c-auris-infection-control.html?CDC_AA_refVal=https%3A%2F%2Fwww.cdc.gov%2Ffungal%2Fdiseases%2Fcandidiasis%2Fc-auris-infection-control.html. Accessed 31 Dec 2019.
88. Centers for Disease Control and Prevention. Core elements of antibiotic stewardship. https://www.cdc.gov/antibiotic-use/core-elements/index.html. Accessed 22 Dec 2022.
89. Snyder GM, Patel PR, Kallen AJ, Strom JA, et al. Antimicrobial use in outpatient hemodialysis units. Infect Control Hosp Epidemiol. 2013;34(4):349–57.
90. D'Agata EM. Antimicrobial use and stewardship programs among dialysis centers. Semin Dial. 2013;26(4):457–64.
91. Apata IW, Kabbani S, Neu AM, Kear TM, et al. Opportunities to improve antibiotic prescribing in outpatient hemodialysis facilities. Am J Kidney Dis. 2020;77(5):757–68.
92. Favero MS, Maynard JE, Petersen NJ, Boyer KM, et al. Letter: Hepatitis-B antigen on environmental surfaces. Lancet. 1973;2(7843):1455.
93. Centers for Disease Control and Prevention. In: H.E.A. Welfare, editor. Control measures for hepatitis B in dialysis centers. Atlanta: Centers for Disease Control; 1977.
94. Alter MJ, Favero MS, Francis DP. Cost benefit of vaccination for hepatitis B in hemodialysis centers. J Infect Dis. 1983;148(4):770–1.
95. Alter MJ, Favero MS, Maynard JE. Impact of infection control strategies on the incidence of dialysis-associated hepatitis in the United States. J Infect Dis. 1986;153(6):1149–51.
96. Centers for Disease Control and Prevention. Viral hepatitis surveillance—United States. https://www.cdc.gov/hepatitis/statistics/SurveillanceRpts.htm. Accessed 31 Dec 2019.
97. Tokars JI, Alter MJ, Miller E, Moyer LA, et al. National surveillance of dialysis associated diseases in the United States—1994. ASAIO J. 1997;43(1):108–19.

98. Mast EE, Margolis HS, Fiore AE, Brink EW, et al. A comprehensive immunization strategy to eliminate transmission of hepatitis B virus infection in the United States: recommendations of the Advisory Committee on Immunization Practices (ACIP) part 1: immunization of infants, children, and adolescents. MMWR Recomm Rep. 2005;54(RR-16):1–31.
99. Mast EE, Weinbaum CM, Fiore AE, Alter MJ, et al. A comprehensive immunization strategy to eliminate transmission of hepatitis B virus infection in the United States: recommendations of the Advisory Committee on Immunization Practices (ACIP) part II: immunization of adults. MMWR Recomm Rep. 2006;55(RR-16):1–33.
100. Rhea S, Moorman A, Pace R, Mobley V, et al. Hepatitis B reverse seroconversion and transmission in a hemodialysis center: a public health investigation and case report. Am J Kidney Dis. 2016;68(2):292–5.
101. Apata IW, Nguyen DB, Khudyakov Y, Mixson-Hayden T, et al. Hepatitis B virus mutant infections in hemodialysis patients: a case series. Kidney Med. 2019;1(6):347–53.
102. Hendrickson B, Kamili S, Timmons T, Iwen PC, et al. Notes from the field: false-negative hepatitis B surface antigen test results in a hemodialysis patient-Nebraska, 2017. MMWR Morb Mortal Wkly Rep. 2018;67(10):311–2.
103. Hoofnagle JH, Di Bisceglie AM. Serologic diagnosis of a cute and chronic hepatitis. Semin Liver Dis. 1991;11(2):73–83.
104. Hochberger S, Althof D, Gallegos de Schrott R, Nachbaur N, et al. Fully automated quantitation of hepatitis B virus (HBV) DNA in human plasma by the COBAS AmpliPrep/COBAS TaqMan system. J Clin Virol. 2006;35(4):373–80.
105. Kaneko S, Miller RH, Di Bisceglie A, Feinstone SM, et al. Hepatitis B virus DNA detection and comparison with hepatitis B surface antigen. Gastroenterol Jpn. 1990;25(Suppl 2):57–61.
106. Levine OS, Vlahov D, Koehler J, Cohn S, et al. Seroepidemiology of hepatitis B virus in a population of injecting drug users. Association with drug injection patterns. Am J Epidemiol. 1995;142(3):331–41.
107. Mezzelani P, Quaglio G, Venturini L, Lugoboni F. The significance of the isolated anti-HBc carrier. A study of 1797 drug addicts. The Intersert Group of Scientific Collaboration. Recenti Prog Med. 1994;85(9):419–24.
108. Bhatti FA, Ullah Z, Salamat N, Ayub M, et al. Anti-hepatitis B core antigen testing, viral markers, and occult hepatitis B virus infection in Pakistani blood donors: implications for transfusion practice. Transfusion. 2007;47(1):74–9.
109. Satake M, Taira R, Yugi H, Hino S, et al. Infectivity of blood components with low hepatitis B virus DNA levels identified in a lookback program. Transfusion. 2007;47(7):1197–205.
110. Silva AE, McMahon BJ, Parkinson AJ, Sjogren MH, et al. Hepatitis B virus DNA in persons with isolated antibody to hepatitis B core antigen who subsequently received hepatitis B vaccine. Clin Infect Dis. 1998;26(4):895–7.
111. Nieto JM, Saab SJCHR. Outcomes of liver transplantation using hepatitis B core-positive liver grafts: implications for prophylaxis. Curr Hepatitis Rep. 2006;5(1):33–9.
112. McMahon BJ, Parkinson AJ, Helminiak C, Wainwright RB, et al. Response to hepatitis B vaccine of persons positive for antibody to hepatitis B core antigen. Gastroenterology. 1992;103(2):590–4.
113. Lai CL, Lau JY, Yeoh EK, Chang WK, et al. Significance of isolated anti-HBc seropositivity by ELISA: implications and the role of radioimmunoassay. J Med Virol. 1992;36(3):180–3.
114. Alter MJ, Ahtone J, Maynard JE. Hepatitis B virus transmission associated with a multiple-dose vial in a hemodialysis unit. Ann Intern Med. 1983;99(3):330–3.
115. Carl M, Francis DP, Maynard JE. A common-source outbreak of hepatitis bin a hemodialysis unit. Dial Transplant. 1983;12:222–9.
116. Centers for Disease Control and Prevention. Outbreaks of hepatitis B virus infection among hemodialysis patients—California, Nebraska, and Texas, 1994. MMWR Morb Mortal Wkly Rep. 1996;45(14):285–9.
117. Fabrizi F, Dixit V, Messa P, Martin P. Transmission of hepatitis B virus in dialysis units: a systematic review of reports on outbreaks. Int J Artif Organs. 2015;38(1):1–7.

118. Hutin YJ, Goldstein ST, Varma JK, O'Dair JB, et al. An outbreak of hospital-acquired hepatitis B virus infection among patients receiving chronic hemodialysis. Infect Control Hosp Epidemiol. 1999;20(11):731–5.
119. Niu MT, Penberthy LT, Alter MJ, et al. Hemodialysis-associated hepatitis B: report of an outbreak. Dial Transplant. 1989;18:542–55.
120. Snydman DR, Bryan JA, London WT, Werner B, et al. Transmission of hepatitis B associated with hemodialysis: role of malfunction (blood leaks) in dialysis machines. J Infect Dis. 1976;134(6):562–70.
121. Snydman DR, Bryan JA, Macon EJ, Gregg MB. Hemodialysis-associated hepatitis: report of an epidemic with further evidence on mechanisms of transmission. Am J Epidemiol. 1976;104(5):563–70.
122. Schillie S, Murphy TV, Sawyer M, Ly K, et al. CDC guidance for evaluating health-care personnel for hepatitis B virus protection and for administering postexposure management. MMWR Recomm Rep. 2013;62(Rr-10):1–19.
123. Centers for Disease Control and Prevention. Infection control requirements for dialysis facilities and clarification regarding guidance on parenteral medication vials. MMWR Morb Mortal Wkly Rep. 2008;57(32):875–6.
124. Kamili S, Krawczynski K, McCaustland K, Li X, et al. Infectivity of hepatitis C virus in plasma after drying and storing at room temperature. Infect Control Hosp Epidemiol. 2007;28(5):519–24.
125. Paintsil E, Binka M, Patel A, Lindenbach BD, et al. Hepatitis C virus maintains infectivity for weeks after drying on inanimate surfaces at room temperature: implications for risks of transmission. J Infect Dis. 2014;209(8):1205–11.
126. World Health Organization. Hepatitis C Fact Sheets. 2022. https://www.who.int/news-room/fact-sheets/detail/hepatitis-c. Accessed 22 Dec 2022.
127. Pol S, Parlati L, Jadoul M. Hepatitis C virus and the kidney. Nat Rev Nephrol. 2019;15(2):73–86.
128. Selvarajah S, Busch MP. Transfusion transmission of HCV, a long but successful road map to safety. Antivir Ther. 2012;17(7 Pt B):1423–9.
129. Alter MJ. The epidemiology of acute and chronic hepatitis C. Clin Liver Dis. 1997;1:559–68.
130. Goodkin DA, Bieber B, Jadoul M, Martin P, et al. Mortality, hospitalization, and quality of life among patients with hepatitis C infection on hemodialysis. Clin J Am Soc Nephrol. 2017;12(2):287–97.
131. Fissell RB, Bragg-Gresham JL, Woods JD, Jadoul M, et al. Patterns of hepatitis C prevalence and seroconversion in hemodialysis units from three continents: the DOPPS. Kidney Int. 2004;65(6):2335–42.
132. Jadoul M, Bieber BA, Martin P, Akiba T, et al. Prevalence, incidence, and risk factors for hepatitis C virus infection in hemodialysis patients. Kidney Int. 2019;95(4):939–47.
133. Centers for Disease Control and Prevention. Testing for HCV infection: an update of guidance for clinicians and laboratorians. MMWR Morb Mortal Wkly Rep. 2013;62(18):362–5.
134. Kidney Disease: Improving Global Outcomes Hepatitis C Work Group. KDIGO 2018 clinical practice guideline for the prevention, diagnosis, evaluation, and treatment of hepatitis C in chronic kidney disease. Kidney Int Suppl (2011). 2018;8(3):91–165.
135. Shimokura G, Chai F, Weber DJ, Samsa GP, et al. Patient-care practices associated with an increased prevalence of hepatitis C virus infection among chronic hemodialysis patients. Infect Control Hosp Epidemiol. 2011;32(5):415–24.
136. Centers for Disease Control and Prevention. CDC urging dialysis providers and facilities to assess and improve infection control practices to stop hepatitis C virus transmission in patients undergoing hemodialysis. https://emergency.cdc.gov/han/han00386.asp. Accessed 31 Dec 2019.
137. Jadoul M, Labriola L, Gordon CE. HCV can and should be eliminated from dialysis units. Am J Kidney Dis. 2021;78(4):487–8.

138. Maduell F, Belmar L, Ugalde J, Laguno M, et al. Elimination of hepatitis C virus infection from a hemodialysis unit and impact of treatment on the control of anemia. Gastroenterol Hepatol. 2019;42(3):164–70.
139. Huang CF, Chiu YW, Yu ML. Patient-centered outreach treatment toward micro-elimination of hepatitis C virus infection in hemodialysis patients. Kidney Int. 2020;97(2):421.
140. Feld JJ, Ward JW. Key elements on the pathway to HCV elimination: lessons learned from the AASLD HCV Special Interest Group 2020. Hepatol Commun. 2021;5(6):911–22.
141. Hu TH, Su WW, Yang CC, Yang CC, et al. Elimination of hepatitis C virus in a dialysis population: a collaborative care model in Taiwan. Am J Kidney Dis. 2021;78(4):511–519 e1.
142. Bhamidimarri KR, Martin P. Finally, safe and effective treatment options for hepatitis C in hemodialysis patients. J Hepatol. 2016;65(1):7–10.
143. Safety, N.T.D. Promoting infection prevention in dialysis facilities hepatitis C testing and monitoring algorithm. https://www.asn-online.org/g/blast/files/NCHHSTP_NTDS-HCV%20Subcommittee%20Algorithm_FINAL%2003.29.19.pdf. Accessed 31 Dec 2019.
144. Kushner T, Serper M, Kaplan DE. Delta hepatitis within the veterans affairs medical system in the United States: prevalence, risk factors, and outcomes. J Hepatol. 2015;63(3):586–92.
145. Chen H-Y, Shen D-T, Ji D-Z, Han P-C, et al. Prevalence and burden of hepatitis D virus infection in the global population: a systematic review and meta-analysis. Gut. 2019;68(3):512–21.
146. Sawinski D, Forde KA, Locke JE, Cohen JB, et al. Race but not hepatitis C co-infection affects survival of HIV(+) individuals on dialysis in contemporary practice. Kidney Int. 2018;93(3):706–15.
147. El Sayed NM, Gomatos PJ, Beck-Sague CM, Dietrich U, et al. Epidemic transmission of human immunodeficiency virus in renal dialysis centers in Egypt. J Infect Dis. 2000;181(1):91–7.
148. Mashragi F, Bernstein RS, Al-Mazroa M, Al-Tawfiq JA, et al. HIV transmission at a Saudi Arabia hemodialysis unit. Clin Infect Dis. 2014;59(6):897–902.
149. Velandia M, Fridkin SK, Cardenas V, Boshell J, et al. Transmission of HIV in dialysis centre. Lancet. 1995;345(8962):1417–22.
150. Centers for Disease Control and Prevention. HIV transmission in a dialysis center—Colombia, 1991–1993. MMWR Morb Mortal Wkly Rep. 1995;44(21):404–5.
151. Branson BM, Handsfield HH, Lampe MA, Janssen RS, et al. Revised recommendations for HIV testing of adults, adolescents, and pregnant women in health-care settings. MMWR Recomm Rep. 2006;55(RR-14):1–17.
152. Archibald LK, Khoi NN, Jarvis WR, Reller LB, et al. Pyrogenic reactions in hemodialysis patients, Hanoi, Vietnam. Infect Control Hosp Epidemiol. 2006;27(4):424–6.
153. Beck-Sague CM, Jarvis WR, Bland LA, Arduino MJ, et al. Outbreak of Gram-negative bacteremia and pyrogenic reactions in a hemodialysis center. Am J Nephrol. 1990;10(5):397–403.
154. Favero MS, Petersen NJ, Carson LA, Bond WW, et al. Gram-negative water bacteria in hemodialysis systems. Health Lab Sci. 1975;12(4):321–34.
155. Gordon SM, Tipple M, Bland LA, Jarvis WR. Pyrogenic reactions associated with the reuse of disposable hollow-fiber hemodialyzers. JAMA. 1988;260(14):2077–81.
156. Hindman SH, Favero MS, Carson LA, Petersen NJ, et al. Pyrogenic reactions during haemodialysis caused by extramural endotoxin. Lancet. 1975;2(7938):732–4.
157. Jackson BM, Beck-Sague CM, Bland LA, Arduino MJ, et al. Outbreak of pyrogenic reactions and Gram-negative bacteremia in a hemodialysis center. Am J Nephrol. 1994;14(2):85–9.
158. Lefton CK. Patients suffer pyrogenic reactions in Philadelphia dialysis units. Nephrol News Issues. 1994;8(12):10.
159. Nystrand R. The microbial world and fluids in dialysis. Biomed Instrum Technol. 2008;42(2):150–9.
160. Petersen NJ, Carson LA, Favero MS. Bacterial endotoxin in new and reused hemodialyzers: a potential cause of endotoxemia. Trans Am Soc Artif Intern Organs. 1981;27:155–60.
161. Pollak VE. Adverse effects and pyrogenic reactions during hemodialysis. JAMA. 1988;260(14):2106–7.

162. Raij L, Shapiro FL, Michael AF. Endotoxemia in febrile reactions during hemodialysis. Kidney Int. 1973;4(1):57–60.
163. Rudnick JR, Arduino MJ, Bland LA, Cusick L, et al. An outbreak of pyrogenic reactions in chronic hemodialysis patients associated with hemodialyzer reuse. Artif Organs. 1995;19(4):289–94.
164. Favero MS, Bland LA. Microbiologic principles applied to reprocessing hemodialyzers. In: Deane N, Wineman R, Bemis J, editors. Guide to reprocessing of hemodialyzers. Boston: Martinus Nijhoff; 1986. p. 63–73.
165. Favero MS, Carson LA, Bond WW, Petersen NJ. Factors that influence microbial contamination of fluids associated with hemodialysis machines. Appl Microbiol. 1974;28(5):822–30.
166. AAMI. Preparation and quality management of fluids for haemodialysis and related therapies—part 1: general requirements. Association for the Advancment of Medical Instrumentation; 2019.
167. AAMI. Preparation and quality management of fluids for haemodialysis and related therapies—part 3: water for haemodialysis related therapies. Association for the Advancment of Medical Instrumentation; 2019.
168. AAMI. Preparation and quality management of fluids for haemodialysis and related therapies—part 5: quality of dialysis fluid for haemodialysis related therapies. Association for the Advancment of Medical Instrumentation; 2019.
169. Centers for Medicare and Medicaid Services. Medicare and Medicaid programs; conditions for coverage for end-stage renal disease facilities. Final rule. Fed Regist. 2008;73(73):20369–484.
170. Stamm JM, Engelhard WE, Parsons JE. Microbiological study of water-softener resins. Appl Microbiol. 1969;18:376–86.
171. Desai N. Basics of base in hemodialysis solution: dialysate buffer production, delivery and decontamination. Indian J Nephrol. 2015;25(4):189–93.
172. Anderson RL, Holland BW, Carr JK. Effect of disinfectants on pseudomonads colonized on the interior surfaces of PVC pipes. Am J Public Health. 1990;80:17–21.
173. Centers for Disease Control and Prevention. Pyrogenic reactions and Gram-negative bacteremia in a hemodialysis center. In: H.a.H. Services, editor. Epidemiologic investigation report. Atlanta: Centers for Disease Control; 1991.
174. Jochimsen EM, Frenette C, Delorme M, Arduino M, et al. A cluster of bloodstream infections and pyrogenic reactions among hemodialysis patients traced to dialysis machine waste-handling option units. Am J Nephrol. 1998;18(6):485–9.
175. Petersen NJ, Boyer KM, Carson LA, Favero MS. Pyrogenic reactions from inadequate disinfection of a dialysis fluid distribution system. Dial Transplant. 1978;7:52–7.
176. Rao CY, Pachucki C, Cali S, Arduino M, et al. An outbreak of phialemonium mold infections in hemodialysis patients: when purified water is Not so Pure-Illinois, 2005. In: 55th Annual Epidemic Intelligence Service Conference. Atlanta: CDC; 2006.
177. Favero MS, Petersen NJ, Boyer KM, Carson LA, et al. Microbial contamination of renal dialysis systems and associated health risks. Trans Am Soc Artif Intern Organs. 1974;20A:175–83.
178. Arduino MJ. Microbiologic quality of water used for hemodialysis. Contemp Dial Nephrol. 1996;17:17–9.
179. Wang SA, Levine RB, Carson LA, Arduino MJ, et al. An outbreak of Gram-negative bacteremia in hemodialysis patients traced to hemodialysis machine waste drain ports. Infect Control Hosp Epidemiol. 1999;20(11):746–51.
180. Backman L, Dumigan DG, Harizaj A, Oleksiw M, et al. A cluster of Gram-Negative bloodstream infections in connecticut hemodialysis patients. Washington, DC: IDWeek; 2019.
181. Centers for Disease Control and Prevention. Dialysis wall boxes and drains. https://www.cdc.gov/dialysis/guidelines/wall-boxes.html. Accessed 31 Dec 2019.
182. AAMI. Water testing methodologies. Arlington: Association for the Advancement of Medical Instrumentation; 2014.
183. Arduino MJ. Heterotrophic plate count and endotoxin assay of hemodialysis fluids. In: Clinical microbiology procedures handbook. ASM Press; 2022.

184. Bland LA, Favero MS, editors. Microbial contamination control strategies for hemodialysis systems. Plant, technology, and safety management series, vol. 3. Oakbrook Terrace: Joint Commission on Accreditation of Healthcare Organizations; 1989.
185. Arduino MJ. What's new in water treatment standards for hemodialysis. Contemp Dial Nephrol. 1997;18:21–4.
186. Petersen NJ, Carson LA, Doto IL, Aguero SM, et al. Microbiologic evaluation of a new glutaraldehyde-based disinfectant for hemodialysis systems. Trans Am Soc Artif Intern Organs. 1982;28:287–90.
187. Townsend TR, Wee SB, Bartlett J. Disinfection of hemodialysis machines. Dial Transplant. 1985;14:274–87.
188. National Institute of Diabetes and Digestive and Kidney Diseases. United States Renal Data System, *USRDS* 2008 Annual Data Report: Atlas of Chronic Kidney Disease and End-Stage Renal Disease in the United States. Bethesda: National Institutes of Health; 2008.
189. Slinin Y, Foley RN, Collins AJ. Clinical epidemiology of pneumonia in hemodialysis patients: the USRDS waves 1, 3, and 4 study. Kidney Int. 2006;70(6):1135–41.
190. Berman SJ, Johnson EW, Nakatsu C, Alkan M, et al. Burden of infection in patients with end-stage renal disease requiring long-term dialysis. Clin Infect Dis. 2004;39(12):1747–53.
191. Centers for Disease Control and Prevention. Pneumococcal ACIP Vaccine Recommendations. https://www.cdc.gov/vaccines/hcp/acip-recs/vacc-specific/pneumo.html. Accessed 23 Dec 2022.
192. Centers for Disease Control and Prevention. Pneumococcal vaccination: summary of who and when to vaccinate. https://www.cdc.gov/vaccines/vpd/pneumo/hcp/who-when-to-vaccinate.html. Accessed 23 Dec 2022.
193. Grohskopf LA, Sokolow LZ, Broder KR, Olsen SJ, et al. Prevention and control of seasonal influenza with vaccines. MMWR Recomm Rep. 2016;65(5):1–54.
194. Gilbertson DT, Unruh M, McBean AM, Kausz AT, et al. Influenza vaccine delivery and effectiveness in end-stage renal disease. Kidney Int. 2003;63(2):738–43.
195. Salgado CD, Giannetta ET, Hayden FG, Farr BM. Preventing nosocomial influenza by improving the vaccine acceptance rate of clinicians. Infect Control Hosp Epidemiol. 2004;25(11):923–8.
196. Saxen H, Virtanen M. Randomized, placebo-controlled double blind study on the efficacy of influenza immunization on absenteeism of health care workers. Pediatr Infect Dis J. 1999;18(9):779–83.
197. Van Buynder PG, Konrad S, Kersteins F, Preston E, et al. Healthcare worker influenza immunization vaccinate or mask policy: strategies for cost effective implementation and subsequent reductions in staff absenteeism due to illness. Vaccine. 2015;33(13):1625–8.
198. Ventura CG, Roque FL, Sousa IQ, Lobo RD, et al. Influenza A (H1N1): outbreak management in a dialysis unit and clinical outcomes of infection in chronic hemodialysis patients. J Bras Nefrol. 2020;42(2):182–90.
199. United States Renal Data System. Epidemiology of kidney disease in the United States. 2022. https://usrds-adr.niddk.nih.gov/2022/suggested-citation. Accessed 23 Dec 2022.
200. Lynch JR, Armistead N, Vinson BB, Howard AD. Correlates of change in health care worker seasonal influenza vaccination rates among dialysis facilities. Am J Infect Control. 2015;43(4):409–11.
201. Segall L, Covic A. Diagnosis of tuberculosis in dialysis patients: current strategy. Clin J Am Soc Nephrol. 2010;5(6):1114–22.
202. Lewinsohn DM, Leonard MK, LoBue PA, Cohn DL, et al. Official American Thoracic Society/Infectious Diseases Society of America/Centers for Disease Control and Prevention clinical practice guidelines: diagnosis of tuberculosis in adults and children. Clin Infect Dis. 2017;64(2):e1–e33.
203. Jensen PA, Lambert LA, Iademarco MF, Ridzon R, et al. Guidelines for preventing the transmission of *Mycobacterium tuberculosis* in health-care settings, 2005. MMWR Recomm Rep. 2005;54(RR-17):1–141.

204. Winthrop KL, Nyendak M, Calvet H, Oh P, et al. Interferon-gamma release assays for diagnosing mycobacterium tuberculosis infection in renal dialysis patients. Clin J Am Soc Nephrol. 2008;3(5):1357–63.
205. Okada RC, Barry PM, Skarbinski J, Chitnis AS. Epidemiology, detection, and management of tuberculosis among end-stage renal disease patients. Infect Control Hosp Epidemiol. 2018;39(11):1367–74.
206. Centers for Disease Control and Prevention. Tuberculosis transmission in a renal dialysis center—Nevada, 2003. MMWR Morb Mortal Wkly Rep. 2004;53(37):873–5.
207. Alberici F, Delbarba E, Manenti C, Econimo L, et al. A report from the Brescia Renal COVID Task Force on the clinical characteristics and short-term outcome of hemodialysis patients with SARS-CoV-2 infection. Kidney Int. 2020;98(1):20–6.
208. Khatri M, Islam S, Dutka P, Carson J, et al. COVID-19 antibodies and outcomes among outpatient maintenance hemodialysis patients. Kidney360. 2021;2(2):263–9.
209. Hsu CM, Weiner DE. COVID-19 in dialysis patients: outlasting and outsmarting a pandemic. Kidney Int. 2020;98(6):1402–4.
210. Meller ME, Pfaff BL, Borgert AJ, Richmond CS, et al. Optimized infection control practices augment the robust protective effect of vaccination for ESRD patients during a hemodialysis facility SARS-CoV-2 outbreak. Am J Infect Control. 2022;50(10):1118–24.
211. Petrilli CM, Jones SA, Yang J, Rajagopalan H, et al. Factors associated with hospital admission and critical illness among 5279 people with coronavirus disease 2019 in New York City: prospective cohort study. BMJ. 2020;369:m1966.
212. Flythe JE, Assimon MM, Tugman MJ, Chang EH, et al. Characteristics and outcomes of individuals with pre-existing kidney disease and COVID-19 admitted to intensive care units in the United States. Am J Kidney Dis. 2021;77(2):190–203 e1.
213. Hsu CM, Weiner DE, Aweh G, Miskulin DC, et al. COVID-19 among US dialysis patients: risk factors and outcomes from a National Dialysis Provider. Am J Kidney Dis. 2021;77(5):748–756 e1.
214. Caplin B, Ashby D, McCafferty K, Hull R, et al. Risk of COVID-19 disease, dialysis unit attributes, and infection control strategy among London in-center hemodialysis patients. Clin J Am Soc Nephrol. 2021;16(8):1237–46.
215. Centers for Disease Control and Prevention. Infection control guidance for healthcare professionals about Coronavirus (COVID-19). https://www.cdc.gov/coronavirus/2019-ncov/hcp/infection-control.html. Accessed 23 Dec 2022.
216. Mahallawi WH, Ibrahim NA, Mumena WA. Effectiveness of COVID-19 vaccines in patients under maintenance hemodialysis. Risk Manag Healthc Policy. 2021;14:5081–8.
217. El Karoui K, Hourmant M, Ayav C, Glowacki F, et al. Vaccination and COVID-19 dynamics in dialysis patients. Clin J Am Soc Nephrol. 2022;17(3):395–402.
218. Ashby DR, Caplin B, Corbett RW, Asgari E, et al. Severity of COVID-19 after vaccination among hemodialysis patients: an observational cohort study. Clin J Am Soc Nephrol. 2022;17(6):843–50.
219. Kallen AJ, Arduino MJ, Patel PR. Preventing infections in patients undergoing hemodialysis. Expert Rev Anti-Infect Ther. 2010;8(6):643–55.
220. Hess S, Bren V. Essential components of an infection prevention program for outpatient hemodialysis centers. Semin Dial. 2013;26(4):384–98.
221. U.S. Department of Health and Human Services, Viral Hepatitis National Strategic Plan for the United States: a roadmap to elimination (2021–2025). 2020.

Arteriovenous Access and Catheter Complications

5

Shashank Sharma, Madeline Miller Drake, Jacob Basil Watson, and Eric Kevin Peden

Complications of Hemodialysis Catheters

Dialysis catheters, typically placed in the central venous system, serve as artificial conduits for immediate renal replacement therapy. Broadly, dialysis catheters have two designations: tunneled and non-tunneled. Non-tunneled dialysis catheters are immediate solutions for urgent or emergent dialysis access. These catheters lack a subcutaneous tunnel and exit the skin at the site of cutaneous puncture. Tunneled dialysis catheters are better solutions for intermediate-term access because they exit the skin away from the central venous access point and possess a felt cuff that lays in the subcutaneous tract. Both catheters can support upwards of 350 mL/min of flow. Many patients and clinicians alike find catheters to be convenient patients do not have to be stuck with large-bore needles, and clinicians have two ports readily available to initiate the dialysis—thereby ridding them of the frustration that comes with fistulas that are difficult to access. However, these catheters are fraught with complications and drawbacks.

Suboptimal Flow

Efficient hemodialysis depends on optimal flow, which is a function of the geometric configuration of the catheter as well as the location of the distal tip. Non-tunneled catheters are generally placed under ultrasound guidance and can have kinks that impede flow. If after a catheter is placed, there are difficulties drawing back blood immediately, they can be addressed with the replacement of the catheter followed by fluoroscopic evaluation. Manufacturers of dialysis catheters often boast kink

S. Sharma · M. M. Drake · J. B. Watson · E. K. Peden (✉)
Department of Vascular Surgery, Houston Methodist Hospital, Houston, TX, USA
e-mail: EKPeden@houstonmethodist.org

S. Z. Fadem et al. (eds.), *Complications in Dialysis*,
https://doi.org/10.1007/978-3-031-44557-6_5

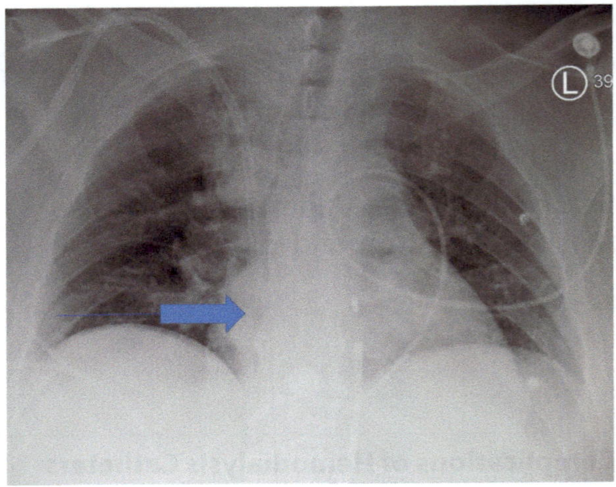

Fig. 5.1 Dialysis catheter with the tip appropriately positioned at the superior vena cava and right atrial junction (blue arrow)

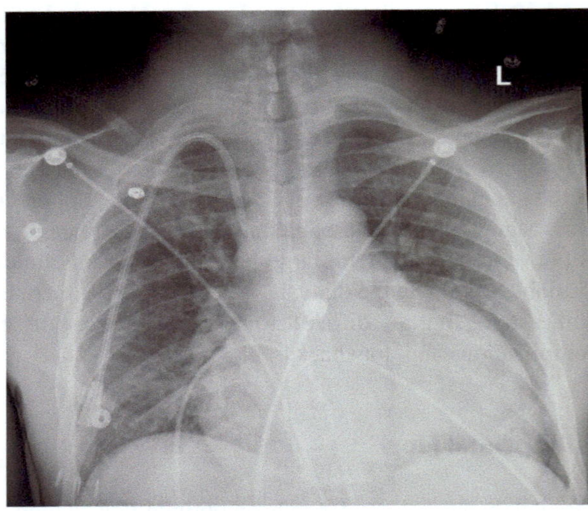

Fig. 5.2 Mispositioned dialysis catheter with the tip in the brachiocephalic vein

resistance as a marketable attribute due to its prevalence. Tunneled catheters tend to be placed under both ultrasound and fluoroscopic guidance. Despite the utilization of dual modalities, tunneled lines are also prone to kinking. Kinks with tunneled lines are most commonly a function of technique in tunneling from the distal skin exit site to the venous access site and are usually resolved with re-tunneling. The importance of the second factor, tip position, cannot be overemphasized. Optimal flow through a dialysis circuit occurs when the tip of the catheter is in the right atrium with the arterial port facing the anterior mediastinum. Figure 5.1 demonstrates the ideal placement with the catheter tip in the right atrium, while Fig. 5.2 shows the catheter tip in the upper SVC.

Infection

The topic of catheter infection is covered in Chap. 2. Two infectious sequelae of chronic catheter presence are worth noting here are metastatic infections, namely endocarditis and disseminated infections. Observational studies note an incidence of metastatic infections at 5–10% [1]. The most frequent and severe complication of catheter-related bloodstream infections is endocarditis, with mortality rates of 22% at 1-month and 50% at 1-year as noted in a Danish study [2]. The most common microbe, *S. aureus*, is reported in approximately a quarter of infections, with the next most common organisms being coagulase-negative staphylococci, enterococci, and *Streptococcus viridans* group [3]. The diagnosis of endocarditis is confirmed with the presence of vegetations on transthoracic echocardiography, and treatment requires immediate catheter removal with a minimum of 6 weeks of intravenous antibiotic course. Similarly, disseminated infections such as vertebral osteomyelitis and spinal epidural abscesses have also been noted in patients with prolonged catheter presence. The diagnosis of these entities is primarily with magnetic resonance imaging and mandates immediate catheter removal. Patients with vertebral osteomyelitis or discitis may require image-guided percutaneous aspiration of the disk space in question if blood cultures are non-diagnostic. A spinal epidural abscess, although uncommon, should have immediate neurosurgical evaluation.

Central Venous Stenoses

Central venous stenoses (CVS) have remained a long-standing challenge for patients requiring dialysis, regardless of conduit, with broad consequences. Common physical exam findings in patients with central venous stenoses are shown in Fig. 5.3 and can include generalized upper extremity and/or facial edema, the presence of prominent chest wall collaterals, and chronic stasis dermatitis. The exact mechanism for the development of stenoses is poorly understood. However, one can imagine that it involves a combination of factors such as inflammation from repetitive endothelial trauma that ultimately leads to smooth muscle proliferation and intimal hyperplasia [4, 5]. Some techniques and decisions do exist to help decrease the development of central venous stenosis. First is ensuring that the catheter tip terminates in the right atrium. Studies have shown that catheters that are placed in the brachiocephalic or subclavian veins lead to higher rates of central venous stenosis [6, 7]. Second is placing an emphasis on placing the catheter via the right internal jugular vein. Unlike the angulated course that the left internal jugular vein takes across the midline to reach the right atrium, the relatively straight central trajectory that the right internal jugular vein offers limits the amount of local trauma experienced by the central veins [8].

It bears mentioning that endovascular interventions in the central venous system, which is a low-flow system, do not provide durable results. Even with faster flows through the central veins that arteriovenous accesses provide, endovascular interventions have a high rate of recurrence with subsequent progression of the degree of

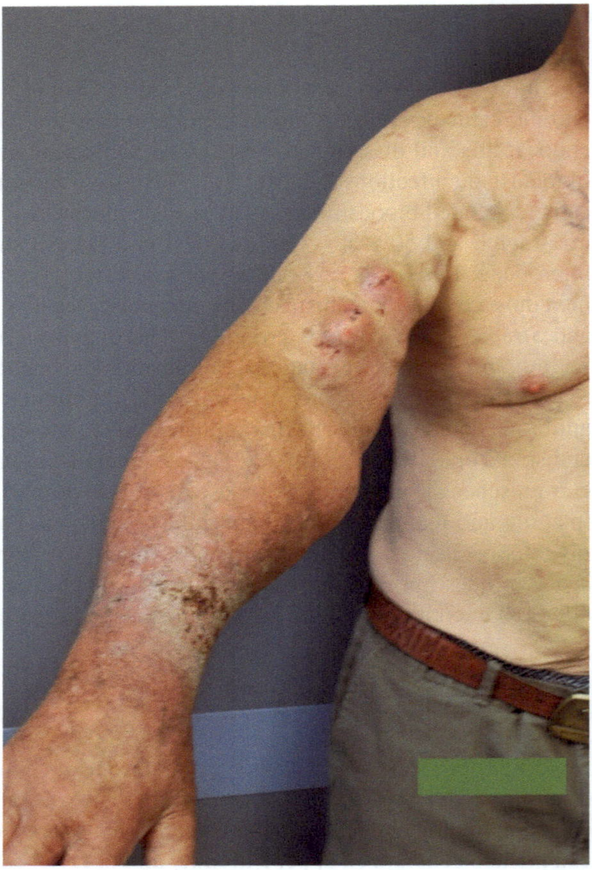

Fig. 5.3 Physical exam findings noted with central venous stenosis. Note the generalized upper extremity, prominent chest wall collaterals, and chronic stasis dermatitis in the forearm

stenosis [9]. Thus, the management of asymptomatic central venous stenosis, with or without the presence of an arteriovenous access, is expectant. Once a lesion becomes symptomatic (e.g., arm swelling), a variety of treatment options exist depending on unique patient factors. First-line treatment for central venous stenoses is generally with percutaneous transluminal angioplasty using non-compliant balloons. There are data that suggest that angioplasty with paclitaxel-coated balloons may have increased freedom from re-intervention; however, no randomized control trials have been conducted to corroborate this finding [10]. Additionally, drug-coated balloons are limited by their size, as the largest diameter commercially available in the United States is 12 mm, and they do not reach the same pressures as non-compliant balloons. Recurrent stenoses or external compression from tumors can warrant the placement of bare metal stents or even covered stent grafts to maintain luminal patency of the central vessels. A growing alternative for patients with recurrent CVS is the placement of a HeRO (Hemodialysis Reliable Outflow) graft (Merit Medical. South Jordan, Utah). Approved by the Food and Drug Administration in 2008, the HeRO graft is a hybrid conduit, the central portion of which is a catheter tip placed under fluoroscopy, thereby bypassing the central stenosis, and the peripheral portion is a polytetrafluoroethylene (PTFE) graft that is surgically implanted to an upper extremity artery. While long-term results are still pending, the HeRO graft has shown reasonable results, with one meta-analysis demonstrating 1-year primary and second patency rate of 21.9% and 59.4%. Kudlaty et al. reported half the infection rates compared to lower extremity grafts [11, 12]. At times, a simpler solution to symptomatic central venous stenosis exists. The symptoms of central venous stenosis are related to an imbalance of the flow in the venous system and the capacity of the residual patent veins and the collateral outflow pathways. Although an exact definition of high flow is not universally agreed upon, if there is high flow in the access peripheral to a central venous stenosis, then simply flow reduction may restore balance and relieve the symptoms. This can be achieved with banding-type procedures or distalization [13, 14]. The most aggressive treatment option, often reserved for patients who have not responded to the above interventions, is surgical venous reconstruction. Our own experience has evolved such that we reserve this for well-functioning autogenous accesses in physiologically fit individuals without other great options [15]. This is usually achieved with an axillary vein to right atrial bypass using a prosthetic graft with good outcomes in carefully selected patients. For some patients, the only realistic option, however, is access ligation and conversion back to catheter-based dialysis.

Clearly, the treatment of CVS needs better and more robust treatment options. The most recent treatment option developed for central venous occlusions is the Surfacer device (Bluegrass Vascular Technologies, San Antonio, Texas). Because femoral vein accesses are associated with an increased risk of infection, malfunction, and thrombosis, the Surfacer device helps recanalize central occlusions and maintain right internal jugular access using an "inside out" technique [16, 17]. This device remains in its infancy and has not been widely adopted.

Complications of Arteriovenous Fistulas and Grafts

Since the adoption of the Fistula First Breakthrough Initiative, the creation of autogenous access with conscious efforts to remove central venous catheters has been noted in the United States [18, 19]. The longevity of arteriovenous (AV) access, whether a graft or autogenous fistula, is a multifaceted topic involving many factors that are unique to every patient, their anatomy, and comorbidities. Meta-analysis performed by Almasri et al. included 875,000 accesses and demonstrated a 2-year primary patency of 55% in fistulas with decreased patency in the diabetic, elderly and female populations [20]. Despite being the Gold Standard for arteriovenous access, fistulae are plagued with a variety of complications, many of which are shared with grafts. Each of the complications that are discussed next is associated with significant morbidity, such as a missed dialysis sessions, placement of tunneled catheters, an inpatient hospital admissions, and at times, death.

Thrombosis

Broadly speaking, the patency of matured access is largely dependent on two factors: inflow and outflow. Any imbalance in these two variables puts the access at higher risk for acute or acute on chronic thrombosis. With regard to arterial inflow, assessment of the feeding artery at the time of access planning is imperative to ensure that the feeding artery is relatively free of proximal atherosclerotic disease and that the fistula does not thrombose due to a low-flow circuit. Another aspect of the inflow disease is the development of intimal hyperplasia at the anastomosis and juxta-anastomotic vein over time. While the exact pathogenesis is poorly understood, it is well established that the connection of a high-pressure arterial system to a low-pressure venous system leads to a combination of abnormal vessel shear stress and endothelial damage leading to impaired flow in the fistula, thereby putting it at a higher risk for thrombosis. From an outflow standpoint, once again, through a poorly understood process, over time the venous outflow develops stenoses that impair flow to the central veins [21].

A distinction exists here between arteriovenous fistulas and grafts in terms of the location of hemodynamically significant lesions: autogenous accesses tend to develop arteriovenous anastomotic and juxta-anastomotic lesions by way of intimal hyperplasia, whereas grafts are more likely to develop intimal hyperplasia, referred to as neointimal hyperplasia, at the outflow anastomosis [22]. Several hypotheses have been offered in the past to try to mitigate this process and decrease the rates of access thrombosis. One agent brought into question was dipyridamole, an antiplatelet agent which concomitantly inhibits vascular smooth muscle cell hyperplasia. It was hypothesized that it could possibly prevent neointimal hyperplasia. Dixon et al. from the Dialysis Access Consortium Study Group performed a multicenter, double-blinded, randomized control trial which demonstrated improved unassisted primary patency in AV grafts among patients who were on dipyridamole and aspirin compared to those who were not, 23% versus 30%, respectively [23]. In an effort to determine if the outcomes noted were because of dipyridamole or aspirin, a secondary cohort analysis was performed which revealed equal improvement in unassisted primary patency between patients on dipyridamole and aspirin versus aspirin alone [24]. Observations of improved unassisted primary patency are also being noted with clopidogrel and the HeRO graft [25]. These data suggest that (neo)intimal hyperplasia may be a platelet-mediated process or at least can be mitigated with the use of antiplatelet therapy.

Thrombosis or loss of clinical patency occurs due to an underlying stenosis over 85% of the time [26]. Impending loss of patency in an AV fistula or graft can be detected using a variety of methods. As always, a good clinical exam by an experienced, qualified clinician proves invaluable. On exam, an ideal mature AV fistula has a thrill present throughout the cardiac cycle, and when the extremity is raised, the fistula will partially collapse. With juxta-anastomotic stenosis, a bounding water-hammer pulse is felt near the arterial anastomosis and a diminished or possibly absent thrill more proximally. A helpful adjunct to assess for inflow disease is known as the "pulse augmentation test," where the examiner occludes the fistula away from the anastomosis and is able to determine the status of the inflow. Similarly, with outflow stenoses pulsatility can be appreciated with the thrill only present in systole. When the extremity raised the fistula proximal to the stenosis collapses while the distal portion remains distended. Swelling of the entire extremity can often be seen with central and proximal stenoses, along with the presence of progressively prolonged bleeding after needle removal. These abnormal physical exam findings warrant further evaluation by a qualified practitioner, with or without imaging, to prevent access thrombosis.

In addition to physical exam findings, dialysis circuit-based surveillance can also be a tool for surveillance and prevent AV access thrombosis. Pressure measurements have proven to be useful in preventing impending thrombosis—AV fistulas and grafts can be at risk of thrombosis when the flows become less than 300 and 500 mL/min, respectively [27]. Kt/*V*, which is used to assess hemodialysis adequacy, can also be used to detect poor flow. Kt/*V* less than 1.2 or a decrease in Kt/*V* by more than 0.2 has been noted to be associated with thrombosis [28]. The utility of acting on abnormal dialysis circuit metrics is unclear with mixed data. Studies suggest monitoring of AV fistulas may lead to improved access patency, but monitoring of AV grafts may lead to increased interventions with no effect on access survival [29, 30].

Once an access has thrombosed, two methods for declotting exist: open and percutaneous. Several percutaneous methods have been described, including but not limited to, mechanical thrombectomy, "lyse and wait," pulse-spray aided pharmacomechanical thrombolysis, and thromboaspiration. The details of these techniques are outside the scope of this chapter. With regard to mechanical thrombectomy, a variety of devices exist on the market and the choice of device is largely user and institution driven. Contraindications to percutaneous include patients with megafistulas; presence of a right to left cardiac shunt; and patients with poor pulmonary or cardiac reserve. Dreaded complications of the percutaneous technique include anastomotic disruption and embolization of clot into the arterial system. When faced with these scenarios, an open surgical approach is preferred, if not emergently required. The open technique is performed by creating an approximately 2-cm skin incision overlying the fistula, obtaining proximal and distal control of the fistula, creating a fistulotomy or graftotomy and evacuating the thrombus using Fogarty balloons, with or without revision of the anastomosis. A completion fistulogram is then performed, and the causative lesion is treated if necessary. While it is accepted that open thrombectomy of AV grafts has greater technical success rates than fistulas—due to difficulties using Fogarty balloons in veins compared to a prosthetic graft—there is no consensus as to which declotting technique is more efficacious and/or more appropriate in which clinical settings [31–33].

Failure of Maturation

The "Rule of 6's," established by the National Kidney Foundation's Kidney Disease Outcomes Quality Initiative (KDOQI), suggests that a fistula can be used when the blood flow has reached >600 mL/min, is at least 6 mm in diameter, and is less than

6 mm in depth. The Hemodialysis Fistula Maturation study, a seven-center prospective cohort study of patients undergoing creation of new single-stage AV fistulas, validated this rule of thumb based on 6-week postoperative AV fistula ultrasounds [34]. Once the Rule of 6's is achieved, some define clinical maturation as successful cannulation with two large-bore needles and adequate hemodialysis for at least 2 weeks. Others define maturation as fistula use for over three quarters of treatments over a month with adequate blood flow and clearance.

One notable downside to AV fistulas that has come to light after the Fistula First initiative is that a significant portion of fistulas created never get successfully used for dialysis. It is important to clarify that, while a 2-year 55% primary patency rate was quoted earlier in the chapter, this statistic applies to fistulas that have successfully matured—fistula non-maturation has been reported as high as 60% in some studies, compared to 15–23% failure to obtain reliable access in grafts. This primary failure, defined as a fistula that fails to mature or is unusable, leads to prolonged catheter use and its inherent disadvantages as described previously [35–37].

The factors that lead to primary failure are poorly understood. It has been posited that non-maturation may be secondary to stenoses in the venous segments and/or competing outflow from side branches. A contemporary approach to accesses that have not matured within the expected 6-week period is the implementation of balloon-assisted maturation and coiling or ligation of side branches. As the name implies, balloon-assisted maturation consists of balloon angioplasty of the vein to improve flow that may be impeded by venous stenoses. Similarly, in hopes of improving the flow through a long segment of vein, venous branches can be coil embolized, functionally serving as surgical ligation of venous side branches. Some interventionists have also put forth that fistulas greater than 6 mm in depth can be easier to access with aggressive angioplasty, thereby forgoing need for surgical a superficialization procedure. Huber et al. performed secondary analysis of the Hemodialysis Fistula Maturation cohort and noted that 37.7% of patients with renal failure underwent interventions to assist maturation with patency rates of 75% at 2 years [38]. These data, while favorable, harbor a significant amount of subjectivity surrounding balloon assisted maturation and its nuances that are not discussed such as length and location of angioplasty, size of balloons, and frequency of ballooning—not to mention the increased cost of coiling and repeat angioplasties compared to simple surgical ligation or revision of anastomosis. Thus, it remains unclear when an access should be abandoned and what the protocols for interventions for maturation should look like.

Several hypotheses to decrease rates of non-maturation have been tested. One notable hypothesis was that prevention of early thrombosis with antiplatelet agents, such as clopidogrel, could help achieve maturation. To address this, Dember et al. performed a multicenter, double-blind, randomized controlled trial which found that while clopidogrel decreased the occurrence of thrombosis of AV fistulas, it did not affect maturation [39]. Another hypothesis is that perhaps failure of maturation is a geometric and hemodynamic phenomenon and primary failure is a function of suboptimal flow. For this, the VasQ device was created—an external scaffold that is surgically placed around the arteriovenous anastomosis at the time of fistula creation to achieve improved geometry at the anastomosis. While still in its early phases, preliminary data from the United Kingdom and Europe appears to be promising, with Shahverdyan et al. reporting no early failures and secondary patency of 90% at 6 months [40].

Infection

Infection of AV accesses is one of the leading causes of access failures. AV grafts are up to 10 times more likely to present with infectious complications compared to fistulas, giving fistulas a clear clinical advantage [41]. The baseline immunocompromised state of uremic and dialysis-dependent patients contributing to this occurrence cannot be understated [42]. Risk factors for access infection include poor patient hygiene, older age, femoral location, diabetes, and a history of bacteremia [43]. Infections can be acquired either at the time of access creation or with repeated access cannulation. The most common causative organisms, in descending order of frequency, are *Staphylococcus aureus*, Coagulase-negative *Staphylococci*, and polymicrobial infections, with organisms such as *Pseudomonas* having the ability to produce proteolytic enzymes which lead to anastomotic disruption and subsequent pseudoaneurysm formation [44, 45].

The diagnosis of an infected AV access is often a clinical one with signs and symptoms including drainage, exposed graft, erythema, and induration, to name a few. Imaging modalities such as duplex ultrasound and CT scans can be used to identify, confirm, or rule out presence of infection. It is worth noting, AV grafts that have failed or have been abandoned do not get surgically excised routinely. Should a patient with thrombosed AV access present with signs of systemic infection from an uncertain source, indium-tagged leukocyte scans, which are highly sensitive, can be obtained to rule out infection [46].

Once a diagnosis of infection has been established, the management of an infected access differs considerably between AV fistulas and grafts. We begin with a focus on autogenous accesses. Broad-spectrum antibiotics should be administered for AV fistula infections, the duration of which depends on the clinical scenario. Once resolution has been achieved, access sites should be monitored for signs of ongoing or reinfection. With the two exceptions, antibiotic therapy tends to be efficacious for treating autogenous access infections, whether in the immediate postoperative period or later. The first is if there are concerns about involvement of the anastomosis, in which case the access should be ligated to avoid formation of a pseudo-aneurysm or frank rupture of the anastomosis. The other scenario is an infection involving a fistula segment with underlying covered stent graft, for which the stent would need to be surgically excised to achieve source control.

Arteriovenous grafts have infection rates anywhere from 3 to 19%, and unlike autogenous fistulas, any infection more extensive than mild cellulitis is unlikely to respond to antibiotic therapy alone [47, 48]. Complete graft excision is often required in cases where the infection involves the entirety of the graft. A thorough surface exam can often clue surgeons to the need for total excision. Other times, extensive purulence or lack of incorporation of the graft will mandate complete excision. In these cases, it is imperative that the entirety of the prosthetic material is removed. To do so, the venous anastomosis must be resected, and the involved vein should either be repaired primarily or with a vein patch. Addressing the arterial anastomosis is more nuanced and challenging, primarily because of concerns for operating in a scarred surgical site with concerns for injury to the artery or nearby median nerve. If the arterial anastomotic area of the graft is not involved, the most common surgery involves leaving a segment of graft attached to the artery as a stump or cuff. If the arterial anastomotic area is involved in the infection, then the entire graft must be removed. If the graft is removed from the artery and the artery is large in diameter, it is reasonable to primarily close the arteriotomy. More often however, the closure of the arteriotomy requires a patch to avoid stenosis the vessel, most commonly with a segment of autogenous vein. Occasionally, arterial bypass through uninfected tissues may be needed for limb preservation. In cases where only a section of the graft is involved or can be safely resected with the remainder of the graft being well-incorporated, segmental excision can be pursued. This is achieved by obtaining proximal and distal control of the graft in healthy, uninvolved areas and tunneling a new graft segment through clean tissues. The infected area can then be resected widely to healthy margins. Depending on the area of accessible graft remaining and the type of graft used for reconstruction, a temporary tunneled dialysis catheter may be needed to allow time for the surgical site to heal prior to attempts at cannulation. While data regarding segmental excision is sparce, Liu et al. recently reported reinfection rates of 16.5% versus 2.3% in complete graft excision versus subtotal excision, respectively [49]. This corroborates findings in previous studies and highlights the importance of judicious source control [45, 49, 50].

An aspect of AV fistula infections that is often under-emphasized by physicians is the cannulation technique. The most common technique for fistula cannulation is the "rope ladder" method, where the point of access is rotated along the length of the fistula. Another is the "area wall" technique, where certain regions are repeatedly cannulated. This method is very commonly used but has been largely discouraged due to the increased incidence of aneurysm formation and its association with access failure [51]. The third technique is the "single site" or "buttonhole" technique, in which a single location is repeatedly cannulated leading to development of an epithelialized and fibrous tract through which a blunt needle is inserted. This method has gained endorsement by several reputable societies for its alleged benefits, such as less pain, improved hemostasis time, and less aneurysmal degeneration [52]. While a decrease in pain is not consistently demonstrated in studies, what does seem to be strongly suggested is a link between the buttonhole method and infectious risk. Five randomized control trials have been published comparing buttonhole to rope ladder methods, of which three have demonstrated a strong relationship between buttonhole and infections, both at the sites of access and bacteremia [53–57]. A 2014 meta-analysis demonstrated over three times higher risk of access infection, likely related to colonization at the buttonhole scab site, with significantly higher rates of bacteremia noted in other reviews [52]. Also of note, the randomized control trial with the longest follow-up reported significantly higher rates of infection which brings into question whether studies have had appropriate follow-up to truly capture the infection risk [56]. The debate remains far from over. Proponents of the buttonhole method cite that while an association with infection has been noted, only one of the five RCTs had a statistically significant difference and there were large variations with what constituted an infection. An analysis of the Swedish Renal Registry, which is a robust dataset and contains over 1300 AV fistulas, failed to demonstrate an increased risk of infection, in line with other Scandinavian data [58, 59]. Generally, however, concern for increased infectious risks with buttonholes has led to steady decline in its usage, except in special circumstances like pediatric populations or home hemodialysis.

Aneurysmal Degeneration

The precise etiology of aneurysmal degeneration of AV fistulas is unclear. Common to most fistulas with aneurysmal changes are high-flow rates, outflow obstruction, and needle access techniques. Aneurysm formation in areas of repeat needling leading to progressive weakening of all the layers of the wall is commonly seen; however, aneurysms can also develop in regions where no cannulation has been previously attempted. Outflow stenoses are commonly seen in aneurysmal fistulas [60]. Furthermore, no standardized definition exists regarding what constitutes a fistula aneurysm, though many classifications and definitions have been proposed [60–62]. Given the lack of reporting standards, the incidence has been noted to be upwards of 60%, with an increased incidence in proximal fistulas involving the cephalic vein [63].

Aneurysm formation is generally a benign process, and some degree of aneurysmal dilation of an AV fistula is expected. Thus, asymptomatic disease should not be treated. Aside from cases of inadequate dialysis, indications for treatment are largely related to bleeding risks as assessed on a physical exam. Standard teaching for what is categorized as an access aneurysm at high risk for rupture is the presence of thinned, depigmented skin with or without the presence of scabs or an ulcer. As with any clinical exam, nuisances exist. One nuance that can help determine the urgency of treatment is the "pinch test" (Fig. 5.4). As fistula aneurysmal disease worsens, the epidermis continues to become tighter, thinner, and the soft tissue layers between the aneurysm wall and the skin become obliterated or displaced. This process of skin thinning and soft tissue displacement occurs at varying rates. Given this variability, fistulas that have ample soft tissue between the aneurysm and the skin, to the point where the skin and soft tissues can be pinched over top of the fistula, do not need to be revised urgently, if at all [64]. Figure 5.5 demonstrates a high-risk aneurysm that did not pass the "pinch test," with skin tinning and scabbing noted over the aneurysm. The dreaded clinical scenario to be avoided with such an access is the unintentional dislodging of the scab with frank hemorrhage. These scenarios are life-threatening and such high-risk findings warrant timely referral to a vascular surgeon for surgical revision.

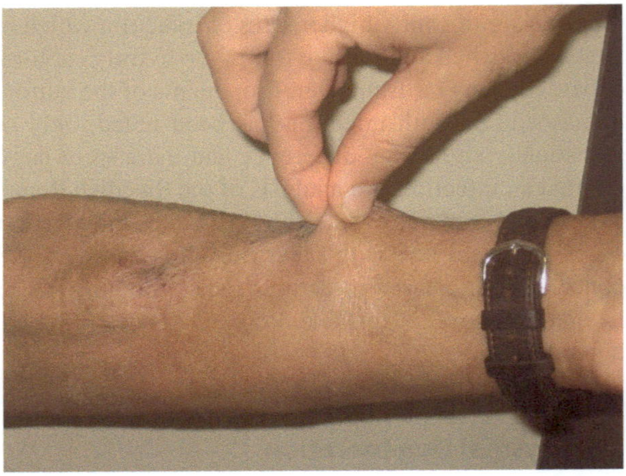

Fig. 5.4 Demonstration of the pinch test. The skin and soft tissues above the aneurysm is tented, suggesting that the aneurysmal degeneration is not an imminent threat to the patient

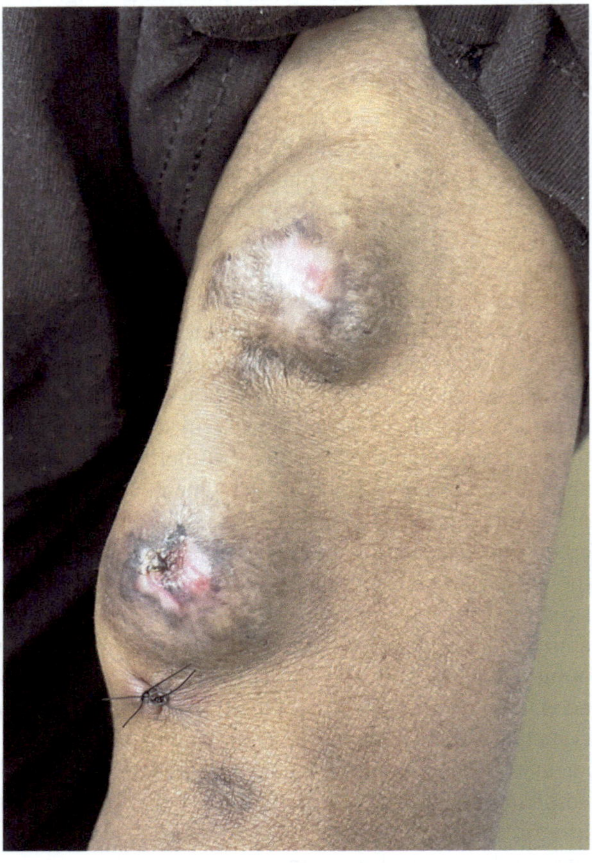

Fig. 5.5 High-risk fistula aneurysm. Note the skin thinning over both aneurysms and the presence of a scab over the lower aneurysm

Revision of aneurysmal fistulas can be very extensive procedures with high degree of subjectivity to its surgical approach. Surgical reconstruction options include, but are not limited to (1) aneurysmorrhaphy (excision of the anterior aneurysm wall with primary suture or stapled closure), (2) ligation with bypass, (3) resection with either end-to-end anastomosis or an interposition graft, and (4) plication (suturing redundant aneurysmal wall to decrease the lumen). Regardless of the reconstruction option employed, one should have a low threshold to obtain a completion fistulogram to assess the quality of reconstruction and the presence of outflow disease not addressed with the reconstruction. Baláž et al. performed a meta-analysis of fistula aneurysmorrhaphy and noted three important findings: (1) 86% of the 597 patients were revised to mitigate bleeding risk while the remainder were for pain and high access flow; (2) an 82% 1-year pooled primary patency rate with low complication rates; and (3) 3% aneurysm recurrence rate [65]. Additionally, the volume flow of the access should be assessed and consideration given to flow reduction, if appropriate.

Similar to aneurysms in fistulas, pseudoaneurysm formation is a common complication seen in AV grafts. As previously mentioned, grafts have the propensity to develop outflow stenosis at the venous anastomosis. These and other outflow lesions result in increased intraluminal pressures, and repeated cannulation of the graft at the same site eventually leads to graft breakdown, thereby leading to pseudoaneurysm formation [66]. The incidence of pseudoaneurysms is largely unknown due to under-recognition. However, it is important to understand the clinical presentation of a pseudoaneurysm due to its increased risk of rupture and become infected over time [67]. Clinically, pseudoaneurysms present as a palpable pulsatile mass with high-risk features similar to fistula aneurysms that help to determine the timeline for intervention. Pseudoaneurysms noted at or near the anastomoses should carry a high suspicion for infection, and the management of this scenario has been discussed previously. Small pseudoaneurysms that clinically do not possess any threat to the fistula or the associated skin and soft tissues can be managed expectantly, with a focus on frequent surveillance for signs of outflow stenosis, either on duplex or physical exam. Large pseudoaneurysms, however, require surgical interventions in addition to treatment of outflow stenoses. Surgical intervention can involve debridement of involved skin and soft tissues with interposition bypass as described in the infectious complications portion of the chapter. One differentiating factor here is that one can be more aggressive about flow restoring reconstruction (e.g., prosthetic bypass conduit, interposition graft) instead of favoring extensive excision since the basis for this complication is trauma rather than infectious. In the endovascular era, the use of covered stent grafts has also become exceedingly more common to treat aneurysms and pseudoaneurysms [68, 69]. Endovascular interventions can be employed for both grafts and fistulas and can help avoid the associated morbidity of open surgery, particularly in re-operative fields. Of course, the tortuous nature of autologous accesses can make it difficult to find suitable landing zones and achieve effective exclusion. While cannulation of stented regions is technically feasible and described in the literature, this practice should ideally be limited and alternative access sites should be chosen to prevent flow-compromising deformation of the stent, stent fracture, or graft infection [70–72]. Long-term outcome data regarding stent graft use in AV access for access degeneration has yet to be reported.

Access-Related Limb Ischemia

Dialysis access-related steal syndrome (DASS), also known as hemodialysis access-induced distal ischemia (HAIDI) or access-related hand ischemia (ARHI), is one of the most dreaded complications in dialysis access surgery. DASS occurs when AV access, which are low-resistance circuits, is created and shunts a clinically significant volume of flow from the higher resistance circuit of the hand. The pathophysiology of steal is the result of a vessel with limited arterial flow supplying two vascular beds with different resistances. This is further exacerbated in the setting of significant atherosclerotic disease proximal or distal to the anastomosis. The size of the anastomosis also plays a large role in the development of DASS as acute cases tend to occur with AV grafts given the graft diameter relative to the artery and fistulas tend to present later as progressive maturation leads to greater shunting [73]. Risk factors most frequently associated with developing symptomatic steal syndrome include distal brachial artery inflow (as opposed to radial artery), female gender, and history of diabetes. Other factors that are commonly attributed include age greater than 60; prior ipsilateral access creation; use of grafts, and previous history of HAIDI [73–75].

DASS presents over a wide spectrum of severities and chronicity. One classification system commonly used to discuss the clinical presentations of DASS divides them over four stages, in order of severity [76]. Stage 1 is asymptomatic retrograde diastolic flow incidentally found on duplex examination; Stage 2A: tolerable pain, paresthesia, or cramping during dialysis or exertion; 2B: intolerable pain, paresthesia, or cramping during dialysis or exertion; Stage 3: rest pain; Stage 4: irreversible tissue necrosis and/or significant loss of hand function. Timing and onset of symptoms can be classified as acute (within hours of creation), subacute (within 30 days), and chronic (greater than 30 days). Figure 5.6 demonstrates severe steal syndrome with an ischemic digit. Given the variability in symptoms, timing, and how one defines a patient to be symptomatic—as subacute and chronic ischemic symptoms are often written off for diabetic neuropathy—the true incidence of symptomatic steal syndrome is largely unknown with reported ranges of 0.25–8% of access created [73]. DASS can be avoided by preferentially using radial artery when able, assessing proximal and distal arteries prior to access creation, and assessing distal arterial flow after access creation at the wrist and hand [73, 74, 76].

Several imaging modalities and diagnostic tests have been studied to help diagnose DASS. Assessment of patients with suspected steal syndrome should include a duplex study and consideration of formal angiography. The duplex study should assess the volume flow of the access, compare the brachial blood pressure in the two arms to rule out inflow arterial disease, assessment of the fistula and arteries of the arm for stenoses. Duplex ultrasonography is commonly used to confirm the presence of steal physiology, namely diastolic or complete reversal of flow in the origin

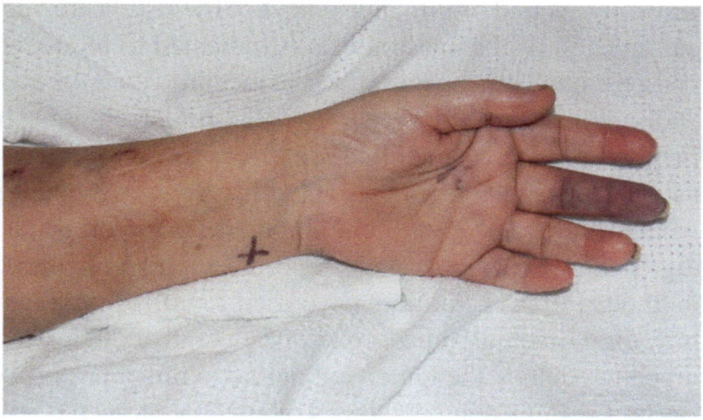

Fig. 5.6 Chronic dialysis access-related steal syndrome leading to ischemic changes to the third digit

artery distal to the anastomosis. However, some degree of distal flow reversal can be seen in anywhere from 75 to 90% of accesses, most of which is asymptomatic [77]. Digital photoplethysmography can also be used as an ischemic digit should reveal nearly monophasic baseline waveforms with significant augmentation upon compression of the outflow. Our vascular lab uses a doubling of digital waveform amplitude with compression of the access to demonstrate a positive steal study. Formal angiography should be considered in patients requiring intervention with imaging from the aortic arch to the digits. This study can uncover proximal inflow disease as well as severe distal arterial pathology. DASS is ultimately a clinical diagnosis, relying on thorough examination of the access itself as well as the distal extremity for neurological and motor deficits. Improvement or resolution of symptoms with compression of the access is highly suggestive of DASS. Once the diagnosis is confirmed, it is important to treat this condition prior to the development of irreversible claw-hand deformities or digit gangrene in cases of severe steal.

Several treatment options exist for the diagnosis of DASS—expectant management, fistula banding, distal revascularization interval ligation (DRIL), revision using distal inflow (RUDI), proximal artery inflow graft (PAI), and ligation. These interventions can be lumped into categories of flow reduction (banding-type procedures and RUDI) and flow redirection (DRIL and PAI). The goals of treatment of steal ideally include preservation of the dialysis access and resolution of the hand symptoms. Stage 1 DASS is typically managed expectantly with the option to use adjuncts such as vasodilators, reduce antihypertensive medication, and physical therapy. Stage 2A can be managed similarly. Patients Stage 2B and above warrant immediate intervention with strong consideration for ligation in patients with Stage 4 disease. Ligation is by far the most definitive treatment to this problem, and sometimes appropriate, but it unfortunately leaves patients without reliable, life-saving dialysis access. Fistula banding, which was developed under the premise that decreased outflow through the fistula would translate to increased distal tissue perfusion, can be performed in many ways. Banding is performed by dissecting over the proximal fistula or graft and tying a suture or felt cuff over a dilator. Banding is ideally performed as close to the anastomosis as possible to avoid creation of a high-pressure segment between the band and the anastomosis. In some patients, the anastomosis and proximal segment of the fistula are very large. In such cases, surgical revision of the anastomosis is indicated to reduce the caliber of the connection and proximal vein segment. More recently, the minimally invasive assisted ligation endoluminal-assisted revision (MILLER) technique has been introduced which involves placing a small balloon across the anastomosis and tying a non-resorbable suture around the vein [78]. The difficulty with banding has been with determining what the adequate degree of banding is to support an access as well as perfusing the digits. Several studies have reported high rates of access thrombosis with these methods [79–81]. Authors have tried to utilize intraoperative digital plethysmography, digit brachial indices, and intraoperative duplex ultrasonography to gauge how much to occlude the lumen but neither adjunct has proven to be reliable [80, 82]. In attempt at improving outcomes of adequate flow reduction and preserved patency, a technique described as "precision banding" has been described with intraoperative flow measurements before and after banding [83]. We believe banding is most appropriate for DASS in the setting of high-flow accesses (>1500 mL/min).

The more widely adopted surgical treatment of DASS is the DRIL technique. This procedure consists of ligation of the native artery distal to the anastomosis and creates a bypass from the proximal aspect of the inflow artery to the distal arterial target. The developers of this method published their long-term data and noted a 1-year patency 96% with decreased numbers for graft conduits [77, 84]. Access preservation rates upwards of 75% have been reported [79, 85]. While efficacious in the near-term, the disadvantage to DRIL technique, which requires ligation of the feeding artery, is the reported risk of bypass occlusion leading to limb ischemia [86]. Thus, our institution to strongly prefer the RUDI and PAI methods. The RUDI technique requires ligation of the fistula and a bypass graft is created to jump from near the area of ligation to a distal artery, thereby creating a more distal inflow. Similarly, with PAI, the fistula is ligated and a bypass is performed to a more proximal artery origin, allowing more blood flow distally through collaterals. Both RUDI and PAI have demonstrated symptom resolution and 1-year primary patency rates comparable to DRIL [85–90]. It is important to note that a subset of patients that develop DASS may have significant peripheral arterial disease impeding antegrade perfusion, the treatment of which can sometimes sufficiently improve perfusion. This can be achieved with endovascular treatment of disease proximal or distal to the anastomosis. Ultimately, treatment algorithms for patients with steal syndrome are based on symptom severity and volume flow of the access.

Excessive Flow

Cardiovascular disease is the leading cause of death in the end-stage renal disease population. A review of the United States Renal Data System (USRDS) data demonstrated the incidence of death of 33, 46, and 57% at 1, 2, and 3 years, respectively, in patients with concomitant heart failure. It has been well established that creation of an AV access results in increased cardiac output, contractility, blood volume, and venous return with subsequent cardiac remodeling in the longer term [91–93]. The clinical consequences of this increased cardiac strain, however, remain unclear. Despite approximately 36% of patients carrying a diagnosis of congestive heart failure (CHF) at the time of dialysis initiation, the prevalence of high-output cardiac failure due to or following access creation is low [94, 95]. Furthermore, the hypothesis that high or excessive flows through a fistula lead to high-output cardiac failure has not been consistently supported [96–98]. Most clinicians speculate that certain individuals with underlying cardiopulmonary risk factors may be at higher risk for developing high-output cardiac failure or worsening of baseline CHF after access creation, but we have been unable to predict this phenomenon reliably.

The recognition of a patient who may be victim to the deleterious effects of a high-flow fistula is made difficult by two primary factors. First, it is often impossible to discern the difference between the intrinsic worsening of heart failure and worsening cardiac function due to flow through a fistula. One exam often described to assess the level of cardiac stress added by a fistula is the Nicoladoni–Branham sign. This test consists of 30–60 s of compression of the arterial anastomosis with a subsequent decrease in heart rate and increased blood pressure. While easily reproducible, this test has not been validated. Second, while high-output cardiac failure is defined as an above-normal cardiac index with signs and symptoms of cardiac failure, there is no universal definition of "excessive flow" in a fistula. MacRae et al. proposed diagnostic metrics of (1) greater than or equal to a 30% ratio of AV access flow to cardiac output and/or (2) access flow rates of greater than 3 L/min, with biannual echocardiogram evaluation. They also note that patients with heart failure not responding to maximal medical therapy should undergo evaluation for AV flow reduction. Due to these two factors, the majority of interventions being performed for high-flow fistulas occur due to frank heart failure symptoms in the setting of flows exceeding an arbitrary threshold [95, 99].

Once high-output cardiac failure due to the presence of an AV fistula is identified, the definitive therapy is ligation of the fistula. This is appropriate in patients who develop symptoms of worsening heart failure in the relatively immediate postoperative period. This obviously comes at the cost of an access. The majority of cases are identified weeks to month out from fistula creation. In these cases, flow reduction procedures such as banding/MILLER technique as previously described have been widely used. As previously stated, these techniques carry a significant risk of over-restricting the inflow leading to thrombosis, and when performed for high-flow accesses, recurrence. A study looking at banding in 50 patients with high-flow accesses reported a recurrence of increased flow in half the patients at 1 year, in-line with other reports [97]. Because brachial origin accesses tend to have higher arterial flow, and thus greater fistula flows, reconstruction with revision using distal inflow (RUDI) is also an option to decrease access flows without sacrificing the access. The durability of this treatment is also unclear, with a Dutch study analyzing 3-year outcomes in RUDI for high-flow accesses noting approximately half of the patients had recurrent high flow [100, 101]. A newer method described to address high flow in aneurysmal fistulas and/or fistulas with wide anastomosis is the graft inclusion technique and relies on the lack of distensibility of PTFE grafts. In this approach, the fistula is opened over the anastomosis and a 4 mm PTFE graft is sewn to the anastomosis and using a 3–4 cm segment of PTFE. The other end is sewn to the venous outflow, and the aneurysm is closed over the graft with resection of the aneurysmal segment. Nojima et al. who reported this technique note a 67.7% secondary patency and note that this technique avoids thrombosis with robust flow suppression [102]. This method has not been widely adopted, and long-term data is still pending.

Unusable Access

Several factors can deem an access unusable. One common scenario is when a fistula matures but is too deep to be accessed, generally greater than 6 mm per the KDOQI guidelines. This is understandably more common in obese patients and can also result from poor tunneling of AV grafts. The management of a deep fistula is primarily surgical. Some authors have employed aggressive balloon angioplasty techniques to the most superficial segments of the fistula and ultrasound-guided liposuction, these methods are not commonly used at present time and carry significant, unique risks [103]. The traditional method for superficialization has been transposition. This involves creating a single longitudinal incision or interrupted incisions overlying the course of the fistula, circumferentially dissecting the fistula, and then placing the fistula in a more superficial location. The new, more superficial location can be created by either developing skin flaps and then a soft tissue pocket for fistula to lay in, or tunneling a new course for the fistula, which requires transection, either a venovenous or an arteriovenous anastomosis of the fistula. Disadvantages to transposition include the morbidity of a long incision, risk of development of stenosis at the "swing segment," where superficial veins transition to the deep venous system, and stenosis at the anastomosis, if performed.

The Minimally Invasive Superficialization technique (MIST) is another option for managing deep fistulas. This technique exposes the fistula through two small transverse incisions with circumferential dissection of the fistula. Once freely dissected and proximal and distal control is obtained, the fistula is transected near the arteriovenous anastomosis and fed to the upper incision. As an optional adjunct to the procedure, a valvulotome is used to ensure no valves are present, and the fistula is then tunneled in a new, superficial tunnel with subsequent venovenous anastomosis. Inkollu et al. reported an average postoperative depth of 3.1 mm with 2-year secondary patency rates of 88.1% and no wound infections using the MIST technique, in line with other reported outcomes [104].

Lipectomy has also been utilized as part of superficialization, where two transverse incisions are made, and the soft tissue overlying the fistula is resected with the creation of skin flaps; the potential space is controlled with a drain. The advantage of this technique is the lack of need for circumferential dissection of the fistula. Theoretical disadvantages include the presence of a significant dead space and a long "valley" where the fat was removed, leading to difficulties cannulating. Bourquelot et al. reported a 3-mm fistula depth with 88% 3-year secondary patency. Notably, venous outflow stenosis was the most common complication in their series [105].

A newer approach to superficialization is described very well by Fontenot et al. [106]. Briefly, this approach requires intermittent transverse incisions throughout the length of the fascia through which skin flaps are made over the length of the fistula. The superficial fascia is then divided over the length of the vein along with the overlying adipose tissue. The fistula is then circumferentially dissected, with care given to not remove any adipose tissue. The superficial fascia and adipose tissue are then reapproximated, creating an adipose bed under the vein with an appropriate thickness skin flap overlying the fistula. Should redundancy of the vein be encountered, it can be addressed by laying the fistula in the most anterolateral aspect of the pocket, but certainly, resection and anastomosis of redundant segments are reasonable solutions. This technique is gaining traction at our institution; however, long-term data have yet to reported by any group. Fontenot et al. reported short-term results in a series of 23 patients noted a cannulation rate of 94.7%, with one case of access thrombosis [106]. We strongly believe that fistula depth is a major source of problematic fistula usability. A simplified approach is an assessment of fistula diameter and depth. If the fistula is deeper than it is big, it should be superficialized.

Besides depth, tortuosity and inadequate flow can also make a fistula unusable. Tortuosity becomes a problem in accesses despite having adequate flows because it can be difficult to cannulate and achieve adequate flows in tortuous fistulas. The management of tortuosity can include techniques outlined for superficialization with the goal of creating an approximately 6 cm straight segment of accessible fistula. Extremely tortuous fistulas may require segmental transection with venovenous anastomosis to achieve the desired linear confirmation or even replacement with a segment of graft.

Inadequate flow is generally defined as flows less than the KDOQI guidelines of 600 mL/min and reason why a fistula may be unusable. A common culprit for low flows is juxta-anastomotic stenoses, with or without anastomotic stenosis. Juxta-anastomotic venous stenoses are defined as a stenosis within the first 3–4 cm arteriovenous anastomosis. These lesions can be managed either surgically or using percutaneous interventions. The surgical treatment for these stenoses is the resection of the vein to a healthy, mature section and creating a new anastomosis proximal to the existing one. Endovascularly, these lesions are addressed by performing balloon angioplasty, which can include both the juxta-anastomotic segment and/or the anastomosis itself. Surgical revision, while at risk of developing repeat stenosis at a new anastomosis site, has been reported to have better 1-year primary patency rate compared to percutaneous balloon angioplasty between (65–88% versus 44–79%); however, limited studies have analyzed this issue specifically [107]. Several practitioners have also reported using drug-coated balloons and cutting balloons for these lesions, with comparable primary patency rates. No randomized trials exist comparing surgical versus endovascular intervention or balloon angioplasty versus drug-coated balloon use. Results from a meta-analysis of 297 patients favored surgical repair (OR 0.53 [0.28–0.98]), but interventionists and surgeons agree that trialing angioplasty and then reserving surgical revision for recurrent lesions are reasonable approaches to treating these lesions [108].

Another reason why a fistula may be deemed unusable is needle infiltration during cannulation attempts. In new fistulas, this commonly occurs because of inexperienced dialysis staff cannulating the fistula. While dialysis centers aim to have an experienced nurse access fistulas the first few times, issues such as staff turnover can lead to less experienced nurses cannulating a new fistula [109]. In older fistulas, infiltration usually occurs due to an underlying factor such as outflow stenosis. While small filtrations can be managed expectantly, large infiltrations warrant diagnostic imaging to determine possible etiology along with a period of "fistula rest" during which dialysis is performed using a tunneled dialysis catheter until the hematoma caused by infiltration can resolve. A study by Allon et al. examined the occurrence of infiltration in their dialysis center and found an incidence rate of 5.2% annually. Infiltration led to increased diagnostic imaging and interventions (e.g., fistulograms, surgical revision; 2.4 per patient), increased duration of catheter dependence, and increased risk of fistula thrombosis (26% of patients) [110].

Conclusion

The gold standard for the treatment of end-stage renal disease remains renal transplantation. However, due to a combination of comorbidities and socioeconomic barriers, thousands of patients remain on some form of dialysis permanently. In this chapter, we have discussed several dialysis access complications, and how to identify and prevent them.

References

1. Farrington CA, Allon M. Complications of hemodialysis catheter bloodstream infections: impact of infecting organism. Am J Nephrol. 2019;50:126–32.
2. Chaudry MS, Carlson N, Gislason GH, Kamper A-L, Rix M, Fowler VG, Torp-Pedersen C, Bruun NE. Risk of infective endocarditis in patients with end stage renal disease. Clin J Am Soc Nephrol. 2017;12:1814–22.
3. Mylonakis E, Calderwood SB. Infective endocarditis in adults. N Engl J Med. 2001;345:1318–30.
4. Yevzlin AS. Hemodialysis catheter-associated central venous stenosis. Semin Dial. 2008;21:522–7.
5. Agarwal AK. Central vein stenosis: current concepts. Adv Chronic Kidney Dis. 2009;16:360–70.
6. Lumsden AB, MJ MD, Isiklar H, Martin LG, Kikeri D, Harker LA, Allen RC. Central venous stenosis in the hemodialysis patient: incidence and efficacy of endovascular treatment. Cardiovasc Surg. 1997;5:504–9.
7. Barrett N, Spencer S, McLvor J, Brown EA. Subclavian stenosis: a major complication of subclavian dialysis catheters. Nephrol Dial Transplant. 1988;3:423–5.
8. Agarwal AK, Patel BM, Haddad NJ. Central vein stenosis: a nephrologist's perspective. Semin Dial. 2007;20:53–62.
9. Levit RD, Cohen RM, Kwak A, et al. Asymptomatic central venous stenosis in hemodialysis patients. Radiology. 2006;238:1051–6.

10. Wee IJY, Yap HY, Ts'ung LT, Qingwei SL, Tan CS, Tang TY, Chong TT. A systematic review and meta-analysis of drug-coated balloon versus conventional balloon angioplasty for dialysis access stenosis. J Vasc Surg. 2019;70:970–979.e3.
11. al Shakarchi J, Houston JG, Jones RG, Inston N. A review on the hemodialysis reliable outflow (HeRO) graft for haemodialysis vascular access. Eur J Vasc Endovasc Surg. 2015;50:108–13.
12. Kudlaty EA, Pan J, Allemang MT, Kendrick DE, Kashyap VS, Wong VL. The end stage of dialysis access: femoral graft or HeRO vascular access device. Ann Vasc Surg. 2015;29:90–7.
13. Jennings WC, Miller GA, Coburn MZ, Howard CA, Lawless MA. Vascular access flow reduction for arteriovenous fistula salvage in symptomatic patients with central venous occlusion. J Vasc Access. 2012;13:157–62.
14. Vaes RHD, van Loon M, Vaes SMM, Cuypers P, Tordoir JH, Scheltinga MR. One-year efficacy of the RUDI technique for flow reduction in high-flow autologous brachial artery-based hemodialysis vascular access. J Vasc Access. 2015;16(Suppl 9):S96–101.
15. Anaya-Ayala JE, Bellows PH, Ismail N, Cheema ZF, Naoum JJ, Bismuth J, Lumsden AB, Reardon MJ, Davies MG, Peden EK. Surgical management of hemodialysis-related central venous occlusive disease: a treatment algorithm. Ann Vasc Surg. 2011;25:108–19.
16. Maya ID, Allon M. Outcomes of tunneled femoral hemodialysis catheters: comparison with internal jugular vein catheters. Kidney Int. 2005;68:2886–9.
17. Razavi MK, Peden EK, Sorial E, Ross JR, Aruny JE, Pflederer TA, Wasse H, Haskal ZJ. Efficacy and safety associated with the use of the Surfacer® Inside-Out® access catheter system: results from a prospective, multicenter Food and Drug Administration-approved investigational device exemption study. J Vasc Access. 2021;22:141–6.
18. Lee T. Fistula first initiative: historical impact on vascular access practice patterns and influence on future vascular access care. Cardiovasc Eng Technol. 2017;8:244.
19. Saran R, Robinson B, Abbott KC, et al. US renal data system 2016 annual data report: epidemiology of kidney disease in the United States. Am J Kidney Dis. 2017;69:A7–8.
20. Almasri J, Alsawas M, Mainou M, Mustafa RA, Wang Z, Woo K, Cull DL, Murad MH. Outcomes of vascular access for hemodialysis: a systematic review and meta-analysis. J Vasc Surg. 2016;64:236–43.
21. Browne LD, Bashar K, Griffin P, Kavanagh EG, Walsh SR, Walsh MT. The role of shear stress in arteriovenous fistula maturation and failure: a systematic review. PLoS One. 2015;10:e0145795.
22. Roy-Chaudhury P, Sukhatme VP, Cheung AK. Hemodialysis vascular access dysfunction: a cellular and molecular viewpoint. J Am Soc Nephrol. 2006;17:1112–27.
23. Dixon BS, Beck GJ, Vazquez MA, et al. Effect of dipyridamole plus aspirin on hemodialysis graft patency. N Engl J Med. 2009;360:2191–201.
24. Dixon BS, Beck GJ, Dember LM, et al. Use of aspirin associates with longer primary patency of hemodialysis grafts. J Am Soc Nephrol. 2011;22:773.
25. Perry JW, Hardy D, Agarwal S, Agarwal G. Safety and efficacy of a modified HeRO dialysis device in achieving early graft cannulation: a single-institution experience. J Vasc Surg Cases Innov Tech. 2017;3:175.
26. Cohen MAH, Kumpe DA, Durham JD, Zwerdlinger SC. Improved treatment of thrombosed hemodialysis access sites with thrombolysis and angioplasty. Kidney Int. 1994;46:1375–80.
27. Neyra NR, Ikizler TA, May RE, Himmelfarb J, Schulman G, Shyr Y, Hakim RM. Change in access blood flow over time predicts vascular access thrombosis. Kidney Int. 1998;54:1714–9.
28. Daugirdas JT. *Kt/V* (and especially its modifications) remains a useful measure of hemodialysis dose. Kidney Int. 2015;88:466–73.
29. Tessitore N, Bedogna V, Poli A, Mantovani W, Lipari G, Baggio E, Mansueto G, Lupo A. Adding access blood flow surveillance to clinical monitoring reduces thrombosis rates and costs, and improves fistula patency in the short term: a controlled cohort study. Nephrol Dial Transplant. 2008;23:3578–84.
30. Moist LM, Churchill DN, House AA, Millward SF, Elliott JE, Kribs SW, Deyoung WJ, Blythe L, Stitt LW, Lindsay RM. Regular monitoring of access flow compared with monitoring of venous pressure fails to improve graft survival. J Am Soc Nephrol. 2003;14:2645–53.

31. Tordoir JHM, Bode AS, Peppelenbosch N, van der Sande FM, de Haan MW. Surgical or endovascular repair of thrombosed dialysis vascular access: is there any evidence? J Vasc Surg. 2009;50:953–6.
32. Lundström UH, Welander G, Carrero JJ, Hedin U, Evans M. Surgical versus endovascular intervention for vascular access thrombosis: a nationwide observational cohort study. Nephrol Dial Transplant. 2022;37:1742–50.
33. Ghaffarian AA, Al-Dulaimi R, Kraiss LW, Sarfati M, Griffin CL, Smith BK, Donald G, Brooke BS. Clinical effectiveness of open thrombectomy for thrombosed autogenous arteriovenous fistulas and grafts. J Vasc Surg. 2018;68(1):189–96. https://doi.org/10.1016/j.jvs.2017.12.050.
34. Robbin ML, Greene T, Allon M, et al. Prediction of arteriovenous fistula clinical maturation from postoperative ultrasound measurements: findings from the hemodialysis fistula maturation study. J Am Soc Nephrol. 2018;29:2735–44.
35. Stoumpos S, Traynor JP, Metcalfe W, Kasthuri R, Stevenson K, Mark PB, Kingsmore DB, Thomson PC. A national study of autogenous arteriovenous access use and patency in a contemporary hemodialysis population. J Vasc Surg. 2019;69:1889–98.
36. Al-Jaishi AA, Oliver MJ, Thomas SM, Lok CE, Zhang JC, Garg AX, Kosa SD, Quinn RR, Moist LM. Patency rates of the arteriovenous fistula for hemodialysis: a systematic review and meta-analysis. Am J Kidney Dis. 2014;63:464–78.
37. Allon M, Robbin ML. Increasing arteriovenous fistulas in hemodialysis patients: problems and solutions. Kidney Int. 2002;62:1109–24.
38. Huber TS, Berceli SA, Scali ST, et al. Arteriovenous fistula maturation, functional patency, and intervention rates. JAMA Surg. 2021;156:1111–9.
39. Dember LM, Beck GJ, Allon M, et al. Effect of clopidogrel on early failure of arteriovenous fistulas for hemodialysis: a randomized controlled trial. JAMA. 2008;299:2164–71.
40. Shahverdyan R, Meyer T, Matoussevitch V. Patency and functionality of radiocephalic arteriovenous fistulas with an external support device (VasQ™): real-world single-center experience. J Vasc Access. 2021;22:166–72.
41. Schild AF, Perez E, Gillaspie E, Seaver C, Livingstone J, Thibonnier A. Arteriovenous fistulae vs. arteriovenous grafts: a retrospective review of 1700 consecutive vascular access cases. J Vasc Access. 2008;9:231–5.
42. Lamarche C, Iliuta IA, Kitzler T. Infectious disease risk in dialysis patients: a transdisciplinary approach. Can J Kidney Health Dis. 2019;6:2054358119839080. https://doi.org/10.1177/2054358119839080.
43. Ryan SV, Calligaro KD, Scharff J, Dougherty MJ, DKW C, Pappas PJ, Gagne PJ, Wickel DJ. Management of infected prosthetic dialysis arteriovenous grafts. J Vasc Surg. 2004;39:73–8.
44. MacRae JM, Dipchand C, Oliver M, et al. Arteriovenous access: infection, neuropathy, and other complications. Can J Kidney Health Dis. 2016;3:2054358116669127. https://doi.org/10.1177/2054358116669127.
45. Kilic A, Arnaoutakis DJ, Reifsnyder T, Black JH, Abularrage CJ, Perler BA, Lum YW. Management of infected vascular grafts. Vasc Med. 2016;21:53–60.
46. Brunner MC, Mitchell RS, Baldwin JC, James DR, Olcott C, Mehigan JT, McDougall IR, Miller DC. Prosthetic graft infection: limitations of indium white blood cell scanning. J Vasc Surg. 1986;3:42–8.
47. Shemesh D, Goldin I, Hijazi J, Zaghal I, Berelowitz D, Verstandig A, Olsha O. A prospective randomized study of heparin-bonded graft (Propaten) versus standard graft in prosthetic arteriovenous access. J Vasc Surg. 2015;62:115–22.
48. Janeckova J, Bachleda P, Utikal P, Jarosciakova J, Orsag J. Arteriovenous grafts' types of indications and their infection rate. Ann Vasc Surg. 2020;69:232–6.
49. Liu RH, Fraser CD, Zhou X, Beaulieu RJ, Reifsnyder T. Complete versus partial excision of infected arteriovenous grafts: does remnant graft material impact outcomes? J Vasc Surg. 2020;71:174–9.

50. Walz P, Ladowski JS. Partial excision of infected fistula results in increased patency at the cost of increased risk of recurrent infection. Ann Vasc Surg. 2005;19:84–9.
51. Parisotto MT, Schoder VU, Miriunis C, Grassmann AH, Scatizzi LP, Kaufmann P, Stopper A, Marcelli D. Cannulation technique influences arteriovenous fistula and graft survival. Kidney Int. 2014;86:790.
52. Wong B, Muneer M, Wiebe N, Storie D, Shurraw S, Pannu N, Klarenbach S, Grudzinski A, Nesrallah G, Pauly RP. Buttonhole versus rope-ladder cannulation of arteriovenous fistulas for hemodialysis: a systematic review. Am J Kidney Dis. 2014;64:918–36.
53. Toma S, Shinzato T, Fukui H, Nakai S, Miwa M, Takai I, Maeda K. A timesaving method to create a fixed puncture route for the buttonhole technique. Nephrol Dial Transplant. 2003;18:2118–21.
54. Vaux E, King J, Lloyd S, Moore J, Bailey L, Reading I, Naik R. Effect of buttonhole cannulation with a polycarbonate PEG on in-center hemodialysis fistula outcomes: a randomized controlled trial. Am J Kidney Dis. 2013;62:81–8.
55. Struthers J, Allan A, Peel RK, Lambie SH. Buttonhole needling of arteriovenous fistulae: a randomized controlled trial. ASAIO J. 2010;56:319–22.
56. MacRae JM, Ahmed SB, Atkar R, Hemmelgarn BR. A randomized trial comparing buttonhole with rope ladder needling in conventional hemodialysis patients. Clin J Am Soc Nephrol. 2012;7:1632–8.
57. Chow J, Rayment G, Miguel SS, Gilbert M. A randomised controlled trial of buttonhole cannulation for the prevention of fistula access complications. J Ren Care. 2011;37:85–93.
58. Grudzinski A, Mendelssohn D, Pierratos A, Nesrallah G. A systematic review of buttonhole cannulation practices and outcomes. Semin Dial. 2013;26:465–75.
59. Staaf K, Fernström A, Uhlin F. Cannulation technique and complications in arteriovenous fistulas: a Swedish Renal Registry-based cohort study. BMC Nephrol. 2021;22:256.
60. Rajput A, Rajan DK, Simons ME, Sniderman KW, Jaskolka JD, Beecroft JR, Kachura JR, Tan KT. Venous aneurysms in autogenous hemodialysis fistulas: is there an association with venous outflow stenosis. J Vasc Access. 2013;14:126–30.
61. Jankovic A, Donfrid B, Adam J, Ilic M, Djuric Z, Damjanovic T, Popovic J, Popovic G, Radojicic Z, Dimkovic N. Arteriovenous fistula aneurysm in patients on regular hemodialysis: prevalence and risk factors. Nephron Clin Pract. 2013;124:94–8.
62. Valenti D, Mistry H, Stephenson M. A novel classification system for autogenous arteriovenous fistula aneurysms in renal access patients. Vasc Endovasc Surg. 2014;48:491–6.
63. Pasklinsky G, Meisner RJ, Labropoulos N, Leon L, Gasparis AP, Landau D, Tassiopoulos AK, Pappas PJ. Management of true aneurysms of hemodialysis access fistulas. J Vasc Surg. 2011;53:1291–7.
64. Lok CE, Huber TS, Lee T, et al. KDOQI clinical practice guideline for vascular access: 2019 update. Am J Kidney Dis. 2020;75(4 Suppl 2):S1–S164. https://doi.org/10.1053/j.ajkd.2019.12.001.
65. Baláž P, Rokošný S, Bafrnec J, Whitley A, O'Neill S. Repair of aneurysmal arteriovenous fistulae: a systematic review and meta-analysis. Eur J Vasc Endovasc Surg. 2020;59:614–23.
66. Charara J, Guidoin R, Gill F, Guzman R. Morphologic assessment of ePTFE graft wall damage following hemodialysis needle punctures. J Appl Biomater. 1990;1:279–87.
67. Ellingson KD, Palekar RS, Lucero CA, et al. Vascular access hemorrhages contribute to deaths among hemodialysis patients. Kidney Int. 2012;82:686–92.
68. Shemesh D, Goldin I, Zaghal I, Berelowitz D, Verstandig AG, Olsha O. Stent graft treatment for hemodialysis access aneurysms. J Vasc Surg. 2011;54:1088–94.
69. Najibi S, Bush RL, Terramani TT, Chaikof EL, Gunnoud AB, Lumsden AB, Weiss VJ. Covered stent exclusion of dialysis access pseudoaneurysms. J Surg Res. 2002;106:15–9.
70. Niyyar VD, Moossavi S, Vachharajani TJ. Cannulating the hemodialysis access through a stent graft—is it advisable? Clin Nephrol. 2012;77:409–12.
71. Asif A, Gadalean F, Eid N, Merrill D, Salman L. Stent graft infection and protrusion through the skin: clinical considerations and potential medico-legal ramifications. Semin Dial. 2010;23:540–2.

72. Wong WK, Su TW, Cheng WL, Yang HT, Wei WC, Ko PJ. Endovascular stent graft repair is an effective and safe alternative therapy for arteriovenous graft pseudoaneurysms. Eur J Vasc Endovasc Surg. 2016;52:682–8.
73. Beathard GA, Spergel LM. Hand ischemia associated with dialysis vascular access: an individualized access flow-based approach to therapy. Semin Dial. 2013;26:287–314.
74. Scheltinga MR, van Hoek F, Bruijninckx CMA. Time of onset in haemodialysis access-induced distal ischaemia (HAIDI) is related to the access type. Nephrol Dial Transplant. 2009;24:3198–204.
75. Huber TS, Larive B, Imrey PB, Radeva MK, Kaufman JM, Kraiss LW, Farber AM, Berceli SA. Access-related hand ischemia and the hemodialysis fistula maturation study. J Vasc Surg. 2016;64:1050–1058.e1.
76. Tordoir JHM, Dammers R, van der Sande FM. Upper extremity ischemia and hemodialysis vascular access. Eur J Vasc Endovasc Surg. 2004;27:1–5.
77. Schanzer H, Eisenberg D. Management of steal syndrome resulting from dialysis access. Semin Vasc Surg. 2004;17:45–9.
78. Goel N, Miller GA, Jotwani MC, Licht J, Schur I, Arnold WP. Minimally invasive limited ligation endoluminal-assisted revision (MILLER) for treatment of dialysis access-associated steal syndrome. Kidney Int. 2006;70:765–70.
79. Leake AE, Winger DG, Leers SA, Gupta N, Dillavou ED. Management and outcomes of dialysis access-associated steal syndrome. J Vasc Surg. 2015;61:754–61.
80. Odland MD, Kelly PH, Ney AL, Andersen RC, Bubrick MP. Management of dialysis-associated steal syndrome complicating upper extremity arteriovenous fistulas: use of intra-operative digital photoplethysmography. Surgery. 1991;110:664–9.
81. Gupta N, Yuo TH, Konig G IV, Dillavou E, Leers SA, Chaer RA, Cho JS, Makaroun MS. Treatment strategies of arterial steal after arteriovenous access. J Vasc Surg. 2011;54:162–7.
82. Wixon CL, Hughes JD, Mills JL. Specialty section: vascular surgery understanding strategies for the treatment of ischemic steal syndrome after hemodialysis access. J Am Coll Surg. 2000;191(3):301–10.
83. Gkotsis G, Jennings WC, Malik J, Mallios A, Taubman K. Treatment of high flow arteriovenous fistulas after successful renal transplant using a simple precision banding technique. Ann Vasc Surg. 2016;31:85–90.
84. Schanzer H, Schwartz M, Harrington E, Haimov M. Treatment of ischemia due to "steal" by arteriovenous fistula with distal artery ligation and revascularization. J Vasc Surg. 1988;7:770–3.
85. Misskey J, Yang C, MacDonald S, Baxter K, Hsiang Y. A comparison of revision using distal inflow and distal revascularization-interval ligation for the management of severe access-related hand ischemia. J Vasc Surg. 2016;63:1574–81.
86. Anaya-Ayala JE, Pettigrew CD, Ismail N, Diez-De Sollano AL, Syed FA, Ahmed FG, Davies MG, Peden EK. Management of dialysis access-associated "steal" syndrome with DRIL procedure: challenges and clinical outcomes. J Vasc Access. 2012;13(3):299–304. https://doi.org/10.5301/jva.5000041.
87. Loh TM, Bennett ME, Peden EK. Revision using distal inflow is a safe and effective treatment for ischemic steal syndrome and pathologic high flow after access creation. J Vasc Surg. 2016;63:441–5.
88. Huber TS, Brown MP, Seeger JM, Lee WA. Midterm outcome after the distal revascularization and interval ligation (DRIL) procedure. J Vasc Surg. 2008;48(4):926–32. https://doi.org/10.1016/J.JVS.2008.05.028.
89. Thermann F, Wollert U. Proximalization of the arterial inflow: new treatment of choice in patients with advanced dialysis shunt-associated steal syndrome? Ann Vasc Surg. 2009;23:485–90.
90. Zanow J, Kruger U, Scholz H. Proximalization of the arterial inflow: a new technique to treat access-related ischemia. J Vasc Surg. 2006;43:1216–21.

91. Guyton AC, Sagawa K. Compensations of cardiac output and other circulatory functions in areflex dogs with large A-V fistulas. Am J Phys. 1961;200:1157–63.
92. Holman E. Abnormal arteriovenous communications. Great variability of effects with particular reference to delayed development of cardiac failure. Circulation. 1965;32:1001–9.
93. Reddy YNV, Obokata M, Dean PG, Melenovsky V, Nath KA, Borlaug BA. Long-term cardiovascular changes following creation of arteriovenous fistula in patients with end stage renal disease. Eur Heart J. 2017;38:1913–23.
94. Stack AG, Bloembergen WE. A cross-sectional study of the prevalence and clinical correlates of congestive heart failure among incident US dialysis patients. Am J Kidney Dis. 2001;38:992–1000.
95. Dixon BS, Lisa N, Jerry F. Hemodialysis vascular access survival: upper-arm native arteriovenous fistula. Am J Kidney Dis. 2002;39:92–101.
96. Pandeya S, Lindsay RM. The relationship between cardiac output and access flow during hemodialysis. ASAIO J. 1999;45:135–8.
97. Basile C, Lomonte C, Vernaglione L, Casucci F, Antonelli M, Losurdo N. The relationship between the flow of arteriovenous fistula and cardiac output in haemodialysis patients. Nephrol Dial Transplant. 2008;23:282–7.
98. Miller GA, Hwang WW. Challenges and management of high-flow arteriovenous fistulae. Semin Nephrol. 2012;32:545–50.
99. MacRae JM, Pandeya S, Humen DP, Krivitski N, Lindsay RM. Arteriovenous fistula-associated high-output cardiac failure: a review of mechanisms. Am J Kidney Dis. 2004;43:e21.1–6.
100. Gerrickens MWM, Vaes RHD, Wiersma V, van Kuijk SMJ, Snoeijs MG, Govaert B, Scheltinga MR. Revision using distal inflow for high flow hemodialysis access alters arterial flow characteristics in the dialysis arm. J Vasc Surg. 2020;71:920–8.
101. Vaes RHD, van Loon M, Vaes SMM, Cuypers P, Tordoir JH, Scheltinga MR. One-year efficacy of the RUDI technique for flow reduction in high-flow autologous brachial artery-based hemodialysis vascular. J Vasc Access. 2015;16:S96–S101. https://doi.org/10.5301/jva.5000357.
102. Nojima T, Motomiya Y. Graft inclusion technique: a new flow reduction procedure for high flow arteriovenous fistulae. Ann Vasc Dis. 2018;11:202–9.
103. Florescu MC, Plumb TJ, Westphal S, Mullane R, Reilly DA. Liposuction used to treat deep vascular accesses for hemodialysis. J Vasc Access. 2021;22:115–20.
104. Inkollu S, Wellen J, Beller Z, Zhang T, Vachharajani N, Shenoy S. Successful use of minimal incision superficialization technique for arteriovenous fistula maturation. J Vasc Surg. 2016;63:1018–25.
105. Bourquelot P, Tawakol JB, Gaudric J, Natário A, Franco G, Turmel-Rodrigues L, van Laere O, Raynaud A. Lipectomy as a new approach to secondary procedure superficialization of direct autogenous forearm radial-cephalic arteriovenous accesses for hemodialysis. J Vasc Surg. 2009;50(2):369–74. https://doi.org/10.1016/J.JVS.2009.03.009.
106. Fontenot DT, Tanious A, Arhuidese I, Chauhan YM, Stafford AM, Illig KA. Arteriovenous access superficialization: a new technique and review of options. Ann Vasc Surg. 2020;69:43–51.
107. Napoli M, Prudenzano R, Russo F, Antonaci AL, Aprile M, Buongiorno E. Juxta-anastomotic stenosis of native arteriovenous fistulas: surgical treatment versus percutaneous transluminal angioplasty. J Vasc Access. 2010;11:346–51.
108. Argyriou C, Schoretsanitis N, Georgakarakos EI, Georgiadis GS, Lazarides MK. Preemptive open surgical vs. Endovascular repair for juxta-anastomotic stenoses of autogenous av fistulae: a meta-analysis. J Vasc Access. 2015;16:454–8. https://doi.org/10.5301/jva.5000444.
109. Harwood LE, Wilson BM, Oudshoorn A. Improving vascular access outcomes: attributes of arteriovenous fistula cannulation success. Clin Kidney J. 2016;9:303.
110. Lee T, Barker J, Allon M. Needle infiltration of arteriovenous fistulae in hemodialysis: risk factors and consequences. Am J Kidney Dis. 2006;47:1020–6.

Anemia in Dialysis Patients

6

Ana Flávia Moura, Joan Araujo Oliveira Moitinho, Lucas G. da Luz, José H. R. Suassuna, and José A. Moura-Neto

Introduction

Anemia is a frequent complication of chronic kidney disease (CKD) [1]. Its prevalence increases with the progression of CKD [2, 3], reaching 90% in some populations on dialysis [4]. Furthermore, anemia is associated with reduced quality of life, cognitive impairment, increased risk of cardiovascular diseases, hospitalization, and mortality [5–7].

Anemia is defined by hemoglobin concentration levels below 13 g/dL among adult males and postmenopausal women and under 12 g/dL among premenopausal women [8]. In general, anemia in CKD patients is normochromic, normocytic, and hypoproliferative [5].

The etiology of anemia in chronic kidney disease is multifactorial. However, the primary cause is erythropoietin (EPO) deficiency. Iron deficiency is also an important pathogenetic mechanism for the development of anemia [9, 10]. Reduced glomerular filtration rate, pro-inflammatory state, frequent blood transfusions, iron load, and vitamin D deficiency lead to increased hepcidin levels. Hepcidin is crucial in reducing iron absorption and release from iron stores [11, 12].

Other factors may contribute to the perpetuation of anemia: bleeding, vitamin B12/folate deficiency, hemoglobinopathies, hypothyroidism, hyperparathyroidism,

A. F. Moura · J. A. Moura-Neto (✉)
Bahiana School of Medicine and Public Health, Salvador, Bahia, Brazil
e-mail: mouraneto@bahiana.edu.br

J. A. O. Moitinho · J. H. R. Suassuna
Clinical and Academic Unit of Nephrology, Hospital Universitário Pedro Ernesto, Faculty of Medical Sciences, Rio de Janeiro State University, Rio de Janeiro, Brazil

L. G. da Luz
Moinhos de Vento Hospital, Porto Alegre, Rio Grande do Sul, Brazil

S. Z. Fadem et al. (eds.), *Complications in Dialysis*,
https://doi.org/10.1007/978-3-031-44557-6_6

underdialysis, infection or inflammation, malignancy, bone marrow disorders, hemolysis, and poor adherence to therapy [5, 13, 14].

Complementary investigations are essential to achieve a differential diagnosis and implement appropriate treatment [15]. The initial assessment includes complete blood count, absolute reticulocyte count, serum ferritin level, serum transferrin saturation (TSAT), serum vitamin B12, and folate levels [15].

At times, additional tests may be necessary, especially in cases where there is no appropriate response to the initial treatment and there is suspect of hyporesponsiveness to erythropoietin [11, 12].

Risks and Complications of Anemia

Anemia is frequently associated with high morbidity and mortality in dialysis patients [16]. In addition, anemia, especially in severe cases, reduces health-related quality of life (HRQOL) [16]. Observational studies suggest that anemia in dialysis patients increases the risk of hospitalization, cardiovascular events such as heart failure, cardiomyopathies, and mortality [17].

A prospective study followed 433 patients from the initiation of ESRD therapy for periods of up to 10 years and analyzed the impact of anemia on echocardiographic abnormalities, cardiac morbidity, and mortality [17]. The study demonstrated that each 1 g/dL decrease in mean hemoglobin level was associated with a 42% increased likelihood of having LV dilatation on a second echocardiogram [17]. In this same study, it was found that each 1 g/dL decreases in mean hemoglobin level while on dialysis therapy was independently associated with the development of either de novo or recurrent cardiac failure (RR = 1.18; $P = 0.008$), de novo cardiac failure (RR = 1.28; $P = 0.048$), recurrent cardiac failure (RR = 1.20; $P = 0.046$), and death while on dialysis therapy (RR = 1.14; $P = 0.024$) [17].

Anemia is also often associated with reduced quality of life. Some typical symptoms of anemic syndrome may explain this impact, such as headache, cognitive impairment, and fatigue, the most common symptom of anemia [18, 19]. Such symptoms interfere with the quality of life by compromising the functional capacity of patients, impairing the sense of well-being.

Targets

Until the end of the 1980s, the treatment of anemia in dialysis patients was based on blood transfusions and, less frequently, androgenic therapies. The perspective of this treatment was altered after 1989 when a large study evaluated the effect of rHuEPO in the correction of anemia among CKD patients. This trial promoted a significant reduction in blood transfusion rates, from 0.52 to 0.03 units per patient, after only 2 months of treatment [20]. In the same year, the FDA approved the use of ESAs. Until then, the main parameter used to monitor treatment was a hematocrit test, with a recommended target between 30 and 33% and a suggestion to discontinue the use of the drug when hematocrit levels were above 36% [21].

Since then several studies have been carried out in order to establish the ideal target to treat anemia in CKD patients. It is known that a hemoglobin target close to that recommended for the general population provides some benefits, such as better quality of life, regression of left ventricular hypertrophy (LVH), better tolerance to physical activity, reduction of CKD progression, and increased survival [22–29]. On the other hand, high hemoglobin levels increase blood viscosity, resulting in a higher risk of thrombotic events and lower solute clearance [30, 31].

The Normal Hematocrit Study (NHS), a breakthrough trial that determined the currently recommended targets for anemia treatment in CKD patients, evaluated dialysis patients with congestive heart failure or ischemic heart disease, comparing high (14.0 g/dL) and low hemoglobin levels (10.0 g/dL). The trial had to be stopped due to the significantly higher rate of adverse events (vascular access thrombosis, acute myocardial infarction, and cardiovascular death) in the high hemoglobin group [30]. Several other clinical trials and metanalyses have confirmed the increased risk of overall mortality and thrombotic events among dialysis patients treated to achieve normal hemoglobin levels, as well as the lack of significant benefits in quality of life [30, 32–35].

Therefore, the main guidelines to manage anemia in CKD patients recommend hemoglobin levels above 9.0 g/dL and suggest keeping it between 10.0 and 12.0 g/dL, with small variations among those guidelines [15, 36–38]. All guidelines contraindicate hemoglobin levels above 12.0 g/dL, due to the increased risk of thrombotic events.

Treatment of Anemia in Dialysis Patients

Iron deficiency is the most common cause of anemia, even among dialysis patients, and is usually present in more than 50% of these patients [15]. The factors associated with iron deficiency in this population are diverse: frequent blood collections, bleeding associated with surgical procedures (vascular accesses) and blood loss in the dialysis circuit, gastrointestinal bleeding, and interference of medications in iron absorption (inhibitors of gastric acid and phosphate binders) [39–41]. Thus, the etiology of anemia should always be investigated, at any stage of CKD, before initiating treatment.

According to the Kidney Disease Improving Global Outcomes (KDIGO), the initial evaluation of anemia in CKD patients includes complete blood count, reticulocyte count, serum ferritin, transferrin saturation (TSAT), serum vitamin B12 and folate levels [15]. More comprehensive assessments can be performed in specific cases, especially if there is a poor response to drug treatment [13, 15].

The treatment of anemia should be initiated whenever the patient presents hemoglobin levels lower than 9.0 g/dL [15, 36–38]. Among the evaluated parameters, serum ferritin and TSAT are the tests used to indicate iron replacement therapies [15]. Once iron deficiency is confirmed, and without contraindications, iron replacement should be initiated, with the intravenous route being preferable for patients on dialysis [42].

Table 6.1 Parameters for indication of IV iron replacement in dialysis patients with hemoglobin <9.0 g/dL

Guidelines	Serum ferritin (ng/mL)	TSAT
KDIGO 2012	≤500	≤30%
European Best Practice 2013	≤300	≤25% *Without ESA: ≤30%
KDOQI 2013	≤500	≤30%
NICE 2015	<100	<20%

*recommendation
IV intravenous, *TSAT* transferrin saturation, *KDIGO* Kidney Disease Improving Global Outcomes, *KDOQI* Kidney Disease Outcomes Quality Initiative, *NICE* National Institute for Health and Care Excellence, *ESA* erythropoiesis-stimulating agents

Table 6.2 Recommended parameters for discontinuation of IV iron replacement in dialysis patients

Guidelines	Serum ferritin	TSAT
KDIGO 2012	>500 ng/mL	>30%
European Best Practice 2013	>500 ng/dL	>30%
KDOQI 2013	No specific recommendation *Maintain replacement when TSAT ≤30%, even when ferritin >500 ng/mL	
NICE 2015	> 800 ng/mL *Evaluate if >500 ng/dL	–

*recommendation
IV intravenous, *TSAT* transferrin saturation, *KDIGO* Kidney Disease Improving Global Outcomes, *KDOQI* Kidney Disease Outcomes Quality Initiative, *NICE* National Institute for Health and Care Excellence

The recommended ferritin and TSAT values to initiate IV iron therapy are similar among the main guidelines. These data are summarized in Table 6.1. In general, the guidelines recommend initiating iron replacement when TSAT <30% and ferritin <500 ng/dL, with small variations among them.

Regarding the parameters for discontinuation of IV iron therapy, there are also a few variations in the recommendations of the main guidelines. However, in general, stopping iron replacement should be considered when ferritin >500 ng/dL. Such recommendations are listed in Table 6.2.

It is worth noting that the consequences associated with the long-term use of IV iron replacement are yet unclear. It is known that aggressive IV iron replacement strategies are associated with increased morbidity and mortality, as well as complications associated with infection and tissue iron accumulation [43, 44].

Intravenous iron therapy should aim to provide the lowest dose capable of replenishing iron stores [45–47]. In addition, the decision regarding the type of IV iron used must be individualized. It should be taken into consideration the main adverse reactions associated with each drug. Preparation and infusion time

Table 6.3 Hemoglobin levels recommended by the main guidelines for treatment of anemia in dialysis patients

Guidelines	Start of ESA (g/dL)	Hemoglobin target (g/dL)	Do not use ESA (g/dL)
KDIGO 2012	<9.0	10.0–12.0	>13.0
European Best Practice 2013	<10.0	10.0–12.0	>13.0
KDOQI 2013	<10.0	10.0–11.0	>13.0
NICE 2015	<10.0	10.0–12.0	>13.0

ESA erythropoiesis-stimulating agents, *KDIGO* Kidney Disease Improving Global Outcomes, *KDOQI* Kidney Disease Outcomes Quality Initiative, *NICE* National Institute for Health and Care Excellence

recommendations by each manufacturer should also be followed in order to reduce the risk of hypersensitivity reactions.

The benefits associated with the use of ESAs are well established and include improvement in quality of life, reduction in blood transfusion rates, and the risk of myocardial ischemia associated with anemia [25–27, 30, 31, 34, 35, 48–50]. However, the risks associated with ESAs should not be forgotten. These include an increased risk of thrombotic events, worsening of arterial hypertension, and potential for tumor progression [25–27, 31, 34, 35, 48–50]. Thus, current guidelines recommend that alternative causes of anemia must be ruled out before initiating the use of ESAs.

In general, the main guidelines advise initiating ESAs for patients with a hemoglobin <10.0 g/dL, avoiding levels as low as 9.0 g/dL, and suggesting maintaining hemoglobin concentration between 10.0 and 12.0 g/dL, with small variations among guidelines. Continued therapy with ESAs is considered inappropriate when hemoglobin >13.0 g/dL [27, 33–35, 51]. Table 6.3 summarizes the recommendations of the main guidelines.

Some patients may have an unsatisfactory response to ESAs. According to KDIGO, hyporesponsiveness can be diagnosed when there is no response after 1 month of treatment with an optimized dose [15]. In turn, KDOQI considers it necessary to observe the patient for at least 2 months before classifying them as hyporesponsive [35]. Regardless of the source used, it is consensual that the diagnosis of hyporesponsiveness to ESAs should only be made after ruling out other causes of anemia. Even in confirmed cases of hyporesponsiveness, it is not advisable to increase the dose of ESAs beyond twice the usual dose [15].

Blood transfusion should be avoided in dialysis patients since it is associated with the risk of viral, bacterial, or parasitic infections [52, 53], as well as a variety of transfusion reactions [53–58]. The cases that most commonly result in the need for blood transfusions are acute severe bleeding, patients with unstable coronary artery disease, the need for urgent preoperative hemoglobin correction, and when ESA therapy is not effective (hemoglobinopathies, bone marrow failure) [15, 36, 59].

Special attention should be given to kidney transplant candidates as blood transfusions increase the risk of sensitization to HLA antigens, resulting in increased waiting time for transplantation and reduced graft survival [52].

Novel Therapies

Hypoxia-Inducible Factor Prolyl Hydroxylase Inhibitors (HIF-PHIs)

HIF-PHIs mimic the cellular response to reduced oxygen levels, with a concomitant increase in HIF activity, which in turn activates endogenous EPO production and stimulate erythropoiesis. HIF-PHIs have also been shown to be effective in indirectly reducing hepcidin levels [60, 61], leading to increased intestinal iron absorption and release of iron from macrophages and hepatocytes [62, 63].

HIF-PHIs are oral medications prescribed in 1–3 times a week regimens. Therefore, they are expected to facilitate therapeutic adherence. Furthermore, this drug class has been shown to be at least as effective and safe in the treatment of anemia in patients on hemodialysis and peritoneal dialysis as medications already used [51, 64–66].

The main adverse effects associated with HIF-PHIs are vascular calcification, increased risk of thrombotic events, increased pulmonary arterial pressure, and hyperkalemia [67, 68]. Roxadustat, daprodustat, and vadadustat are all part of this new class [62, 63, 69–71].

Direct Analogues of rEPO

rEPO analogues, such as darbepoetin alfa and methoxy polyethylene glycol-epoetin beta (methoxy PEG-epoetin beta) have shown good response in the treatment of anemia. These medications are extended-release molecules referred to as 'biobetter,' and their prolonged presence in the bloodstream is partly because of a reduced binding affinity to Epo receptor molecules (EpoR) [72] and are also. The half-life of methoxy PEG-epoetin beta, in its intravenous presentation, is 130–140 h [73]. One of the greatest advantage of the "biobetters" is to allow the reduction of the EPO dose below the commonly used ratio of 1:200 [73].

Other Therapies

Some innovative therapeutic possibilities are being studied to treat anemia in CKD patients. Sotatercept and luspatercept are recombinant human fusion proteins capable of binding and inhibiting activin, and other members of the TGF-β superfamily are also involved in erythropoiesis [74, 75]. The mechanism of action underlying the increased production and release of mature erythrocytes is poorly understood. GATA-2 inhibitors that act by depressing EPO synthesis, antihepcidin drugs, and ferroportin agonists/stabilizers may also contribute in the future to the better management of anemia in CKD [76–78].

Anemia and Special Conditions in Dialysis Patients

Anemia and Surgical Clearance

The preoperative care of ESKD patients aims to reduce the need for blood transfusions and avoid the immunological risk of a future kidney transplant. For surgical planning, there is no recommendation of KDIGO guidelines to aim a higher target preoperatively than the standard for patients with CKD [15, 79]. Reassessments of ESA and iron stocks should be performed, as well as a search for bleeding and causes of ESA resistance if the target is not achieved. A postoperative increase of iron and ESA doses might be necessary to allow correction of surgery-induced anemia [80]. Urgent surgery is one of the few situations where the KDIGO suggests red cell transfusion, mainly with Hb is <7 g/dL [15].

Sickle Cell Disease in Dialysis Patients

Previous data suggest that the use of ESAs in sickle cell disease patients is associated with an increase in veno-occlusive episodes. However, other studies did not confirm this assumption, and nowadays most guidelines recommend associating ESA with hydroxyurea in the worsening of SCD-related anemia among ESKD patients [81]. Using ESAs reduces the need for transfusion but does not eliminate it. SCD patients are an exception since the hemoglobin target might not exceed 10.0 mg/dL in order to avoid an increase in viscosity. Probably, hemoglobin levels between 8.0 and 9.0 mg/dL might be the optimal range [82]. When feasible, co-management with a hematologist is recommended.

Myelodysplastic Syndrome in Dialysis Patients

In case of no bleeding and resistance to ESAs, the clinical reasoning will lead to hematologic dysplasia and neoplasia.

Myelodysplastic syndromes (MDS) are a heterogeneous group of acquired clonal disorders defined by ineffective hematopoiesis with dysplasia in one or several hematopoietic cell lineages leading to cytopenia. They can also worsen anemia in ESKD patients [83]. The disease can be categorized into low- and high risk based on prognosis [84]. Most MDS respond to ESA [85]. It is interesting to note that patients who had a diagnosis of MDS before entering dialysis seem to have better outcomes compared with those diagnosed after initiating renal replacement therapy [86].

The incidence of MDS seems to increase over time among dialysis patients. This is hypothetically related to chronic exposure to TNF and other cytokines [87]. KDIGO categorize MDS as a particular case considering that not every MDS has responded to ESA [15]. However, those that do respond can take more than a month to increase hemoglobin levels.

It is also a fact that MDS patients might need higher doses of ESA. Hypoxia-inducible factor prolyl hydroxylase inhibitors (HIF-PHIs) might be a new option for these cases [88].

Anemia and Malignancies in Dialysis Patients

There is also a special recommendation about anemia and CKD related to cancer, myeloma, lymphoma, and amyloidosis in dialysis patients regarding the effect of ESA in this special population. Treating anemia with erythropoietin is one of the few pharmacological interventions that reduce the severity of fatigue in this population [89]. Unsurprisingly, when we look at CKD patients, the level of evidence decreases.

A post-hoc analysis of the TREAT study has shown higher mortality among patients with malignancy who underwent an ESA treatment [90]. Based on this data, the American Society of Hematology (ASH) and KDIGO advise great caution when using ESAs on these patients, especially when the cure is the anticipated outcome [15, 91]. ASH suggests avoiding the initiation of ESA therapy in patients with malignancy and Hb levels ≥10.0 g/dL. It also recommends discontinuing the therapy if there is no response in 6–8 weeks. KDIGO suggests initiating ESA therapy before Hb concentration levels fall below 8.0 mg/dL. However, there is an exception, even in the context of neoplasia, that EPO can be used as adjuvant therapy without evidence of an increase in mortality, such as in small-cell lung cancer [92]. As a general recommendation, the National Comprehensive Cancer Network (NCCN) suggests an individualized approach and the avoidance of ESA use in patients receiving active therapy. On the other hand, the use of ESAs should be considered in lieu of transfusions to treat severe anemia [93].

Acute Hemolysis

A small degree of hemolysis occurs during hemodialysis without causing significant anemia [94, 95]. However, acute hemolysis associated with hemodialysis is a rare complication, and it can be associated with considerable morbidity and mortality [96, 97]. Hemolysis can manifest itself through nausea, vomiting, and even severe symptoms such as precordial pain, back pain, arterial hypertension, dyspnea, and cyanosis, as well as cherry-red blood in the venous line [95]. Several factors can lead to hemolytic disease in dialysis patients, and these causes are listed in Table 6.4 [93, 94, 97–101].

Table 6.4 Causes of hemolytic disease in dialysis patients

Patient related	Dialysate related	Mechanical
Sickle cell anemia	Contamination by formaldehyde, peracetic acid, sodium hypochlorite, chloramines, copper, zinc, nitrate, and nitrite	Kinks or narrowing in hemodialysis circuit
Hereditary spherocytosis	Heated dialysate (failure of heating system, thermostat, and temperature gauge)	High blood flow through small-caliber needles
Autoimmune hemolytic anemia	Hypo-osmolar dialysate	Poor needle positioning
Malignant hypertension	Use of hypotonic solutions when priming	Partially obstructed catheter
Hypersplenism		
Mechanical valves		
G6PD deficiency		

Laboratory diagnosis should be confirmed with hematocrit, potassium, lactate dehydrogenase, haptoglobin, reticulocyte count, bilirubin, and Coombs test [95, 97]. Dialysis should be stopped immediately if hemolysis is suspected. The blood should not be returned to the patient due to the risk of severe hyperkalemia. Support measures such as oxygen supply and maintenance of hemodynamic stability may be required [94–96].

Conclusion

Anemia in dialysis patients is associated with increased morbidity and mortality. The use of recombinant erythropoietin significantly modified the treatment of anemia, reducing the need for frequent blood transfusions and leading to a significant improvement in quality of life. The association of CKD with other comorbidities is an additional challenge in the management of these patients.

Over the past few years, several studies have been carried out aiming to establish ideal hemoglobin levels and appropriate iron replacement, in order to reduce adverse effects caused by treatment. Among the new treatments being studied, hypoxia-inducible factor prolyl hydroxylase inhibitors appear to be the most promising in the management of anemia in CKD patients.

References

1. McClellan WM, Flanders WD, Langston RD, Jurkovitz C, Presley R. Anemia and renal insufficiency are independent risk factors for death among patients with congestive heart failure admitted to community hospitals: a population-based study. J Am Soc Nephrol. 2002;13(7):1928–36.
2. Minutolo R, Provenzano M, Chiodini P, Borrelli S, Garofalo C, Andreucci M, Liberti ME, Bellizzi V, Conte G, De Nicola L, Collaborative Study Group on the Conservative Treatment of CKD of the Italian Society of Nephrology. New-onset anemia and associated risk of ESKD

and death in non-dialysis CKD patients: a multicohort observational study. Clin Kidney J. 2022;15(6):1120–8.

3. Palaka E, Grandy S, van Haalen H, et al. The impact of CKD anaemia on patients: incidence, risk factors, and clinical outcomes: a systematic literature review. Int J Nephrol. 2020;2020:7692376.
4. Chen N, Hao C, Liu BC, Lin H, Wang C, Xing C, Liang X, Jiang G, Liu Z, Li X, Zuo L, Luo L, Wang J, Zhao MH, Liu Z, Cai GY, Hao L, Leong R, Wang C, Liu C, Neff T, Szczech L, Yu KP. Roxadustat treatment for anemia in patients undergoing long-term dialysis. N Engl J Med. 2019;381(11):1011–22.
5. Babitt JL, Lin HY. Mechanisms of anemia in CKD. J Am Soc Nephrol. 2012;23:1631–4.
6. Li S, Foley RN, Collins AJ. Anemia and cardiovascular disease, hospitalization, end stage renal disease, and death in older patients with chronic kidney disease. Int Urol Nephrol. 2005;37(2):395–402.
7. Soni RK, Weisbord SD, Unruh ML. Health-related quality of life outcomes in chronic kidney disease. Curr Opin Nephrol Hypertens. 2010;19(2):153–9.
8. Anonymous. Nutritional anaemias. Report of a WHO scientific group. World Health Organ Tech Rep Ser. 1968;405:5–37.
9. Bruce G, Schulga P, Reynolds BC. Use of erythropoiesis-stimulating agents in children with chronic kidney disease: a systematic review. Clin Kidney J. 2022;15(8):1483–505.
10. Zadrazil J, Horak P. Pathophysiology of anemia in chronic kidney diseases: a review. Biomed Pap Med Fac Univ Palacky Olomouc Czech Repub. 2015;159(2):197–202.
11. Coyne DW. Hepcidin: clinical utility as a diagnostic tool and therapeutic target. Kidney Int. 2011;80(3):240–4.
12. Panwar B, Gutiérrez OM. Disorders of iron metabolism and anemia in chronic kidney disease. Semin Nephrol. 2016;36(4):252–61.
13. Elliott J, Mishler D, Agarwal R. Hyporesponsiveness to erythropoietin: causes and management. Adv Chronic Kidney Dis. 2009;16(2):94–100.
14. Nangaku M, Mimura I, Yamaguchi J, Higashijima Y, Wada T, Tanaka T. Role of uremic toxins in erythropoiesis-stimulating agent resistance in chronic kidney disease and dialysis patients. J Ren Nutr. 2015;25(2):160–3.
15. KDIGO Anemia Work Group. KDIGO clinical practice Guideline for anemia in chronic kidney disease. Kidney Int Suppl. 2012;2(4):279–335.
16. Locatelli F, Pisoni RL, Combe C, et al. Anaemia in haemodialysis patients of five European countries: association with morbidity and mortality in the dialysis outcomes and practice patterns study (DOPPS). Nephrol Dial Transplant. 2004;19:121–32.
17. Foley RN, Parfrey PS, Harnett JD, Kent GM, Murray DC, Barre PE. The impact of anemia on cardiomyopathy, morbidity, and mortality in end-stage renal disease. Am J Kidney Dis. 1996;28(1):53–61. https://doi.org/10.1016/s0272-6386(96)90130-4.
18. Pecorelli S. Suboptimal hemoglobin levels: do they impact patients and their therapy? Semin Oncol. 2000;27(suppl 4):1–3.
19. Holzner B, Kemmler G, Greil R, et al. The impact of hemoglobin levels on fatigue and quality of life in cancer patients. Ann Oncol. 2002;13(6):965–73.
20. Eschbach JW, Abdulhadi MH, Browne JK, Delano BG, Downing MR, Egrie JC, et al. Recombinant human erythropoietin in anemic patients with end-stage renal disease. Results of a phase III multicenter clinical trial. Ann Intern Med. 1989;111(12):992–1000.
21. Procrit [package insert]. Thousand Oaks: Amgen Inc.; 1993.
22. Kuriyama S, Tomonari H, Yoshida H, Hashimoto T, Kawaguchi Y, Sakai O. Reversal of anemia by erythropoietin therapy retards the progression of chronic renal failure, especially in nondiabetic patients. Nephron. 1997;77(2):176–85.
23. Silberberg JS, Rahal DP, Patton DR, Sniderman AD. Role of anemia in the pathogenesis of left ventricular hypertrophy in end-stage renal disease. Am J Cardiol. 1989;64(3):222–4.

24. National Kidney Foundation Anemia Working Group. NKF-DOQI clinical practice guidelines for the treatment of anemia of chronic renal failure. National Kidney Foundation-dialysis outcomes quality initiative. Am J Kidney Dis. 1997;30(4 Suppl 3):S192–240.
25. Auer J, Simon G, Stevens J, Griffiths P, Howarth D, Anastassiades E, et al. Quality of life improvements in CAPD patients treated with subcutaneously administered erythropoietin for anemia. Perit Dial Int. 1992;12(1):40–2.
26. Paganini EP. In search of an optimal hematocrit level in dialysis patients: rehabilitation and quality-of-life implications. Am J Kidney Dis. 1994;24(1 Suppl 1):S10–6.
27. Revicki DA, Brown RE, Feeny DH, Henry D, Teehan BP, Rudnick MR, et al. Health-related quality of life associated with recombinant human erythropoietin therapy for predialysis chronic renal disease patients. Am J Kidney Dis. 1995;25(4):548–54.
28. Ritz E, Zeier M, Schneider P, Jones E. Cardiovascular mortality of patients with polycystic kidney disease on dialysis: is there a lesson to learn? Nephron. 1994;66(2):125–8.
29. Silberberg J, Racine N, Barre P, Sniderman AD. Regression of left ventricular hypertrophy in dialysis patients following correction of anemia with recombinant human erythropoietin. Can J Cardiol. 1990;6(1):1–4.
30. Foley RN, Curtis BM, Parfrey PS. Hemoglobin targets and blood transfusions in hemodialysis patients without symptomatic cardiac disease receiving erythropoietin therapy. Clin J Am Soc Nephrol. 2008;3(6):1669–75.
31. Junor BJ. Hematocrit above 30% in continuous ambulatory peritoneal dialysis patients treated with erythropoietin is harmful. Perit Dial Int. 1993;13(Suppl 2):S535–7.
32. Drueke TB, Locatelli F, Clyne N, Eckardt KU, Macdougall IC, Tsakiris D, et al. Normalization of hemoglobin level in patients with chronic kidney disease and anemia. N Engl J Med. 2006;355(20):2071–84.
33. Singh AK, Szczech L, Tang KL, Barnhart H, Sapp S, Wolfson M, et al. Correction of anemia with epoetin alfa in chronic kidney disease. N Engl J Med. 2006;355(20):2085–98.
34. Coyne DW. The health-related quality of life was not improved by targeting higher hemoglobin in the Normal hematocrit trial. Kidney Int. 2012;82(2):235–41.
35. Phrommintikul A, Haas SJ, Elsik M, Krum H. Mortality and target haemoglobin concentrations in anaemic patients with chronic kidney disease treated with erythropoietin: a meta-analysis. Lancet. 2007;369(9559):381–8.
36. Locatelli F, Barany P, Covic A, De Francisco A, Del Vecchio L, Goldsmith D, et al. Kidney disease: improving global outcomes guidelines on anaemia management in chronic kidney disease: a European Renal Best Practice position statement. Nephrol Dial Transplant. 2013;28(6):1346–59.
37. Kliger AS, Foley RN, Goldfarb DS, Goldstein SL, Johansen K, Singh A, et al. KDOQI US commentary on the 2012 KDIGO clinical practice Guideline for anemia in CKD. Am J Kidney Dis. 2013;62(5):849–59.
38. Padhi S, Glen J, Pordes BA, Thomas ME, Guideline Development Group. Management of anaemia in chronic kidney disease: summary of updated NICE guidance. BMJ. 2015;350:h2258.
39. Ganz T. Hepcidin and iron regulation, 10 years later. Blood. 2011;117(17):4425–33.
40. Rosenblatt SG, Drake S, Fadem S, Welch R, Lifschitz MD. Gastrointestinal blood loss in patients with chronic renal failure. Am J Kidney Dis. 1982;1(4):232–6.
41. Sargent JA, Acchiardo SR. Iron requirements in hemodialysis. Blood Purif. 2004;22(1):112–23.
42. Shepshelovich D, Rozen-Zvi B, Avni T, Gafter U, Gafter-Gvili A. Intravenous versus oral iron supplementation for the treatment of anemia in CKD: an updated systematic review and meta-analysis. Am J Kidney Dis. 2016;68(5):677–90.
43. Li X, Cole SR, Kshirsagar AV, Fine JP, Sturmer T, Brookhart MA. Safety of dynamic intravenous iron administration strategies in hemodialysis patients. Clin J Am Soc Nephrol. 2019;14(5):728–37.
44. Macdougall IC, White C, Anker SD, Bhandari S, Farrington K, Kalra PA, et al. Randomized trial comparing proactive, high-dose versus reactive, low-dose intravenous iron supple-

mentation in hemodialysis (PIVOTAL): study design and baseline data. Am J Nephrol. 2018;48(4):260–8.
45. Gabrielsen JS, Gao Y, Simcox JA, Huang J, Thorup D, Jones D, et al. Adipocyte iron regulates adiponectin and insulin sensitivity. J Clin Invest. 2012;122(10):3529–40.
46. Wish JB, Aronoff GR, Bacon BR, Brugnara C, Eckardt KU, Ganz T, et al. Positive iron balance in chronic kidney disease: how much is too much and how to tell? Am J Nephrol. 2018;47(2):72–83.
47. Wlazlo N, van Greevenbroek MM, Ferreira I, Jansen EH, Feskens EJ, van der Kallen CJ, et al. Iron metabolism is associated with adipocyte insulin resistance and plasma adiponectin: the Cohort on Diabetes and Atherosclerosis Maastricht (CODAM) study. Diabetes Care. 2013;36(2):309–15.
48. Bazeley J, Wish JB. The evolution of target hemoglobin levels in anemia of chronic kidney disease. Adv Chronic Kidney Dis. 2019;26(4):229–36.
49. Krapf R, Hulter HN. Arterial hypertension induced by erythropoietin and erythropoiesis-stimulating agents (ESAs). Clin J Am Soc Nephrol. 2009;4(2):470–80.
50. Tonia T, Mettler A, Robert N, Schwarzer G, Seidenfeld J, Weingart O, et al. Erythropoietin or darbepoetin for patients with cancer. Cochrane Database Syst Rev. 2012;12:Cd003407.
51. Sugahara M, Tanaka T, Nangaku M. Prolyl hydroxylase domain inhibitors as a novel therapeutic approach against anemia in chronic kidney disease. Kidney Int. 2017;92(2):306–12.
52. Brenner N, Kommalapati A, Ahsan M, Ganguli A. Red cell transfusion in chronic kidney disease in the United States in the current era of erythropoiesis stimulating agents. J Nephrol. 2020;33(2):267–75.
53. Tanhehco YC, Berns JS. Red blood cell transfusion risks in patients with end-stage renal disease. Semin Dial. 2012;25(5):539–44.
54. Alam A, Lin Y, Lima A, Hansen M, Callum JL. The prevention of transfusion-associated circulatory overload. Transfus Med Rev. 2013;27(2):105–12.
55. Carson JL, Guyatt G, Heddle NM, Grossman BJ, Cohn CS, Fung MK, et al. Clinical practice guidelines from the AABB: red blood cell transfusion thresholds and storage. JAMA. 2016;316(19):2025–35.
56. Kleinman S, Caulfield T, Chan P, Davenport R, McFarland J, McPhedran S, et al. Toward an understanding of transfusion-related acute lung injury: statement of a consensus panel. Transfusion. 2004;44(12):1774–89.
57. Oakley FD, Woods M, Arnold S, Young PP. Transfusion reactions in pediatric compared with adult patients: a look at rate, reaction type, and associated products. Transfusion. 2015;55(3):563–70.
58. Tobian AA, King KE, Ness PM. Transfusion premedications: a growing practice not based on evidence. Transfusion. 2007;47(6):1089–96.
59. Obrador GT, Macdougall IC. Effect of red cell transfusions on future kidney transplantation. Clin J Am Soc Nephrol. 2013;8(5):852–60.
60. Dhillon S. Roxadustat: first global approval. Drugs. 2019;79(5):563–72.
61. Locatelli F, Fishbane S, Block GA, Macdougall IC. Targeting hypoxia-inducible factors for the treatment of anemia in chronic kidney disease patients. Am J Nephrol. 2017;45(3): 187–99.
62. Besarab A, Chernyavskaya E, Motylev I, Shutov E, Kumbar LM, Gurevich K, et al. Roxadustat (FG-4592): correction of anemia in incident dialysis patients. J Am Soc Nephrol. 2016;27(4):1225–33.
63. Besarab A, Provenzano R, Hertel J, Zabaneh R, Klaus SJ, Lee T, et al. Randomized placebo-controlled dose-ranging and pharmacodynamics study of roxadustat (FG-4592) to treat anemia in nondialysis-dependent chronic kidney disease (NDD-CKD) patients. Nephrol Dial Transplant. 2015;30(10):1665–73.
64. Akizawa T, Iwasaki M, Yamaguchi Y, Majikawa Y, Reusch M. Phase 3, randomized, double-blind, active-comparator (darbepoetin alfa) study of oral Roxadustat in CKD patients with anemia on hemodialysis in Japan. J Am Soc Nephrol. 2020;31(7):1628–39.

65. Chen N, Hao C, Liu BC, Lin H, Wang C, Xing C, et al. Roxadustat treatment for anemia in patients undergoing long-term dialysis. N Engl J Med. 2019;381(11):1011–22.
66. Akizawa T, Otsuka T, Reusch M, Ueno M. Intermittent oral dosing of roxadustat in peritoneal dialysis chronic kidney disease patients with anemia: a randomized, phase 3, multicenter, open-label study. Ther Apher Dial. 2020;24(2):115–25.
67. Mokas S, Lariviere R, Lamalice L, Gobeil S, Cornfield DN, Agharazii M, et al. Hypoxia-inducible factor-1 plays a role in phosphate-induced vascular smooth muscle cell calcification. Kidney Int. 2016;90(3):598–609.
68. Sanghani NS, Haase VH. Hypoxia-inducible factor activators in renal anemia: current clinical experience. Adv Chronic Kidney Dis. 2019;26(4):253–66.
69. Haase VH. Regulation of erythropoiesis by hypoxia-inducible factors. Blood Rev. 2013;27(1):41–53.
70. Flamme I, Oehme F, Ellinghaus P, Jeske M, Keldenich J, Thuss U. Mimicking hypoxia to treat anemia: HIF-stabilizer BAY 85-3934 (Molidustat) stimulates erythropoietin production without hypertensive effects. PLoS One. 2014;9(11):e111838.
71. Holdstock L, Meadowcroft AM, Maier R, Johnson BM, Jones D, Rastogi A, et al. Four-week studies of oral hypoxia-inducible factor-prolyl hydroxylase inhibitor GSK1278863 for treatment of anemia. J Am Soc Nephrol. 2016;27(4):1234–44.
72. Jelkmann W. Physiology and pharmacology of erythropoietin. Transfus Med Hemother. 2013;40(5):302–9. https://doi.org/10.1159/000356193.
73. Hörl WH. Differentiating factors between erythropoiesis-stimulating agents: an update to selection for anaemia of chronic kidney disease. Drugs. 2013;73:117–30.
74. Carrancio S, Markovics J, Wong P, Leisten J, Castiglioni P, Groza MC, et al. An activin receptor IIA ligand trap promotes erythropoiesis resulting in a rapid induction of red blood cells and haemoglobin. Br J Haematol. 2014;165(6):870–82.
75. Jelkmann W. Activin receptor ligand traps in chronic kidney disease. Curr Opin Nephrol Hypertens. 2018;27(5):351–7.
76. Locatelli F, Del Vecchio L, Luise MC. Current and future chemical therapies for treating anaemia in chronic kidney disease. Expert Opin Pharmacother. 2017;18(8):781–8.
77. López-Gómez JM, Abad S, Vega A. New expectations in the treatment of anemia in chronic kidney disease. Nefrología (English Edition). 2016;36(3):232–6.
78. Schmid H, Jelkmann W. Investigational therapies for renal disease-induced anemia. Expert Opin Investig Drugs. 2016;25(8):901–16.
79. Nasr R, Chilimuri S. Preoperative evaluation in patients with end-stage renal disease and chronic kidney disease. Health Serv Insights. 2017;10:117863291771302.
80. Trainor D, Borthwick E, Ferguson A. Perioperative management of the hemodialysis patient. Semin Dial. 2011;24(3):314–26.
81. Han J, Zhou J, Kondragunta V, Zhang X, Molokie RE, Gowhari M, et al. Erythropoiesis-stimulating agents in sickle cell anaemia. Br J Haematol. 2017;182(4):602–5. https://doi.org/10.1111/bjh.14846.
82. Boyle SM, Jacobs B, Sayani FA, Hoffman B. Management of the dialysis patient with sickle cell disease. Semin Dial. 2015;29(1):62–70.
83. Arber DA, Orazi A, Hasserjian R, Thiele J, Borowitz MJ, Le Beau MM, et al. The 2016 revision to the World Health Organization classification of myeloid neoplasms and acute leukemia. Blood. 2016;127(20):2391–405.
84. Pfeilstöcker M, Tuechler H, Sanz G, Schanz J, Garcia-Manero G, Solé F, et al. Time-dependent changes in mortality and transformation risk in MDS. Blood. 2016;128(7):902–10.
85. Santini V. Clinical use of erythropoietic stimulating agents in myelodysplastic syndromes. Oncologist. 2011;16(S3):35–42.
86. Ayari H, Pasquier F, Karoui KE, Sallée M, Faguer S, Krummel T, et al. Myelodysplastic syndrome in hemodialysis patients. Kidney Int Rep. 2019;4(8):1175–8.
87. Chang M-Y, Lin S-F, Wu S-C, Yang W-C. Myelodysplastic syndrome: the other cause of anemia in end-stage renal disease patients undergoing dialysis. Sci Rep. 2020;10(1):15557.

88. Hara R, Goto N, Furuya D, Kitahara T, Numata H, Watanabe S, et al. The effect of roxadustat on transfusion-dependent myelodysplastic syndrome complicated by chronic kidney disease. Case Rep Oncol. 2021;14(3):1574–9.
89. Tomlinson D, Robinson PD, Oberoi S, Cataudella D, Culos-Reed N, Davis H, et al. Pharmacologic interventions for fatigue in cancer and transplantation: a meta-analysis. Curr Oncol. 2018;25(2):152–67.
90. Pfeffer MA, Burdmann EA, Chen C-Y, Cooper ME, de Zeeuw D, Eckardt K-U, et al. A trial of darbepoetin alfa in type 2 diabetes and chronic kidney disease. N Engl J Med. 2009;361(21):2019–32.
91. Rizzo JD, Brouwers M, Hurley P, Seidenfeld J, Arcasoy MO, Spivak JL, et al. American Society of Clinical Oncology/American Society of Hematology clinical practice guideline update on the use of epoetin and darbepoetin in adult patients with cancer. J Clin Oncol. 2010;28(33):4996–5010.
92. Pirker R, Ramlau RA, Schuette W, Zatloukal P, Ferreira I, Lillie T, et al. Safety and efficacy of darbepoetin alfa in previously untreated extensive-stage small-cell lung cancer treated with platinum plus etoposide. J Clin Oncol. 2008;26(14):2342–9.
93. NCCN Clinical Practice Guidelines in Oncology (NCCN Guidelines®) Cancer-and Chemotherapy-Induced Anemia. NCCN.org. https://oncolife.com.ua/doc/nccn/Cancer-and_Chemotherapy-Induced_Anemia.pdf. Accessed 22 Nov 2019.
94. Saha M, Allon M. Diagnosis, treatment, and prevention of hemodialysis emergencies. Clin J Am Soc Nephrol. 2017;12(2):357–69.
95. Greenberg KI, Choi MJ. Hemodialysis emergencies: core curriculum 2021. Am J Kidney Dis. 2021;77(5):796–809.
96. Yoon J, Thapa S, Chow RD, Jaar BG. Hemolysis as a rare but potentially life-threatening complication of hemodialysis: a case report. BMC Res Notes. 2014;28(7):475.
97. Tharmaraj D, Kerr PG. Haemolysis in haemodialysis. Nephrology (Carlton). 2017;22(11):838–47.
98. Fluck S, McKane W, Cairns T, Fairchild V, Lawrence A, Lee J, Murray D, Polpitiye M, Palmer A, Taube D. Chloramine-induced haemolysis presenting as erythropoietin resistance. Nephrol Dial Transplant. 1999;14(7):1687–91.
99. Orringer EP, Mattern WD. Formaldehyde-induced hemolysis during chronic hemodialysis. N Engl J Med. 1976;294(26):1416–20. https://doi.org/10.1056/NEJM197606242942602.
100. Duffy R, Tomashek K, Spangenberg M, Spry L, Dwyer D, Safranek TJ, Ying C, Portesi D, Divan H, Kobrenski J, Arduino M, Tokars J, Jarvis W. Multistate outbreak of hemolysis in hemodialysis patients traced to faulty blood tubing sets. Kidney Int. 2000;57(4):1668–74.
101. Malinauskas RA. Decreased hemodialysis circuit pressures indicating postpump tubing kinks: a retrospective investigation of hemolysis in five patients. Hemodial Int. 2008;12(3):383–93.
102. Besarab A, Bolton WK, Browne JK, Egrie JC, Nissenson AR, Okamoto DM, et al. The effects of normal as compared with low hematocrit values in patients with cardiac disease who are receiving hemodialysis and epoetin. N Engl J Med. 1998;339(9):584–90.

Chronic Kidney Disease-Bone and Mineral Disease

7

Tushar Bajaj and Stuart M. Sprague

Introduction

Chronic kidney disease-mineral bone disease (CKD-MBD) is frequently encountered during the management of patients with chronic kidney disease (CKD). The systemic phenomenon of CKD-MBD results in derangements in mineral metabolism, disturbances in bone mineralization, or renal osteodystrophy and extraskeletal calcification, resulting in significant morbidity and mortality, especially cardiovascular complications. The kidneys are an integral part of maintaining mineral homeostasis, especially phosphorus and calcium. Disruption of this homeostasis due to progressive kidney failure can lead to changes in circulating concentrations of hormones that regulate mineral metabolism. The pathophysiology is complex (Fig. 7.1); however, it begins with a decreased glomerular filtration rate that leads to phosphate retention, resulting in increased fibroblastic growth factor-23 (FGF23). FGF23 and further phosphate retention lead to decreases in calcitriol (1,25-dihydroxycholecalciferol), which ultimately results in a decrease in serum ionized calcium and an increase in parathyroid hormone (PTH). The decrease in calcitriol increases skeletal resistance to PTH, which further decreases serum calcium, resulting in further increases in PTH. The increase in PTH will further increase FGF-23. Klotho, a gene mainly expressed in the cell surface membrane of proximal and distal renal tubules is an essential co-receptor for the binding of FGF23 to its receptors. CKD-associated decreases in Klotho result in the inactivity of FGF23 to inhibit PTH production, thus

T. Bajaj
Department of Medicine, University of Chicago Pritzker School of Medicine, Chicago, IL, USA

S. M. Sprague (✉)
Division of Nephrology and Hypertension, Department of Medicine, Northshore University Health System, University of Chicago Pritzker School of Medicine, Evanston, IL, USA
e-mail: ssprague@northshore.org

S. Z. Fadem et al. (eds.), *Complications in Dialysis*,
https://doi.org/10.1007/978-3-031-44557-6_7

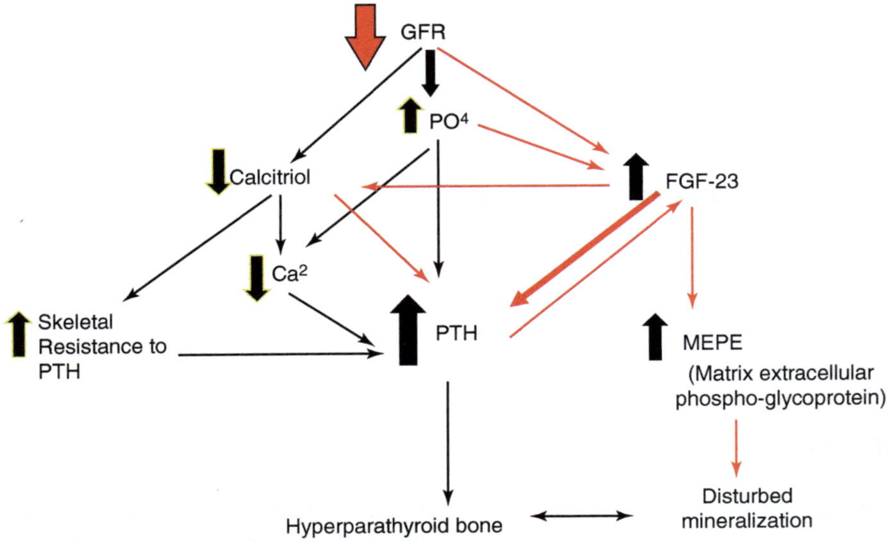

Fig. 7.1 Pathophysiology of CKD-MBD. A cascade of events take place once the glomerular filtration rate decreases, resulting in changes in minerals, hormones, vitamins, and peptides. Initially, retention of phosphate triggers an increase in FGF23 and a decrease in calcitriol. In addition, PTH increases, stimulating FGF23 and attempting to stimulate calcitriol production. The net effect of the increase in PTH causes an increase in bone turnover that further stimulates the release of phosphate and calcium from the bone. In addition, FGF23 stimulates matrix proteins that result in altered mineralization of bone

resulting in further increases in PTH. As the kidney fails to respond to increasing levels of PTH, and due to the downregulation of vitamin D receptors (VDR), therapy should be focused on normalizing biochemical and hormonal abnormalities to limit their complications. Furthermore, mineral and endocrine functions are critically important in maintaining bone modeling, remodeling, and mineralization. The abnormalities in calcium and phosphate metabolism increase the risk of extraskeletal calcifications resulting in calcific uremic arteriolopathy and vascular calcifications. The importance of managing these disturbances is important due to numerous studies which have shown associations between this imbalance of hormones and minerals leading to increased cardiovascular disease, fractures, and mortality.

Parathyroid Hormone

Parathyroid hormone is synthesized in the chief cells of the parathyroid glands and is essential for the maintenance of serum calcium concentration and the regulation of phosphorus metabolism. It also has direct actions on the bone and kidney as well as indirect actions on the gastrointestinal tract [1, 2]. Parathyroid gland secretion has seasonal and circadian fluctuations as well as spontaneous secretion characterized by the ultradian rhythm with tonic and pulsatile components [3]. The synthesis and secretion of PTH are controlled by the calcium-sensing receptor, (CaSR) which is normally expressed at high levels on the surface of the parathyroid chief cells, regulating calcium homeostasis by CaSR-regulated inhibition of PTH secretion. This is an inverse relationship; the reduction in extracellular ionized calcium concentration acts as a signal for PTH production and secretion. However, when extracellular ionized calcium concentration is high, there is stimulation of the CaSR and a reduction in PTH production and secretion. Furthermore, PTH secretion can be stimulated by an increase in serum phosphate concentrations either directly or indirectly by a reduction in calcium levels [4]. Additionally, as there is a VDR in the parathyroid gland, calcitriol is the main regulator of PTH secretion and parathyroid cell proliferation [5]. Parathyroid glands also express FGF receptors, but the role of FGF23 on the parathyroid gland in normal physiology remains to be understood. Recent studies suggest that the cofactor klotho is required for FGF23 receptor to activate downstream effects [6].

The direct action of PTH on the kidney is to stimulate calcium reabsorption in the distal tubule by activating specific ion channels, TRPV5, and increase phosphate excretion in the proximal tubule mainly by regulating sodium-coupled cotransporters via both PKA and PKC-dependent pathways [7, 8]. PTH is also an important regulator of active vitamin D as it stimulates the conversion of 25-hydroxyvitamin D to 1,25-dihydroxyvitamin D (calcitriol) by transcriptional activation (CYP27B1 gene) of 25-hydroxyvitamin D 1 α-hydroxylase. Calcitriol enhances intestinal calcium and phosphate uptake [9]. PTH has an important role in modulating bone remodeling and binds to PTH1R (parathyroid hormone receptor type 1) on cells of the osteoblastic lineage. This stimulates a variety of factors, ultimately leading to increased proliferation of mesenchymal stem cells that are committed into the osteoblast lineage and to enhanced osteoblast differentiation and activity with new bone matrix production and, ultimately, mineralization of bone tissue [10]. PTH stimulation of osteoblastic cells also produces tumor necrosis factor-related cytokine, receptor activator of nuclear factor κB (RANK) ligand (RANKL), which is a critical stimulator of osteoclast production and action, as well as the soluble RANKL decoy receptor, osteoprotegerin (OPG) [11]. PTH increases the production of RANKL and inhibits the production of OPG, leading to increased osteoclastic bone resorption. This leads to the release of calcium and phosphate as a result of the degradation of hydroxyapatite. PTH is a potent stimulator of bone turnover which can lead to a net increase in bone formation or a net increase in bone resorption [10]. Primary, secondary, and tertiary hyperparathyroidism can occur in patients with CKD.

Primary hyperparathyroidism (PHPT) is an endocrine disorder characterized by elevated or inappropriately normal levels of PTH and hypercalcemia. This results from the excessive secretion of PTH from one or more of the parathyroid glands, which can be a solitary adenoma (80% of cases), four-gland hyperplasia (10–15%), multiple adenomas (5%), or parathyroid cancer (<1%) [12]. The underlying cause of sporadic PHPT is unknown in a majority of cases, and the genetic pathogenesis also remains unclear; however, ionizing radiation in childhood is a risk factor, as is chronic lithium use. Lithium decreases the sensitivity of the parathyroid glands to calcium [13, 14]. Two genes that have been documented as contributing to the development of PHPT are MEN1 (which encodes menin) and CCND1 (which encodes cyclin D1). The pathophysiology of PHPT is the loss of normal feedback suppression of serum calcium concentrations upon the synthesis and secretion of PTH either due to increased parathyroid cell mass and/or a reduction in the number of CaSR proteins on the parathyroid cells [15]. Diagnosis is established biochemically with elevated serum calcium and simultaneous elevated intact PTH concentrations. Furthermore, levels of PTH that are inappropriately normal (>20 pg/mL) in a patient with hypercalcemia are consistent with a diagnosis of PHPT. Non-parathyroid causes of hypercalcemia (malignancy, granulomatous disease) are associated with suppressed PTH concentrations [12]. Parathyroid imaging has a limited role in the diagnosis of PHPT; imaging studies are used to assist the parathyroid surgeon in identifying the anatomic position of the abnormal gland(s) when planning for parathyroidectomy. PHPT can be a symptomatic multi-system disorder classified by renal, skeletal, neurological, gastrointestinal, and psychiatric manifestations, as well as increased mortality [16]. These manifestations include nephrolithiasis, nephrocalcinosis, polyuria, polydipsia, osteitis fibrosa cystica, anorexia, constipation, peptic ulcer disease, pancreatitis, muscle weakness, mental disturbances, and fatigue [16, 17]. The vast majority of patients are asymptomatic and are identified due to a routine laboratory check for hypercalcemia. Parathyroidectomy remains the only cure for PHPT and is recommended in all symptomatic patients and in patients who are asymptomatic but have evidence of subclinical end-organ effects or risk of disease progression [18]. The criteria for asymptomatic patients at initial evaluation include age less than 50 years, serum calcium concentration greater than or equal to 1 mg/dL above the upper limit of normal, eGFR less than 60 mL/min, 24 h urinary calcium of greater than 400 mg/day, increased biochemical stone profile risk, presence of nephrolithiasis or nephrocalcinosis, osteoporosis (DEXA spine, hip, and forearm) T-Score less than or equal to −2.5, or presence of a vertebral fracture.

Secondary hyperparathyroidism (SHP) occurs when the parathyroid glands respond secondarily to a stimulus of hypocalcemia (CKD, malabsorption, vitamin D deficiency) and reacts by increasing PTH secretion. When secondary hyperparathyroidism is longstanding, and serum calcium is high, the stimulated parathyroid glands assume a quasi-autonomous role; this is termed tertiary or refractory hyperparathyroidism. The initially proposed pathophysiology of secondary hyperparathyroidism was thought to be due to decreased renal function leading to hyperphosphatemia. The elevated serum phosphorus would bind with calcium to create calcium phosphate salts, which along with decreased activation of vitamin D by 1 α-hydroxylase would lead to reduced concentrations of calcitriol, and hypocalcemia. Recent data has identified FGF-23 as an important role in the early pathogenesis of SHP [19]. FGF-23 is discussed in detail later in this chapter, but it is secreted mainly by osteocytes and osteoblasts. Synthesis and release of FGF-23 are stimulated by calcitriol, phosphate, PTH, and calcium. FGF-23, with its co-receptor α Klotho, functions to induce phosphaturia, inhibits calcitriol synthesis by

Table 7.1 Hyperparathyroidism comparison with levels of PTH, calcium, phosphorus, 25-OH vitamin D, and calcitriol

Hyperparathyroidism	PTH	Calcium	Phosphorus	25 Vitamin D	Calcitriol
Primary	↑ →	↑	↓	↑	↑↓
Secondary	↑	↓ →	↓↑	↓	↓
Tertiary	↑↑	↑	↑	↓	↓

inhibiting 1 α-hydroxylase, catabolizes active vitamin D sterols by stimulating 24 hydroxylases, eventually leading to further hypocalcemia and stimulation of the parathyroid gland [20]. Tertiary hyperparathyroidism occurs when there is extensive hypertrophy of parathyroid glands with a monoclonal expansion of parathyroid cells in which the set point of the CaSRs has been altered such that semi-autonomous secretion of PTH occurs despite hypercalcemia. Table 7.1 demonstrates the different categories of hyperparathyroidism with levels of serum PTH, calcium, phosphorus, 25 OH vitamin D, and calcitriol. In addition, there is a decrease in VDR expression in nodules, resulting in the inability of calcitriol to inhibit PTH production and release. The number of available therapeutic options for the management of secondary and tertiary hyperparathyroidism has increased but control of PTH, calcium, phosphate, and calcitriol are paramount. A significant portion of patients may still require parathyroidectomy to prevent fractures, cardiovascular events, or improve survival.

The administration of different phosphate binder classes with moderate to severe CKD results in distinct changes in vitamin D metabolism. In general, serum phosphate and vitamin D metabolite concentrations are often thought of as separate potential therapeutic targets; however, some studies have demonstrated that there is considerable overlap in the treatment of these parameters [21]. In one recent analysis, the effects of three phosphate binders (lanthanum, sevelamer, and calcium acetate) on circulating vitamin D metabolites in a post hoc analysis of the Phosphate Normalization Trial demonstrated that when compared to placebo, calcium acetate increased clearance of 25(OH)D3 to 24,25(OH)2D3 and decreased 25(OH)D3 activation to 1,25(OH)2D3, whereas sevelamer carbonate decreased 25(OH)D3 clearance. Lanthanum carbonate did not significantly change the yield of studied metabolites [21]. The U.S. FDA has approved extended-release calcifediol, a 25-hydroxyvitamin D3 (prohormone of calcitriol), for the treatment of secondary hyperparathyroidism in adults with stage 3–4 (not 5) CKD and vitamin D insufficiency (serum total 25-hydroxyvitamin D <30 ng/mL). Vitamin D receptor activators (VDRA, calcitriol, and paricalcitol) are available to treat hyperparathyroidism associated with vitamin D deficiency from decreased production of calcitriol.

The advent of calcimimetics has extended the armamentarium against SHP treatment. The cloning of the calcium-sensing receptor led to the discovery of multiple compounds capable of modulating its function in different organ tissues, specifically the introduction of cinacalcet hydrochloride [22]. Cinacalcet works by increasing the sensitivity of the calcium-sensing receptor to extracellular calcium, shifting the Ca-PTH concentration-response curves to the left, and reducing the "set point" for the Ca-regulated PTH secretion [23–25]. Cinacalcet decreases the secretion of PTH in a dose-dependent manner and diminishes calcium concentration; therefore, it is currently indicated for the treatment of SHP in dialysis patients. It has also been shown to reduce hypercalcemia in patients with parathyroid carcinoma and in selected cases of primary hyperparathyroidism. The only other medication approved by the FDA in the U.S. is etelcalcetide, an intravenous calcimimetic agent, for treating secondary hyperparathyroidism in adult patients with CKD on hemodialysis. Etelcalcetide is a synthetic peptide that allosterically activates the CaSR in the extracellular domain of the receptor. The CaSR is located on the parathyroid chief cells, and by binding to it, etelcaletide enhances its activation by extracellular calcium, which results in decreased PTH secretion [26, 27].

Calcium

Calcium is the most abundant mineral in the human body, and most of the body's calcium is sequestered in the skeleton [28]. Calcium metabolism is regulated through hormonal control of a three-tissue axis of the kidney, intestine, and bone to tightly control serum ionized calcium (the free cation in the extracellular fluid) within a narrow range. Intestinal calcium absorption occurs through two components. The first is a saturable, transcellular active transport/facilitated diffusion component, which is largely regulated by calcitriol acting through the transcriptional actions of the VDR. The second is an unsaturable, paracellular, passive diffusion component that is considered unregulated and linearly related to dietary calcium load [29]. Active calcium absorption is highest in the proximal small intestine, followed by the large intestine, which parallels the abundance of VDR expression [29]. Therefore, calcium intake is an important factor affecting calcium absorption because when calcium intake is low, elevations in PTH and subsequent increases in calcitriol act to increase the active absorption of calcium. However, when the calcium intake is insufficient, there is an increase in bone turnover, with bone calcium reserve utilized to maintain serum calcium within a normal range. Conversely, high calcium intake will suppress PTH and conversion of 25 vitamin D to calcitriol, thereby lowering active calcium absorption.

In CKD, calcitriol concentrations are decreased due to the effects of FGF23 decreasing the conversion of vitamin D to its active state by inhibiting 1 α-hydroxylase enzyme. Therefore, these patients are at risk for low calcium absorption due to decreased calcitriol and low active calcium transport [30]. From stage 3 CKD onwards, calcium excretion in the kidney is diminished, and a positive calcium balance occurs because the intestinal absorption is greater than the kidney's capacity for its excretion. In healthy individuals, the recommended dietary calcium allowance is approximately 1 g/day; however, in CKD, the precise dose has not been determined. Present data suggest a more moderate target in CKD patients, around 800–1000 mg/day [30].

As patients progress from CKD to dialysis, hypocalcemia can occur from increased serum phosphorus and decreased renal production of calcitriol. Increased serum phosphorus may also bind with calcium and deposit into bones and other soft tissues, while decreased calcitriol can decrease gastrointestinal absorption. Patients with acute and severe hypocalcemia (<7.5 mg/dL), neurological manifestations, or stridor should first receive intravenous calcium and then oral calcium [31]. In patients with chronic hypocalcemia, oral calcium and vitamin D preparations should be used. In addition to nutritional vitamin D, both extended-release calcifediol and calcitriol are the preferred formulations due to their rapid action [32].

In CKD, treatment of secondary hyperparathyroidism with calcitriol and calcium-based phosphate binders can produce hypercalcemia and over suppression of PTH, which results in an adynamic bone that cannot buffer calcium and phosphate levels, increasing the risk of vascular calcification [33]. Another cause of hypercalcemia is prolonged stimulation of the parathyroid gland leading to autonomous PTH hypersecretion (tertiary hyperparathyroidism) [34]. The first step in treatment is to perform medication reconciliation, including over-the-counter medications, and to avoid calcium-containing drugs. As mentioned previously, the treatment for tertiary hyperparathyroidism is primarily surgical. Acute hypercalcemia in chronic disease is unusual and can be primary hyperparathyroidism, underlying malignancy, or a myriad of other conditions.

In ESRD, the choice of dialysate calcium depends on several factors, including dietary habits, drug treatment, parathyroid levels, vitamin D levels, type and severity of bone disease, and presence or absence of arterial calcification. The goal is to maintain a neutral calcium balance in adult patients however, due to the advent of calcitriol combined with oral calcium, many centers have adopted to use a lower dialysate calcium concentration to minimize hypercalcemia. Most patients in ESRD are in a positive calcium balance despite lower dialysate calcium which is likely contributing to extensive vascular calcification [35]. Ideally, the dialysate calcium would be adapted to each patient's needs; however, this is not feasible in most dialysis settings.

Phosphorus

Phosphorus is a critical mineral that is important for multiple biological and biochemical reactions to the maintenance of life. In large cross-sectional studies, it remains constant at approximately 3.8 mg/dL in subjects with normal kidney function [36]. Due to the interaction of PTH, FGF23, and vitamin D, as well as the interplay between the gastrointestinal tract, bone, and kidneys, serum phosphorus generally stays within a normal range until the GFR falls to below 30 mL/min/1.72 m^2, at which point phosphate concentrations start to rise. Multiple studies have demonstrated a correlation between serum phosphate concentrations with a higher-than-normal range predicting a higher risk of adverse events, including the development of cardiovascular and cerebrovascular events [37, 38].

Dietary intake of phosphorus varies by country. The amount of absorption depends on the type of phosphorus: 30–70% of the phosphorus found naturally in the foods is absorbable, whereas 100% of the phosphorus from inorganic phosphate additives is absorbable [39, 40]. The dietary recommendation for phosphorus in maintaining bone homeostasis in adults without kidney disease is 3000 mg/day (upper intake level), and with kidney disease 1000 mg/day (upper intake level) [41, 42].

The glomerulus filters between 3700 and 6100 mg/day of phosphorus with a net renal excretion between 600 and 1500 mg/day. Furthermore, 85% of phosphate reabsorption occurs within the proximal tubule [43]. As renal function continues to decline in advanced CKD and end-stage disease requiring dialysis, serum phosphate concentrations continue to rise, leading to hyperphosphatemia.

The approach to treating hyperphosphatemia includes dietary and lifestyle modification, drug treatment with phosphate binders, and dialysis. In terms of diet, the first step would be to avoid phosphorus-rich foods and be cognizant of food additives, poor labeling of phosphorus content, and phosphorus-containing medications. A Cochrane review assessed the value of dietary interventions for preventing and treating CKD-MBD; however, the review only identified two randomized controlled trials showing that a targeted low phosphate intake led to a modest 0.18 mmol/L (−0.56 mg/dL) decrease in the serum phosphate. The review concluded that there is limited low-quality evidence to indicate that dietary interventions positively affect serum phosphate control [44].

There are various phosphate binders on the market ranging from calcium-containing phosphate binders, polymeric phosphate binders, magnesium-containing phosphate binders, lanthanum carbonate, ferric citrate, sucroferric oxyhydroxide, as well as new compounds in development such as tenapanor. Tenapanor is a novel medication that inhibits gastrointestinal exchange and reduces paracellular phosphate transport in the intestine. Table 7.2 has the characteristics of oral phosphate binders with their mechanism of action, advantages, and disadvantages. Palmer et al. performed a network meta-analysis on adults with CKD. In reviewing 77 randomized trials where allocation to phosphate binders was included, there was no evidence that any drug class lowered mortality or cardiovascular events when compared to a placebo. Furthermore, when compared to calcium, sevelamer reduced all-cause mortality (OR 0.39 95% CI 0.21–0.74), while treatments effects of lanthanum, iron, and colestilan were not significant [45]. All phosphate binders lowered serum phosphorus concentrations to a greater extent than placebo, with iron (sucroferric oxyhydroxide) ranked as the best treatment. Lower risks of hypercalcemia were seen in sevelamer and lanthanum when compared to calcium [45]. Additionally, in a Cochrane review, sevelamer reduced all-cause mortality in dialysis patients by

Table 7.2 Phosphate binders with their mechanism of action advantages and disadvantages

Phosphate binder	Mechanism of action	Advantages	Disadvantages
Aluminum hydroxide	Forms insoluble phosphate complexes in the gut	Inexpensive, calcium free, binds phosphate at wide range of pH	No safe dose established, potential adverse effects from aluminum accumulation, requires regular monitoring of serum aluminum
Calcium carbonate	Forms insoluble calcium phosphate complexes in the gut	Moderately effective, relatively inexpensive	Hypercalcemia, large doses required to be effective, possible vascular calcification, unpalatable
Calcium acetate	Forms insoluble calcium phosphate complexes in the gut	Moderately effective, more effective than calcium carbonate, relatively inexpensive	Hypercalcemia, large doses required to be effective, possible vascular calcification, unpalatable
Sevelamer hydrochloride	An anion exchange resin	Calcium free, lipid-lowering effect	High pill burden, contribute to acidosis, binds fat-soluble vitamins, gastrointestinal adverse effects
Sevelamer carbonate	An anion exchange resin	Calcium free, lipid-lowering effect	High pill burden, binds fat-soluble vitamins, gastrointestinal adverse effects
Lanthanum carbonate	Forms insoluble phosphate complexes in the gut	Low pill burden, high efficacy, works in wide range of pH, no negative changes on bone histology	Expensive, gastrointestinal adverse effects
Sucroferric oxyhydroxide	A ligand exchange iron-based compound	Low pill burden, works in wide range of pH, minimal systemic absorption	Expensive, gastrointestinal adverse effects
Ferric citrate	Forms insoluble ferric phosphate complexes in the gut	Calcium free	Expensive, gastrointestinal adverse effects, may increase iron stores

50–60% versus calcium, whereas all other comparisons either did not reach statistical significance or were not tested. No drug class lowered cardiovascular events or cardiovascular mortality when compared to placebo [46].

Recent ESRD data from the Dialysis Outcomes and Practice Patterns Study (DOPPS) shows that >40% of ESRD patients had serum phosphate levels >5.5 mg/dL and >70% had levels >4.6 mg/dL [47]. Phosphorus removal with thrice-weekly hemodialysis, at 4 h per session, is approximately 3000 mg/week [48]. There are multiple randomized clinical trials that have demonstrated intensive hemodialysis to reduce serum phosphate concentrations, including the Frequent Hemodialysis Network trial that examined nocturnal and daily intensive hemodialysis which both decreased serum phosphorus and led to binder discontinuation in a large subset of patients. However, the studies did not have any meaningful effects on serum calcium and PTH concentrations [48]. Ganesh et al. were one of the earliest groups to demonstrate the effect of hyperphosphatemia on cardiovascular and mortality outcomes. A 2-year follow-up of 12,833 hemodialysis patients, looking at random serum phosphorus samples, demonstrated a higher mortality risk in patients with a serum phosphate >6.5 mg/dL compared with ≤6.5 mg/dL. Deaths resulting from coronary artery disease had a relative risk (RR) of 1.41 ($P < 0.0005$). The RR of sudden death was 1.2 ($P < 0.01$), infection 1.20 ($P < 0.05$), and unknown causes 1.25; ($P < 0.05$) [49]. Furthermore, they demonstrated that patients in the high phosphate group had an increased relative risk of death from other cardiac and cerebrovascular causes of death [49]. In another study, Block et al. evaluated the associations of mineral metabolism, mortality, and morbidity in HD patients, with data collected from 40,538 HD patients. After adjusting for case mix and laboratory variables, serum phosphorus concentrations >5.0 mg/dL were associated with an increased relative risk of death [50]. In DOPPS, 25,588 patients with ESRD on HD for longer than 180 days at 925 facilities were studied to identify adjusted hazard ratios for all-cause and cardiovascular mortality, with the greatest risk of mortality found for serum phosphorus concentrations greater than 7.0 mg/dL [51].

Fibroblast Growth Factor 23

FGF-23 is produced by osteoblasts and osteocytes and induces a negative phosphate balance by functioning as a phosphaturic peptide as well as a counterregulatory hormone for calcitriol, resulting in reduced intestinal absorption of phosphate. The inhibition of calcitriol also leads to secondary hyperparathyroidism development. FGF-23 inhibits PTH production and secretion, which opposes the progression of secondary hyperparathyroidism [52–54]. However, a decrease in the FGF23 co-receptor Klotho with progressive renal disease results in the inability of FGF23 to effectively decrease PTH secretion as CKD progresses. Recent studies have explored the effects of FGF-23 on the cardiovascular system. In animal and observational human studies, there is a link between elevated FGF-23 levels and multiple cardiovascular outcomes, including hypertension, left ventricular hypertrophy, and cardiovascular events and mortality [55]. FGF-23 and its co-receptor α-Klotho are key factors in underlying mechanisms that integrate accelerated atherosclerosis, vascular calcification, mineral disorders, and osteodystrophy [56].

α-Klotho

There are two basic forms of the α-klotho protein, a membrane-bound peptide and a soluble protein generated from extracellular domain cleavage by 2 membrane-anchored proteases [57]. Soluble a-klotho, via glucosidase or sialidase activity, acts to suppress growth factor signaling, protects from oxidative stress, and regulates a variety of ion channels and transporters [58, 59]. The co-receptor even has a key role in phosphate metabolism as a phosphaturic factor (independent of its role as a co-receptor of FGF-23), via direct actions on NaPi-2a to modulate renal phosphate excretion [60]. Unlike FGF-23, a-Klotho concentrations in CKD show a progressive decrease in parallel with reduced renal function with studies demonstrating urinary Klotho is reduced at a very early-stage CKD Stages 1 and 2 and is progressively lowered with declining eGFR [57]. Studies are still under investigation if α-klotho levels are associated with any adverse clinical outcomes. Emerging evidence from clinical and basic studies reveals that CKD is a state of endocrine and renal Klotho deficiency, which may serve as an early biomarker and pathogenic contributor to chronic progression and complications in CKD, including vascular calcification, cardiac hypertrophy, and secondary hyperparathyroidism [61]. Supplementation of exogenous Klotho and/or upregulation of endogenous Klotho production by using renin angiotensin system inhibitors, HMG CoA reductase inhibitors, vitamin D analogs, peroxisome proliferator-activated receptors-gamma agonists, or anti-oxidants may confer renoprotection from oxidation and suppression of renal fibrosis, and prevent or alleviate complications in CKD [61]. Klotho is a highly promising candidate on the horizon as an early biomarker and perhaps as a novel therapeutic agent for CKD.

Vascular Calcification

Vascular calcification is an active, highly regulated, and complex biological process that is mediated by genetics, epigenetics, dysregulated forms of matrix mineral metabolism, hormones, and the activation of cellular signaling pathways [62]. Dysregulated mineral metabolism and elevated levels of circulating calcium and phosphate are key factors for the initiation and progression of vascular calcification in CKD, and vascular calcification is the result of this pathological deposition of calcium phosphate mineral in soft tissues that decreases the elasticity of blood vessels and elevates blood pressure. This mineral deposition has been described as calciprotein particles—circulating complexes of proteins, calcium, and phosphate. The primary calciprotein particles are amorphic and solid-phase. They disperse as colloids in the circulation to eliminate mineral crystal formation, guard against calcification, and help maintain blood mineral homeostasis. Calciprotein particles are complexes of phosphate, calcium, and proteins. Primary calciprotein particles are amorphic and solid-phase calcium phosphate that bind to serum fetuin-A protein and calcium-regulatory proteins, disperse as colloids in the circulation to eliminate mineral crystal formation, and guard against ectopic calcification [63]. This defense mechanism maintains blood mineral homeostasis and inhibits calcification. In vascular calcification, the balance between the primary calciprotein particle formation and absorption is dysregulated. These calciprotein particles may undergo a transition to the crystalline (secondary calciprotein) phase [63]. Secondary calciprotein particles are stretched particles that contain predominantly hydroxyapatite surrounding proteins. Vascular smooth muscle cells undergo transdifferentiation to osteoblast-like cells and extrude matrix vesicles that contain proteins similar to osteoblastic vesicles. When these proteins are secreted by vascular smooth muscle cells, an osteogenic environment is created and results in vascular calcification [63, 64].

In physiological circumstances, the active mineralization inhibitors such as matrix Gla protein, pyrophosphate, fetuin-A, osteoprotegerin, adenosine, bone morphogenetic protein 7, and osteopontin protect blood vessels from the formation of stable hydroxyapatite crystals. However, a decline in these inhibitors, along with elevated levels of active inducers, leads to a high prevalence of vascular calcification in CKD [65, 66]. Patients with CKD can develop calcification in both the media and intimal layers of the vessel wall; however, medial calcification is more common, especially in pediatric patients [67]. The switch to an osteogenic and/or chondrogenic-like phenotype is characterized by the expression of Runx2 (also known as core-binding factor a-1 CBFA1), SRY-Box 9 (SOX9), Msh Homeobox 2 (MSX2), and Osterix. These are all important transcription factors for both intimal and medial vascular calcification [68]. The transdifferentiation of vascular smooth muscle cells into osteo-/chondrogenic-like cells is coordinated by a complex network of intracellular signaling pathways like nuclear factor kappa beta (NF-Kβ), receptor activator of NF-Kβ (RANK)/RANK ligand (RANKL), Wnt-β-catenin, mitogen-activated protein kinase (MAPK) p38, calcium-induced signaling, and nitric oxide-plasminogen activator inhibitor-1 (PAI-1) pathways [69–72]. The transdifferentiation can, moreover, be mediated by extracellular signal-regulated kinases 1/2 (ERK1/2) pathways [71].

Elastin Degradation

Elastin is a key constituent of the extracellular matrix in elastic arteries. It is secreted by vascular smooth muscle cells as a soluble monomer, tropoelastin, which interacts with fibrillin or microfibril-associated glycoprotein, and is oriented into alignment for cross-linking by lysyl oxidase. This structure provides elastin with extensive tensile strength critical for contractile function. The process of elastin degradation is facilitated by proteases upregulated in CKD. These include cathepsin-s and matrix metalloproteinases. Disruption of elastin in the aortic wall causes an increase in the expression level of transforming growth factor (TGF-β). TGF-β is involved in osteoblast differentiation and increases arterial stiffness [73, 74].

Uremic Toxins

The accumulation of uremic toxins (phosphate, advanced glycation end products, indoxyl sulfate, IL-1B, IL-6, TNF-a), as well as uremia-related factors (malnutrition, hyperhomocysteinemia, and anemia) may also directly enhance vascular calcification in CKD patients [62]. In CKD, the influx of urea and other toxins causes an alteration in the gut microbiome in which a diminished number of beneficial bacteria are associated with an increase in uremic toxin-producing bacteria. The degradation of cellular tight junctions and intestinal inflammation enables these gut-derived uremic toxins to translocate into the bloodstream and cause extensive oxidative stress. This oxidative stress is damaging to the kidney, cardiovascular system, bone-mineral, erythropoiesis, and endocrine systems [75]. One of the uremic toxins, indoxyl sulfate, has been shown in rats to stimulate vascular smooth muscle cell proliferation mediated by MAPK activation in vitro. In another study, stimulation of the aortic expression of (pro)renin receptor and renin/prorenin through an OAT3-mediated uptake leads to the production of reactive oxygen species and activation of AhR and NF-Kβ p65 in vascular smooth muscle cells [76, 77]. This indoxyl sulfate-induced activation of (pro)renin receptor promotes cell proliferation and tissue factor expression in vascular smooth muscle cells [77].

Inducers and Inhibitors of Vascular Calcification

An imbalance between inducers and inhibitors of vascular calcification occurs in CKD and chronic dialysis patients, including factors such as c-reactive protein, Wnt1, KEAP1/NRF2/P62 signaling, CDC42, osteopontin, sclerostin, chemerin, PiT-2, autophagy, protein carbamylation, magnesium carbonate, and zinc. C-Reactive protein, an important promoter of vascular inflammation, has been found to promote osteo-/chondrogenic transdifferentiation, and aggravated phosphate-induced osteo-/chondrogenic transdifferentiation, and calcification of primary human aortic smooth muscle cells [78]. Wnt1, a ligand of Wnt/β-catenin signaling, promotes pro-angiogenesis and reduces myocardial infarction. However, it has also been shown to reduce vascular calcification by regulating the expression of ANKH, a PPi transport regulator [79]. KEAP1 (Kelch-like ECH-associated protein 1)/NF-E2-related factor 2 (NRF2) signaling has been shown to play an important role in protecting cells from oxidative stress. The activation of this signaling pathway has been shown to lessen vascular calcification [80]. Cell division cycle 42 (CDC42), a Rac1 family member GTPase, is essential for cartilage development during endochondral bone formation, CDC42 has been shown to contribute to vascular calcification through a mechanism involving AKT signaling [81].

Osteopontin, an anti-calcific protein, is a multifunctional phosphoprotein and member of the small integrin-binding ligand N-linked glycoproteins family that was initially discovered as a major non-collagenous component of cortical bone. It is produced by multiple cell types in bone and plays an integral role in bone remodeling by osteoclast adhesion and bone resorption [82, 83]. Paloian et al. tested whether osteopontin protected against high phosphate load-induced nephrocalcinosis and vascular calcification in mice and found that endogenous osteopontin does play a critical role, yet further studies are yet to be conducted [84]. Sclerostin, an antagonist of Wnt signaling, is a potential contributor to vascular calcification and has a positive association with bone mineral density [85]. Chemerin, an adipokine that signals through G protein-coupled receptor ChemR23, has been shown to protect against vascular calcification by reducing phosphate-induced calcification as well as increased MGP (Matrix GLA Protein) expression [86]. Autophagy is an endogenous response of vascular smooth muscle cells to protect from calcification in uremia. Frauscher et al. demonstrated induction of autophagy by rapamycin which protected cells and mice from uremic media calcification, possibly by inhibiting osteogenic transdifferentiation [87]. Protein carbamylation is a posttranslational modification that can occur non-enzymatically in the presence of high concentrations of urea. A study by Mori et al. demonstrated that protein carbamylation exacerbates vascular calcification by decreasing ectonucleotide pyrophosphate/phosphodiesterase 1 expression, owing to carbamylation of mitochondrial proteins and oxidative stress [88].

An increasing number of studies report a close relationship between serum magnesium concentration and cardiovascular disease risk in the general population [89]. In end-stage renal disease, an association was found between serum magnesium and survival [89]. Hypomagnesemia was identified as a strong predictor for cardiovascular disease in these patients [89]. Magnesium carbonate as a phosphate binder could reduce calcification severity in CKD mice by increasing the expression of Pit-1 in the intestine. Furthermore, magnesium itself could prevent vascular calcification by extracellular phosphate binding and inhibit extracellular Ca-apatite crystal formation [90–92]. Magnesium also prevents the activity of Wnt/beta-catenin and reverses the osteogenic-like transformation of vascular smooth muscle cells [93]. Magnesium serum levels are reduced with long-term proton pump inhibitor treatment, and this may explain the association between proton pump inhibitors and vascular calcification; however, further studies are needed [94].

Plasma levels of zinc are significantly lower in CKD. Zinc supplementation improves phosphate-induced osteo-/chondrogenic transdifferentiation of vascular smooth muscle cells. It also reduces vascular calcification by TNFAIP3-dependent suppression of the NF-κB pathway [95, 96]. Furthermore, zinc can be an effective biomineral for the prevention of vascular smooth muscle cell mineralization in response to high phosphate and PHI FG4592. It may also reduce the calcification associated with atherosclerosis [97].

Fetuin-A

Fetuin-A is a glycoprotein that is secreted into the circulatory system by adipose tissue and the liver. It acts as a prominent protective factor in preventing vascular calcification in patients with CKD and ESRD [98, 99]. Low fetuin-A levels are independently associated with aortic calcifications and a higher risk of cardiovascular vents and mortality [100]. Fetuin-A inhibits in vitro vascular smooth muscle cell calcification induced by elevated concentrations of extracellular mineral ions in a concentration-dependent manner by inhibiting apoptosis and caspase cleavage [101]. Previous studies have identified intracellular vesicles as the nidus for mineral nucleation, and the presence of fetuin-A in vesicles abrogated their ability to nucleate basic calcium phosphate. In addition, fetuin-A enhanced phagocytosis of vesicles by vascular smooth muscle cells [101]. Observations such as these provide evidence that the uptake of serum protein fetuin-A by vascular smooth muscle cells is a key event in the inhibition of vesicle-mediated vascular smooth muscle cell calcification. Strategies in the future aimed at maintaining normal circulating levels of fetuin-A may prove beneficial in patients with ESRD.

Role of Vitamin D

The role of vitamin D has yet to be fully elucidated and remains controversial, with many studies suggesting that vitamin D excess is associated with extensive calcification, whereas others reporting that vitamin D deficiency promotes calcification. Some trials suggest that long-term supplementation provides protective effects [102]. Deficiency is predominantly caused by a lack of sunlight exposure and synthesis in the skin. This leads to inadequate production of calcifediol which results in reduced downstream effects. Correction of deficiency generally involves direct supplementation of calcifediol. Toxicity has not been associated with excessive sunlight exposure but rather with abnormal supplementation. The overproduction of inactive cholecalciferol in the skin does not result in the overproduction of calcifediol. Excess supplementation leads to the saturation of free calcifediol levels that exceed vitamin D binding protein binding capacity. This induces gene expression and functional changes in target cells [103, 104]. Supplementation is an accepted form of treatment for vitamin D deficiency; however, the process should be closely monitored to ensure appropriate levels rather than toxicity. Both stimulation and ablation of VDR signaling promote different types of calcifications, such as arterial atherosclerotic calcification and medial calcification, indicating that VDR signaling itself impacts VC by regulating gene expression programs within target tissues [105–108]. Current evidence from experimental studies suggests a biphasic response of vitamin D activity, with either excess or deficient levels of vitamin D potentially leading to deleterious calcification outcomes [109, 110].

Role of Vitamin K

Vitamin K is a fat-soluble vitamin naturally occurring in two forms; vitamin K1 (phylloquinone) and vitamin K2 (menaquinones, the latter of which is the most potent form and longer half-life). Vitamin K1 is predominantly found in green leafy vegetables and plant oils such as canola, olive, and soybean, whereas vitamin K2 is present in fermented foods, milk products, and meat. Vitamin K has been shown in several in vitro and in vivo studies to have anti-inflammatory action [111]. Clinical studies have showed that vitamin K status is negatively associated with circulating levels of inflammatory markers. Plasma K1 levels were inversely associated with IL-6 and CRP in a cross-sectional study conducted with 379 healthy men and women. No significant changes in the levels of inflammatory biomarkers were observed in the 3-year follow-up of patients supplemented with vitamin K1 [112]. In another cross-sectional analysis of the Framingham Offspring Study, plasma levels of vitamin K1 and its intake were inversely associated with overall circulating markers of inflammation, including CD40 ligand and IL-6 [113]. It is likely that vitamin K may prevent inflammatory vascular diseases, including atherosclerosis and vascular calcification, through its anti-inflammatory actions on vascular cells [111]. As vitamin K has clear associations with slower progression of systemic calcification, its inhibition by warfarin is central to long-term effects in the vasculature of warfarin users [114]. Most CKD patients, including those on renal replacement therapy, have vitamin K2 deficiency. The dephosphorylated and uncarboxylated matrix Gla protein level, a marker of vitamin K2 status, is decreased by vitamin K2 supplementation in CKD patients, but there is no unequivocal proof that it influences arterial calcification progression and bone complications [115].

Calcific Uremic Arteriopathy

Calcific uremic arteriopathy (CUA), previously referred to as calciphylaxis, is a rare, life-threatening syndrome of vascular calcification characterized by the occlusion of microvessels in the subcutaneous adipose tissue and dermis. It results in intensely painful, ischemic skin lesions [116]. The pathogenesis of CUA remains uncertain; however, histologic analysis suggests that calcified narrowed microvessels lead to chronic, low-grade ischemia. Further occlusion of vessels induced by endothelial injury. Microthrombosis results in infarction [117, 118]. Development of microvascular calcifications is likely to be an active, cell-mediated process that depends on the balance between promoters and inhibitors of calcification with serum samples from patients with CUA show impaired inhibition of calcium phosphate precipitation. This is probably a result of a deficiency of calcification inhibitors (matrix G1a protein, carboxylated matrix G1A protein, fetuin-A) [116, 118–120]. Risk factors include female sex, obesity, diabetes mellitus, vitamin K antagonists, and ESRD [116]. Predominant involvement of subcutaneous panniculus and aggregation of lesions in body areas with abundant adipose tissue, such as the abdomen and thighs, suggest a role of adipocytes in the pathogenesis of calciphylaxis [116]. Furthermore, mature adipocytes exposed to high phosphate levels calcify and unidirectionally induce the calcification of vascular smooth muscle cells, probably through the release of adipokines [121].

The initial skin manifestations may include induration, plaques, nodules, livedo, or purpura [122, 123]. The pain is somatic and can precede the appearance of skin lesions [124]. Furthermore, the pain may initially fluctuate in intensity; however, characteristically remains severe during the disease and is frequently accompanied by tactile hyperesthesia [124]. Initial lesions rapidly progress to stellate, malodorous ulcers with black eschars. Sepsis can originate from the resultant wounds and is considered the most common cause of death [122, 123, 125–127]. The skin biopsy is the standard method for confirmation of a clinically suspected CUA. A biopsy is not needed for a patient with ESRD, and the classic presentation of a painful necrotic ulcer covered with a black eschar [116, 128]. A biopsy should be strongly considered if a patient has early atypical lesions or if calciphylaxis is suspected in a patient without ESRD. A biopsy is contraindicated for acral, penile, or infected lesions [116]. A biopsy can be considered invasive, time-consuming, and destructive because the presence of calcified and blocked vessels restricts blood flow to the debrided area, and the sites do not heal well. There are also the risks of propagating new lesions, ulceration, superimposed infection, induction of necrosis, and bleeding [129]. A punch biopsy is safer than a large excisional biopsy but has limited depth and can be non-diagnostic. The yield can be improved with a double-punch technique wherein a second punch is inserted through the center of the first to retrieve deeper subcutaneous tissue and by biopsy of an active lesion margin rather than a central or necrotic area [116].

Pain management can be challenging in these patients, and pain relief may be unresponsive to high-dose opioids. In refractory cases, concomitant treatment with gabapentin, ketamine, or spinal anesthetic agents can be used [124]. Wound care is important to remove exudate and necrotic tissue and prevent infection. Surgical wound debridement is a controversial procedure in these cases and should be considered on a case-by-case basis. Evidence suggests that wounds with non-infected, stable, and dry eschars with limited tissue involvement are better managed with chemical rather than surgical debridement and the aim of surgical debridement involves the removal of necrosed tissues (without interfering with the adjacent healthy tissue) to facilitate wound healing [130–132]. In a retrospective analysis of 34 patients with CUA (predominantly with peripheral disease), hyperbaric oxygen therapy was associated with complete healing in half of the patients after 44 sessions of therapy administered over a period of 2 months [133]. It is important to eliminate or minimize risk factors; therefore, warfarin should be discontinued, hypercalcemia and hyperphosphatemia should be corrected, intake of vitamin D and calcium should be eliminated, and high levels of dialysate calcium should be avoided [116].

An important pharmacotherapeutic agent studied in CUA is sodium thiosulfate. Sodium thiosulfate is an agent with antioxidant and vasodilatory properties that also inhibits adipocyte calcification and blocks the ability of adipocytes to induce the calcification of vascular smooth muscle cells [121, 134]. While this may be the most common intervention to treat CUA, it is an off-label indication. Its use in CUA was first described in 2004 in a case report, and there is no prospective trial data on this agent [135]. Intraperitoneal administration has been used, but its effectiveness is unclear, and it increases the risk of chemical peritonitis [136, 137]. Intralesional administration has been described to aid in the resolution of calciphylaxis lesions [138].

In patients with ESRD, the hemodialysis or peritoneal dialysis prescription should be optimized to achieve the recommended KDOQI goals of adequacy. Limited data has been published on the option of increasing length or frequency of hemodialysis to accelerate wound healing, converting peritoneal dialysis patients to hemodialysis, or kidney transplantation to treat and possibly completely resolve CUA [139, 140].

Bone Disease

Bone is a mineralized connective tissue that exhibits four types of cells: osteoblasts, bone lining cells, osteocytes, and osteoclasts [141, 142]. The bone has important functions in the body, including locomotion, support, and protection of soft tissues, calcium and phosphate storage, and harboring of bone marrow [143, 144]. Bone is a highly dynamic organ in which bone remodeling is a highly complex process in which old bone is replaced by new bone through a cycle comprised of three phases: initiation of bone resorption by osteoclasts, the transition from resorption to new bone formation, and the bone formation by osteoblasts [145, 146]. Normal bone remodeling is necessary for fracture healing and skeleton adaptation to mechanical use as well as for calcium homeostasis; however, an imbalance of bone resorption and formation results in several bone diseases [147].

Bone mineralization is initiated in matrix vesicles; the small extracellular vesicles derived from osteoblasts and chondrocytes, in which calcium and inorganic phosphate are taken up by matrix vesicles and form hydroxyapatite crystals that propagate on collagen fibrils to mineralize the extracellular matrix [148]. The chemical structure of bone minerals implies that the extracellular levels of ionic calcium and inorganic phosphate are two critical determinants of bone mineralization, and data from patients and animal models of human diseases clearly demonstrates that the reduction of systemic phosphate levels with or without any alteration of the calcium levels leads to osteomalacia with the characteristic increase of unmineralized osteoid volume [149]. This importance of systemic levels of mineral ions was demonstrated by impairment in the calcitriol signaling pathway in which mutations in 25, hydroxy D3–1 α-hydroxylase or inactivating mutations in the vitamin D receptor impair the absorption of calcium and phosphate in the gut. These mutations also reduce the mobilization of these ions from the bone by restricting bone resorption [150–152].

The World Health Organization (WHO) has defined osteoporosis as a progressive systemic skeletal disease characterized by low bone mass and microarchitectural deterioration of bone tissue, with a consequential increase in bone fragility and susceptibility to fracture [153]. Differentiations among the disorders of osteoporosis or CKD-MBD are dependent on the measurement of specific biochemical markers, including serum PTH and/or quantitative bone histomorphometry. Furthermore, the WHO proposes a dual-energy X-ray absorptiometry-BMD T-score ≤ -2.5 as an operational diagnostic threshold for osteoporosis. The major fracture risk estimation tools, Fracture Risk Assessment Tool (FRAX), the Garvan Calculator, and QFracture differ in important ways as they include different risk factors, encode into an estimation model differently, and report different outputs. Age and sex are included in all three instruments. Age is a powerful fracture risk factor, and its importance is more apparent in QFracture and Garvan than FRAX, because only FRAX considers the competing risk of death. The FRAX model yields lower fracture risk in the eldest individuals because mortality occurs before the fracture. In QFracture and Garvan, the fracture risk increases exponentially with age.

Furthermore, the female sex approximately doubles fracture risk which is reflected in all three models.

Disruptions in mineral metabolism and bone microarchitecture occur early during CKD and worsen with the progressive decline in kidney function so that at the time of initiation of dialysis, up to 50% of patients have had a fracture [154–159]. CKD and fracture risk are not isolated to only ESRD. Recent data obtained as part of the Third National Health and Nutrition Examination Survey reported that among 6270 men and women, there was an approximately twofold increased the risk of hip fractures among those with an eGFR <60 mL/min compared to those with eGFR >60 mL/min [160]. The incidence of fractures is higher in patients with ESRD on dialysis. In a large retrospective study using data from the United States Renal Data System (USRDS), the relative risk of hip fracture was increased in both men (RR = 4.44 95% CI 4.16–4.75) and women (RR = 4.40 95% CI 4.17–4.64) with CKD5 on dialysis compared with the general population [161]. The gold standard for diagnosis and classification of CKD-MBD is a bone biopsy with quantitative bone histomorphometry; however, the routine use of bone biopsy to evaluate fracture risk among patients with CKD is neither feasible nor appropriate, and recent research has focused on studying the associations between noninvasive assessments of fracture risk and fracture [162, 163].

In a majority of patients with CKD, renal excretion of net acid falls sufficiently when the glomerular filtration rate is reduced to approximately 30% of normal. This causes metabolic acidosis [164]. Metabolic acidosis may affect changes in bone by directly inducing the dissolution of bone, stimulating osteoclast-mediated bone resorption, inhibiting osteoblast-mediated bone formation, and altering the serum concentrations or the biological actions of PTH and vitamin D [165]. As a consequence, in some patients with normal kidney function, osteoporosis and osteomalacia have been reported that are linked in part to metabolic acidosis [165]. Also, in patients with CKD before and after initiation of dialysis, the severity of metabolic acidosis appears to have a bearing on the presence and degree of hyperparathyroidism, osteitis fibrosa, and osteomalacia [165]. Taken as a whole, these data suggest that correction of the metabolic acidosis of CKD may have a beneficial effect on the bone disease observed in these patients [165].

Renal osteodystrophy is an alteration of bone morphology in patients with CKD; it is one measure of the skeletal component of the systemic disorder of CKD-MBD that is quantifiable by histomorphometry of bone biopsy [166]. The evaluation and definitive diagnosis of renal osteodystrophy require a bone biopsy. Although histomorphometry is not essential for clinical diagnosis, one should be performed in research studies [166]. The bone turnover, mineralization, and volume (TMV) classification scheme provides a clinically relevant description of the underlying bone pathology as assessed by histomorphometry, which in turn helps define the pathophysiology, and thereby guide therapy [166].

Turnover reflects the rate of skeletal remodeling, which is normally the coupled process of bone resorption and bone formation [166]. It is assessed with histomorphometry by dynamic measurements of osteoblast function using the technique of double-tetracycline labeling [166]. Bone formation rates and activation frequency represent acceptable parameters for assessing bone turnover. When bone formation rate is reported, the referent (bone surface, area, volume, or tissue volume) should be specified [166]. Bone turnover is mainly affected by hormones, cytokines, mechanical stimuli, and growth factors that influence the recruitment, differentiation, and activity of osteoclasts and osteoblasts [166].

Mineralization reflects how well bone collagen becomes calcified during the formation phase of skeletal remodeling [166]. It is assessed with histomorphometry by static measurements of osteoid volume and osteoid thickness and by dynamic, tetracycline-based measurements of mineralization lag time and osteoid maturation time [166]. Causes of impaired mineralization include inadequate vitamin D, malnutrition, mineral deficiency, acidosis, or bone aluminum toxicity [166].

Volume indicates the amount of bone per unit volume of tissue [166]. It is assessed with histomorphometry by static measurements of bone volume in cancellous bone [166]. Determinants of bone volume in the general population and CKD patients include age, gender, race, genetic factors, nutrition, endocrine disorders, mechanical stimuli, toxicities, neurological function, vascular supply, growth factors, and cytokines [166].

Adynamic, or low turnover, bone disease, first described in the 1980s, is defined by a faulty rate of collagen synthesis and mineralization [167]. An example of this would be low bone turnover without osteoid accumulation. This is different from osteomalacia, in which there is low-turnover disease. However, the defect in mineralization exceeds the defects in bone formation, leading to relative osteoid excess. In adynamic bone disease, there are few or no osteoblasts, minimal or no peritrabecular fibrosis, a substantially low bone formation rate. The number of remodeling sites is also low [167]. Risk factors are multifactorial and include elderly individuals, diabetes, high calcium load, vitamin D excess, overzealous treatment of hyperparathyroidism, low parathyroid hormone levels, parathyroidectomy, systemic inflammation, calcimimetics, and bisphosphonates [168, 169]. The pathophysiology includes bone formation rate less than 97–108 $\mu m^2/mm^2/day$, osteoid volume less than 12–15%, and no (minimal) fibrosis [167]. One of the most common symptoms is skeletal pain; furthermore, bone alkaline phosphatase is the most useful parameter for bone formation as elevated levels exclude adynamic bone disease while low PTH levels distinguish it from high turnover CKD-MBD [170–172].

The chief management strategy aims to increase PTH synthesis in low-turnover bone disease are as follows

(a) Switch from calcium-containing phosphate binders to non-calcium/non-aluminum-containing binders.
(b) Evaluate daily dietary calcium intake and reduce it to 1200 mg (1000 mg for men aged 19–70 and women aged 19–50).
(c) Stop/reduce active vitamin D medications.

(d) Lower dialysate calcium to 1.25 mmol/L or below.
(e) Teriparatide (recombinant human PTH approved for the treatment of patients at high risk for fracture).
(f) Abaloparatide (PTH-related peptide analogue).
(g) Romosozumab (monoclonal antibody that binds and inhibits sclerostin) [167, 173–177].

Osteitis fibrosa cystica, or high turnover bone disease, is a skeletal disorder caused by an overproduction of PTH from overactive parathyroid glands and is the late manifestation of hyperparathyroidism [178]. The presentation is usually bone pain. Characteristic radiologic findings include subperiosteal bone resorption in middle phalanges and distal radius, thinning of distal clavicle, bone cyst formation, "salt and pepper" pattern of the skull, brown tumor involving the bones, and generalized osteopenia [178]. The pathophysiology includes PTH attaching to receptors on osteoblasts, which results in the expression of RANK ligand-receptor activator, then RANK ligand attaches to RANK on precursors of the osteoclasts, promoting osteoclast formation, and activated osteoclasts cause bone resorption, cortical bone destruction, and fibrous cysts formation [178].

Treatment aims for the management of hyperparathyroidism and high bone turnover disease are as follows

(a) By correcting the underlying metabolic abnormalities (non-calcium based binder, vitamin D receptor analog, calcimimetic).
(b) Parathyroidectomy [178].

A mixed osteodystrophy includes components of the high turnover osteitis fibrosa and low turnover mineralization defects (as seen in osteomalacia) [179]. An example of the above bone disorders with the TMV classification can be seen in Fig. 7.2.

CKD-MBD is a major complication in dialysis patients but begins early in the course of the disease. It describes a complex syndrome of mineral disturbances, hormonal changes, renal osteodystrophy, and bone disorders which can lead to several complications, including vascular calcification, cardiovascular morbidity and mortality, calciphylaxis, and bone fractures. The pathophysiology is complex, with multiple inducers and inhibitors of signaling regulation as well as some pathways which remain uncertain. In the last two decades, therapeutic options have increased, and many new novel agents are under investigation. In order to optimize the evidence behind CKD-MBD therapy, there is a necessity for more high-quality and large-scale randomized controlled interventional trials.

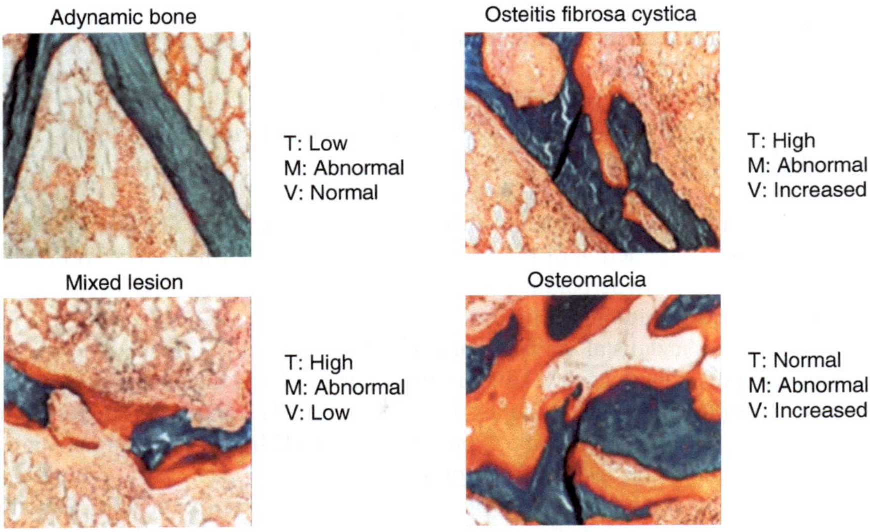

Fig. 7.2 Classification of renal osteodystrophy. An illustration of adynamic bone, osteitis fibrosa cystica, mixed lesion, and osteomalacia using both the old classification of renal osteodystrophy as well as the newer CKD-MBD TMV classification

Management Pearls for Clinicians

- Treatment for primary and tertiary hyperparathyroidism is primarily surgical.
- Vitamin D receptor activators (calcitriol and paricalcitol) are available for the treatment of hyperparathyroidism associated with vitamin D deficiency from decreased production of calcitriol.
- Cinacalcet, a calcimimetic, is indicated for the treatment of secondary hyperparathyroidism in dialysis patients.
- Extended-release calcifediol can be used in the treatment of secondary hyperparathyroidism in adults with stage 3–4 (not 5) CKD and vitamin D insufficiency.
- There are many phosphate binders available; however, individual consideration should be made due to different mechanisms of action, advantages and disadvantages of each, and patient preference.
- A biopsy is not needed for a patient with ESRD with the classic presentation of a painful necrotic ulcer covered with a black eschar for the diagnosis of CUA.
- CUA management includes pain management, wound care to remove exudate and necrotic tissue, sodium thiosulfate, and hyperbaric oxygen therapy.
- Pain management can be challenging in patients with CUA, and relief may be unresponsive to high-dose opioids. Consider concomitant treatment with gabapentin, ketamine, or spinal anesthetic agents.

- Magnesium serum levels are reduced with long-term proton pump inhibitor (PPI) treatment.
- Supplementation is an accepted form of treatment for vitamin D deficiency; however, the process should be closely monitored to ensure appropriate levels rather than toxicity.
- In low turnover bone disease, the treatment strategy aims to increase PTH synthesis by switching calcium-containing phosphate binders to non-calcium binders, reducing dietary calcium intake, stopping/reducing vitamin D medications, lowering dialysate calcium, or medications (teriparatide, abaloparatide, romosozumab).
- Hyperparathyroidism and high turnover bone disease can be managed by correcting underlying metabolic abnormalities and parathyroidectomy.

References

1. Hanley DA, Watson PH, Hodsman AB, Dempster DW. Pharmacological mechanisms of therapeutics: parathyroid hormone. In: Bilezikian J, Raisz LG, Martin TJ, editors. Principles of bone biology, vol. 2. Elsevier; 2008. p. 1661–95.
2. Civitelli R, Ziambaras K. Calcium and phosphate homeostasis: concerted interplay of new regulators. J Endocrinol Investig. 2011;34:3–7.
3. Chiavistelli S, Giustina A, Mazziotti G. Parathyroid hormone pulsatility: physiological and clinical aspects. Bone Res. 2015;3:14049. https://doi.org/10.1038/boneres.2014.49.
4. Bringhurst FR, Demay MB, Kronenberg HM. Hormones and disorders of mineral metabolism. In: Kronenberg HM, Melmed S, Polonsky KS, Larsen PR, editors. Williams textbook of endocrinology, vol. 1. Saunders Elsevier; 2008. p. 1203–68.
5. Carling T, Rastad J, Akerström G, Westin G. Vitamin D receptor (VDR) and parathyroid hormone messenger ribonucleic acid levels correspond to polymorphic VDR alleles in human parathyroid tumors. J Clin Endocrinol Metab. 1998;83(7):2255–9. https://doi.org/10.1210/jcem.83.7.4862.
6. Martin A, David V, Quarles LD. Regulation and function of the FGF23/klotho endocrine pathways. Physiol Rev. 2012;92(1):131–55. https://doi.org/10.1152/physrev.00002.2011.
7. van Abel M, Hoenderop JG, van der Kemp AW, et al. Coordinated control of renal Ca^{2+} transport proteins by parathyroid hormone. Kidney Int. 2005;68:1708–21.
8. Cha SK, Wu T, Huang CL. Protein kinase C inhibits caveolae-mediated endocytosis of TRPV5. Am J Physiol Ren Physiol. 2008;294:F1212–21.
9. Brenza HL, Kimmel-Jehan C, Jehan F, et al. Parathyroid hormone activation of the 25-hydroxyvitamin D3–1alpha-hydroxylase gene promoter. Proc Natl Acad Sci U S A. 1998;95:1387–91.
10. Goltzman D. Physiology of parathyroid hormone. Endocrinol Metab Clin N Am. 2018;47(4):743–58. https://doi.org/10.1016/j.ecl.2018.07.003.
11. Boyle WJ, Simonet WS, Lacey DL. Osteoclast differentiation and activation. Nature. 2003;423(6937):337–42. https://doi.org/10.1038/nature01658.
12. Walker MD, Silverberg SJ. Primary hyperparathyroidism. Nat Rev Endocrinol. 2018;14(2):115–25. https://doi.org/10.1038/nrendo.2017.104.
13. Rao SD, et al. Hyperparathyroidism following head and neck irradiation. Arch Intern Med. 1980;140:205–7.
14. Bendz H, Sjodin I, Toss G, Berglund K. Hyperparathyroidism and long-term lithium therapy—a cross-sectional study and the effect of lithium withdrawal. J Intern Med. 1996;240:357–65.

15. Brown EM. Role of the calcium-sensing receptor in extracellular calcium homeostasis. Best Pract Res Clin Endocrinol Metab. 2013;27:333–43.
16. Cope O. The study of hyperparathyroidism at the Massachusetts General Hospital. N Engl J Med. 1966;274:1174–82.
17. Albright F, Aub J, Bauer W. Hyperparathyroidism: common and polymorphic condition as illustrated by seventeen proven cases in one clinic. JAMA. 1934;102:1276.
18. Bilezikian JP, et al. Guidelines for the management of asymptomatic primary hyperparathyroidism: summary statement from the Fourth International Workshop. J Clin Endocrinol Metab. 2014;99:3561–9.
19. Elias RM, Dalboni MA, Coelho ACE, Moysés RMA. CKD-MBD: from the pathogenesis to the identification and development of potential novel therapeutic targets. Curr Osteoporos Rep. 2018;16:693–702.
20. Shimada T, Hasegawa H, Yamazaki Y, Muto T, Hino R, Takeuchi Y, et al. FGF-23 is a potent regulator of vitamin D metabolism and phosphate homeostasis. J Bone Miner Res. 2004;19:429–35.
21. Ginsberg C, Zelnick LR, Block GA, Chertow GM, Chonchol M, Hoofnagle A, Kestenbaum B, de Boer IH. Differential effects of phosphate binders on vitamin D metabolism in chronic kidney disease. Nephrol Dial Transplant. 2020;35(4):616–23. https://doi.org/10.1093/ndt/gfaa010.
22. Rroji M, Spasovski G. Calcimimetics versus parathyroidectomy: what is preferable? Int Urol Nephrol. 2018;50(7):1271–5. https://doi.org/10.1007/s11255-018-1838-5.
23. Brown EM. Extracellular Ca^{2+} sensing, regulation of parathyroid cell function, and role of Ca^{2+} and other ions as extracellular (first) messengers. Physiol Rev. 1991;71(2):371–411. https://doi.org/10.1152/physrev.1991.71.2.371.
24. Nemeth EF, Steffey ME, Hammerland LG, Hung BC, Van Wagenen BC, DelMar EG, Balandrin MF. Calcimimetics with potent and selective activity on the parathyroid calcium receptor. Proc Natl Acad Sci U S A. 1998;95:4040–5.
25. Bover J, Aguilar A, Venegas R, Jofré R. Calcimiméticos en la enfermedad renal crónica estadio 5D. In: Cannata-Andía JB, editor. Alteraciones del metabolismo óseo y mineral en la enfermedad renal crónica: avances en patogenia, diagnóstico y tratamiento; 2010. p. 209–27.
26. Parsabiv (etelcalcetide) prescribing information. Thousand Oaks: Amgen, Inc.; 2017.
27. Chen P, Olsson Gisleskok P, Perez-Ruixo JJ, et al. Population pharmacokinetics and pharmacodynamics of the calcimimetic etelcalcetide in chronic kidney disease and secondary hyperparathyroidism receiving hemodialysis. CPT Pharmacometr Syst Pharmacol. 2016;5:484–94.
28. Baird GS. Ionized calcium. Clin Chim Acta. 2011;412(9–10):696–701. https://doi.org/10.1016/j.cca.2011.01.004.
29. Hill Gallant KM, Spiegel DM. Calcium balance in chronic kidney disease. Curr Osteoporos Rep. 2017;15(3):214–21. https://doi.org/10.1007/s11914-017-0368-x.
30. Perwad F, Zhang MY, Tenenhouse HS, Portale AA. Fibroblast growth factor 23 impairs phosphorus and vitamin D metabolism in vivo and suppresses 25-hydroxyvitamin D-1alpha-hydroxylase expression in vitro. Am J Physiol Ren Physiol. 2007;293(5):F1577–83. https://doi.org/10.1152/ajprenal.00463.2006.
31. Rao MN, Shoback DM. Hypocalcemia. In: Feingold KR, Anawalt B, Boyce A, et al., editors. Endotext. South Dartmouth: MDText.com, Inc.; 2000.
32. Sprague SM, Silva A, Al-Saghir F, Damle R, Tabash SP, Petkovich M, Messner EJ, White JA, Melnick JZ, Bishop CW. Modified-release calcifediol safely suppresses PTH levels in patients with secondary hyperparathyroidism associated with vitamin D insufficiency in chronic kidney disease stages 3 and 4: a randomized controlled trial. Am J Nephrol. 2014;40:535–45. https://doi.org/10.1159/000369939.
33. Brown AJ, Slatopolsky E. Drug insight: vitamin D analogs in the treatment of secondary hyperparathyroidism in patients with chronic kidney disease. Nat Clin Pract Endocrinol Metab. 2007;3(2):134–44. https://doi.org/10.1038/ncpendmet0394.
34. Jamal SA, Miller PD. Secondary and tertiary hyperparathyroidism. J Clin Densitom. 2013;16(1):64–8.

35. O'Neill WC. Targeting serum calcium in chronic kidney disease and end-stage renal disease: is normal too high? Kidney Int. 2016;89(1):40–5. https://doi.org/10.1016/j.kint.2015.10.001.
36. Suki WN, Moore LW. Phosphorus regulation in chronic kidney disease. Methodist Debakey Cardiovasc J. 2016;12(4 Suppl):6–9. https://doi.org/10.14797/mdcj-12-4s1-6.
37. Dominguez JR, Kestenbaum B, Chonchol M, . et al. Relationships between serum and urine phosphorus with all-cause and cardiovascular mortality: the Osteoporotic Fractures in Men (MrOS) Study. Am J Kidney Dis 2013; 61(4): 555–563
38. Weinman EJ, Light PD, Suki WN. Gastrointestinal phosphate handling in CKD and its association with cardiovascular disease. Am J Kidney Dis. 2013;62(5):1006–11.
39. Lemann JJ. Calcium and phosphate metabolism: an overview in health and in calcium stone formers. In: Coe F, Favus M, Pak C, Parks J, Preminger G, editors. Kidney stones: medical and surgical management. Philadelphia: Lippincott-Raven; 1996. p. 259–88.
40. Cupisti A, Kalantar-Zadeh K. Management of natural and added dietary phosphorus burden in kidney disease. Semin Nephrol. 2013;33(2):180–90.
41. Health.gov [Internet]. Rockville, MD: Office of Disease Prevention and health promotion; 2016. July Dietary Guidelines for Americans 2015–2020, 8th Edition [cited 2016 Jul 22].
42. National Kidney Foundation. K/DOQI clinical practice guidelines for bone metabolism and disease in chronic kidney disease. Am J Kidney Dis. 2003;42(4 Suppl 3):S1–S201.
43. Blaine J, Chonchol M, Levi M. Renal control of calcium, phosphate, and magnesium homeostasis [Erratum in: Clin J Am Soc Nephrol. 2015 Oct 7;10(10):1886–7.]. Clin J Am Soc Nephrol. 2015;10(7):1257–72. https://doi.org/10.2215/CJN.09750913.
44. Liu Z, Su G, Guo X, Wu Y, Liu X, Zou C, Zhang L, Yang Q, Xu Y, Ma W. Dietary interventions for mineral and bone dis- order in people with chronic kidney disease. Cochrane Database Syst Rev. 2015;9:CD010350.
45. Palmer SC, Gardner S, Tonelli M, Mavridis D, Johnson DW, Craig JC, French R, Ruospo M, Strippoli GF. Phosphate-binding agents in adults with CKD: a network meta-analysis of randomized trials [Erratum in: Am J Kidney Dis. 2017 Sep;70(3):452.]. Am J Kidney Dis. 2016;68(5):691–702. https://doi.org/10.1053/j.ajkd.2016.05.015.
46. Ruospo M, Palmer SC, Natale P, Craig JC, Vecchio M, Elder GJ, Strippoli GF. Phosphate binders for preventing and treating chronic kidney disease-mineral and bone disorder (CKD-MBD). Cochrane Database Syst Rev. 2018;8:CD006023.
47. Serum phosphorus (most recent), categories. DOPPS Practice Monitor. 2020. https://www.dopps.org/OurStudies/DOPPSPracticeMonitor.aspx.
48. Copland M, Komenda P, Weinhandl ED, McCullough PA, Morfin JA. Intensive hemodialysis, mineral and bone disorder, and phosphate binder use. Am J Kidney Dis. 2016;68(5S1):S24–32. https://doi.org/10.1053/j.ajkd.2016.05.024.
49. Ganesh SK, Stack AG, Levin NW, Hulbert-Shearon T, Port FK. Association of elevated serum PO_4, Ca × PO_4 product, and parathyroid hormone with cardiac mortality risk in chronic hemodialysis patients. J Am Soc Nephrol. 2001;12(10):2131–8.
50. Block GA, Klassen PS, Lazarus JM, Ofsthun N, Lowrie EG, Chertow GM. Mineral metabolism, mortality, and morbidity in maintenance hemodialysis. J Am Soc Nephrol. 2004;15(8):2208–18. https://doi.org/10.1097/01.ASN.0000133041.27682.A2.
51. Tentori F, Blayney MJ, Albert JM, et al. Mortality risk for dialysis patients with different levels of serum calcium, phosphorus, and PTH: the Dialysis Outcomes and Practice Patterns Study (DOPPS). Am J Kidney Dis. 2008;52(3):519–30. https://doi.org/10.1053/j.ajkd.2008.03.020.
52. Kovesdy CP, Quarles LD. Fibroblast growth factor-23: what we know, what we don't know, and what we need to know. Nephrol Dial Transplant. 2013;28(9):2228–36.
53. Wolf M. Forging forward with 10 burning questions on FGF23 in kidney disease. J Am Soc Nephrol. 2010;21(9):1427–35.
54. Wesseling-Perry K, Jüppner H. The osteocyte in CKD: new concepts regarding the role of FGF23 in mineral metabolism and systemic complications. Bone. 2013;54(2):222–9.
55. Batra J, Buttar RS, Kaur P, Kreimerman J, Melamed ML. FGF-23 and cardiovascular disease: review of literature. Curr Opin Endocrinol Diabetes Obes. 2016;23(6):423–9. https://doi.org/10.1097/MED.0000000000000294.

56. Gupta M, Orozco G, Rao M, Gedaly R, Malluche HH, Neyra JA. The role of alterations in alpha-klotho and FGF-23 in kidney transplantation and kidney donation. Front Med (Lausanne). 2022;9:803016. https://doi.org/10.3389/fmed.2022.803016.
57. Hu MC, Kuro-o M, Moe OW. Secreted klotho and chronic kidney disease. Adv Exp Med Biol. 2012;728:126–57.
58. Kuro-o M. Klotho and aging. Biochim Biophys Acta. 2009;1790(10):1049–58.
59. Hu MC, Kuro-o M, Moe OW. The emerging role of Klotho in clinical nephrology. Nephrol Dial Transplant. 2012;27(7):2650–7.
60. Hu MC, Shi M, Zhang J, Pastor J, Nakatani T, Lanske B, Razzaque MS, Rosenblatt KP, Baum MG, Kuro-o M, Moe OW. Klotho: a novel phosphaturic substance acting as an autocrine enzyme in the renal proximal tubule. FASEB J. 2010;24(9):3438–50. https://doi.org/10.1096/fj.10-154765.
61. Hu MC, Kuro-o M, Moe OW. Klotho and chronic kidney disease. Contrib Nephrol. 2013;180:47–63. https://doi.org/10.1159/000346778.
62. Zununi Vahed S, Mostafavi S, Hosseiniyan Khatibi SM, Shoja MM, Ardalan M. Vascular calcification: an important understanding in nephrology. Vasc Health Risk Manag. 2020;16:167–80. https://doi.org/10.2147/VHRM.S242685.
63. Pérez-Hernández N, Aptilon-Duque G, Blachman-Braun R, et al. Vascular calcification: current genetics underlying this complex phenomenon. Chin Med J. 2017;130(9):1113–21. https://doi.org/10.4103/0366-6999.204931.
64. Bowman MAH, McNally EM. Genetic pathways of vascular calcification. Trends Cardiovasc Med. 2012;22(4):93–8. https://doi.org/10.1016/j.tcm.2012.07.002.
65. Schurgers LJ, Barreto DV, Barreto FC, et al. The circulating inactive form of matrix gla protein is a surrogate marker for vascular calcification in chronic kidney disease: a preliminary report. Clin J Am Soc Nephrol. 2010;5(4):568–75. https://doi.org/10.2215/CJN.07081009.
66. Smith ER, Ford ML, Tomlinson LA, Rajkumar C, McMahon LP, Holt SG. Phosphorylated fetuin-A-containing calciprotein particles are associated with aortic stiffness and a procalcific milieu in patients with pre-dialysis CKD. Nephrol Dial Transplant. 2012;27(5):1957–66.
67. Shroff RC, McNair R, Figg N, et al. Dialysis accelerates medial vascular calcification in part by triggering smooth muscle cell apoptosis. Circulation. 2008;118(17):1748–57. https://doi.org/10.1161/CIRCULATIONAHA.108.783738.
68. Lang F, Leibrock C, Pelzl L, et al. Therapeutic interference with vascular calcification-lessons from klotho-hypomorphic mice and beyond. Front Endocrinol (Lausanne). 2018;9:207. https://doi.org/10.3389/fendo.2018.00207.
69. Kanno Y, Into T, Lowenstein CJ, Matsushita K. Nitric oxide regulates vascular calcification by interfering with TGF-signalling. Cardiovasc Res. 2008;77(1):221–30. https://doi.org/10.1093/cvr/cvm049.
70. Cai T, Sun D, Duan Y, et al. WNT/beta-catenin signaling promotes VSMCs to osteogenic transdifferentiation and calcification through directly modulating Runx2 gene expression. Exp Cell Res. 2016;345(2):206–17. https://doi.org/10.1016/j.yexcr.2016.06.007.
71. Lee GL, Yeh CC, Wu JY, et al. TLR2 promotes vascular smooth muscle cell chondrogenic differentiation and consequent calcification via the concerted actions of osteoprotegerin suppression and IL-6-mediated RANKL induction. Arterioscler Thromb Vasc Biol. 2019;39(3):432–45. https://doi.org/10.1161/ATVBAHA.118.311874.
72. Osako MK, Nakagami H, Shimamura M, et al. Cross-talk of receptor activator of nuclear factor-κB ligand signaling with renin–angiotensin system in vascular calcification. Arterioscler Thromb Vasc Biol. 2013;33(6):1287–96. https://doi.org/10.1161/ATVBAHA.112.301099.
73. Gauthier-Bastien A, Ung RV, Lariviere R, Mac-Way F, Lebel M, Agharazii M. Vascular remodeling and media calcification increases arterial stiffness in chronic kidney disease. Clin Exp Hypertens. 2014;36(3):173–80. https://doi.org/10.3109/10641963.2013.804541.
74. Pai AS, Giachelli CM. Matrix remodeling in vascular calcification associated with chronic kidney disease. J Am Soc Nephrol. 2010;21(10):1637–40. https://doi.org/10.1681/ASN.2010040349.

75. Lau WL, Savoj J, Nakata MB, Vaziri ND. Altered microbiome in chronic kidney disease: systemic effects of gut-derived uremic toxins. Clin Sci (Lond). 2018;132(5):509–22. https://doi.org/10.1042/CS20171107.
76. Yamamoto H, Tsuruoka S, Ioka T, et al. Indoxyl sulfate stimulates proliferation of rat vascular smooth muscle cells. Kidney Int. 2006;69(10):1780–5. https://doi.org/10.1038/sj.ki.5000340.
77. Yisireyili M, Saito S, Abudureyimu S, et al. Indoxyl sulfate-induced activation of (pro)renin receptor promotes cell proliferation and tissue factor expression in vascular smooth muscle cells. PLoS One. 2014;9(10):e109268. https://doi.org/10.1371/journal.pone.0109268.
78. Henze LA, Luong TTD, Boehme B, et al. Impact of C-reactive protein on osteo-/chondrogenic transdifferentiation and calcification of vascular smooth muscle cells. Aging (Albany NY). 2019;11(15):5445–62. https://doi.org/10.18632/aging.102130.
79. Chen B, Zhao Y, Han D, et al. Wnt1 inhibits vascular smooth muscle cell calcification by promoting ANKH expression. J Mol Cell Cardiol. 2019;135:10–21. https://doi.org/10.1016/j.yjmcc.2019.07.00.
80. Wei R, Enaka M, Muragaki Y. Activation of KEAP1/NRF2/P62 signaling alleviates high phosphate-induced calcification of vascular smooth muscle cells by suppressing reactive oxygen species production. Sci Rep. 2019;9(1):10366. https://doi.org/10.1038/s41598-019-46824-2.
81. Li Z, Wu J, Zhang X, et al. CDC42 promotes vascular calcification in chronic kidney disease. J Pathol. 2019;249(4):461–71. https://doi.org/10.1002/path.5334.
82. Oldberg A, Franzen A, Heinegard D. Cloning and sequence analysis of rat bone sialoprotein (osteopontin) cDNA reveals an Arg–Gly–Asp cell-binding sequence. Proc Natl Acad Sci U S A. 1986;83:8819–23.
83. Standal T, Borset M, Sundan A. Role of osteopontin in adhesion, migration, cell survival and bone remodeling. Exp Oncol. 2004;26:179–84.
84. Paloian NJ, Leaf EM, Giachelli CM. Osteopontin protects against high phosphate-induced nephrocalcinosis and vascular calcification. Kidney Int. 2016;89(5):1027–36. https://doi.org/10.1016/j.kint.2015.12.046.
85. Kuo TH, Lin WH, Chao JY, et al. Serum sclerostin levels are positively related to bone mineral density in peritoneal dialysis patients: a cross-sectional study. BMC Nephrol. 2019;20(1):266. https://doi.org/10.1186/s12882-019-1452-5.
86. Carracedo M, Witasp A, Qureshi AR, et al. Chemerin inhibits vascular calcification through ChemR23 and is associated with lower coronary calcium in chronic kidney disease. J Intern Med. 2019;286(4):449–57. https://doi.org/10.1111/joim.12940.
87. Frauscher B, Kirsch AH, Schabhuttl C, et al. Autophagy protects from uremic vascular media calcification. Front Immunol. 2018;9:1866. https://doi.org/10.3389/fimmu.2018.01866.
88. Mori D, Matsui I, Shimomura A, Hashimoto N, Matsumoto A, Shimada K, Yamaguchi S, Oka T, Kubota K, Yonemoto S, Sakaguchi Y, Takahashi A, Shintani Y, Takashima S, Takabatake Y, Hamano T, Isaka Y. Protein carbamylation exacerbates vascular calcification. Kidney Int. 2018;94(1):72–90. https://doi.org/10.1016/j.kint.2018.01.033.
89. Ter Braake AD, Shanahan CM, de Baaij JHF. Magnesium counteracts vascular calcification: passive interference or active modulation? Arterioscler Thromb Vasc Biol. 2017;37(8):1431–45. https://doi.org/10.1161/ATVBAHA.117.309182.
90. Louvet L, Metzinger L, Buchel J, Steppan S, Massy ZA. Magnesium attenuates phosphate-induced deregulation of a microRNA signature and prevents modulation of Smad1 and osterix during the course of vascular calcification. Biomed Res Int. 2016;2016:7419524. https://doi.org/10.1155/2016/7419524.
91. Ter Braake AD, Tinnemans PT, Shanahan CM, Hoenderop JGJ, de Baaij JHF. Magnesium prevents vascular calcification in vitro by inhibition of hydroxyapatite crystal formation. Sci Rep. 2018;8(1):2069. https://doi.org/10.1038/s41598-018-20241-3.
92. Kaesler N, Goettsch C, Weis D, et al. Magnesium but not nicotinamide prevents vascular calcification in experimental uraemia. Nephrol Dial Transplant. 2019;35(1):65–73. https://doi.org/10.1093/ndt/gfy410.

93. Montes de Oca A, Guerrero F, Martinez-Moreno JM, et al. Magnesium inhibits Wnt/beta-catenin activity and reverses the osteogenic transformation of vascular smooth muscle cells. PLoS One. 2014;9(2):e89525. https://doi.org/10.1371/journal.pone.0089525.
94. Fusaro M, Noale M, Tripepi G, Giannini S, D'Angelo A, Pica A, Calò LA, Miozzo D, Gallieni M. Long-term proton pump inhibitor use is associated with vascular calcification in chronic kidney disease: a cross-sectional study using propensity score analysis. Drug Saf. 2013;36(8):635–42. https://doi.org/10.1007/s40264-013-0062-6.
95. Nagy A, Petho D, Gall T, et al. Zinc inhibits HIF-prolyl hydroxylase inhibitor-aggravated VSMC calcification induced by high phosphate. Front Physiol. 2019;10:1584. https://doi.org/10.3389/fphys.2019.01584.
96. Voelkl J, Tuffaha R, Luong TTD, et al. Zinc inhibits phosphate-induced vascular calcification through TNFAIP3-mediated suppression of NF-kappaB. J Am Soc Nephrol. 2018;29(6):1636–48. https://doi.org/10.1681/ASN.2017050492.
97. Shin MY, Kwun IS. Zinc restored the decreased vascular smooth muscle cell viability under atherosclerotic calcification conditions. Prev Nutr Food Sci. 2014;19(4):363–6. https://doi.org/10.3746/pnf.2014.19.4.363.
98. Akbari M, Nayeri H, Nasri H. Association of fetuin-A with kidney disease; a review on current concepts and new data. J Nephropharmacol. 2019;8(2):e14.
99. Dai L, Qureshi AR, Witasp A, Lindholm B, Stenvinkel P. Early vascular ageing and cellular senescence in chronic kidney disease. Comput Struct Biotechnol J. 2019;17:721–9. https://doi.org/10.1016/j.csbj.2019.06.015.
100. Maréchal C, Schlieper G, Nguyen P, et al. Serum fetuin-A levels are associated with vascular calcifications and predict cardiovascular events in renal transplant recipients. Clin J Am Soc Nephrol. 2011;6(5):974–85. https://doi.org/10.2215/CJN.06150710.
101. Reynolds JL, Skepper JN, McNair R, Kasama T, Gupta K, Weissberg PL, Jahnen-Dechent W, Shanahan CM. Multifunctional roles for serum protein fetuin-A in inhibition of human vascular smooth muscle cell calcification. J Am Soc Nephrol. 2005;16(10):2920–30. https://doi.org/10.1681/ASN.2004100895.
102. Wang J, Zhou JJ, Robertson GR, Lee VW. Vitamin D in vascular calcification: a double-edged sword? Nutrients. 2018;10(5):652. https://doi.org/10.3390/nu10050652.
103. Norman PE, Powell JT. Vitamin D and cardiovascular disease. Circ Res. 2014;114:379–93. https://doi.org/10.1161/CIRCRESAHA.113.301241.
104. Holick MF, MacLaughlin JA, Doppelt SH. Regulation of cutaneous previtamin D3 photosynthesis in man: skin pigment is not an essential regulator. Science. 1981;211:590–3. https://doi.org/10.1126/science.6256855.
105. Bas A, Lopez I, Perez J, Rodriguez M, Aguilera-Tejero E. Reversibility of calcitriol-induced medial artery calcification in rats with intact renal function. J Bone Miner Res. 2006;21:484–90. https://doi.org/10.1359/JBMR.051211.
106. Schmidt N, Brandsch C, Kuhne H, Thiele A, Hirche F, Stangl GI. Vitamin D receptor deficiency and low vitamin D diet stimulate aortic calcification and osteogenic key factor expression in mice. PLoS One. 2012;7:e35316. https://doi.org/10.1371/journal.pone.0035316.
107. Mizobuchi M, Finch J, Martin D, Slatopolsky E. Differential effects of vitamin D receptor activators on vascular calcification in uremic rats. Kidney Int. 2007;72:709–15. https://doi.org/10.1038/sj.ki.5002406.
108. Noonan W, Koch K, Nakane M, Ma J, Dixon D, Bolin A, Reinhart G. Differential effects of vitamin D receptor activators on aortic calcification and pulse wave velocity in uraemic rats. Nephrol Dial Transplant. 2008;23:3824–30. https://doi.org/10.1093/ndt/gfn375.
109. Zittermann A, Schleithoff SS, Koerfer R. Vitamin D and vascular calcification. Curr Opin Lipidol. 2007;18:41–6. https://doi.org/10.1097/MOL.0b013e328011c6fc.
110. Ellam T, Hameed A, ul Haque R, Muthana M, Wilkie M, Francis SE, Chico TJ. Vitamin D deficiency and exogenous vitamin D excess similarly increase diffuse atherosclerotic calcification in apolipoprotein E knockout mice. PLoS One. 2014;9:e88767. https://doi.org/10.1371/journal.pone.0088767.

111. Shioi A, Morioka T, Shoji T, Emoto M. The inhibitory roles of vitamin K in progression of vascular calcification. Nutrients. 2020;12(2):583. https://doi.org/10.3390/nu12020583.
112. Shea MK, Dallal GE, Dawson-Hughes B, Ordovas JM, O'Donnell CJ, Gundberg CM, Peterson JW, Booth SL. Vitamin K, circulating cytokines, and bone mineral density in older men and women. Am J Clin Nutr. 2008;88:356–63. https://doi.org/10.1093/ajcn/88.2.356.
113. Shea MK, Booth SL, Massaro JM, Jacques PF, D'Agostino RB Sr, Dawson-Hughes B, Ordovas JM, O'Donnell CJ, Kathiresan S, Keaney JF Jr, et al. Vitamin K and vitamin D status: associations with inflammatory markers in the Framingham Offspring Study. Am J Epidemiol. 2008;167:313–20. https://doi.org/10.1093/aje/kwm306.
114. Elango K, Javaid A, Khetarpal BK, Ramalingam S, Kolandaivel KP, Gunasekaran K, Ahsan C. The effects of warfarin and direct oral anticoagulants on systemic vascular calcification: a review. Cell. 2021;10(4):773. https://doi.org/10.3390/cells10040773.
115. Grzejszczak P, Kurnatowska I. Role of vitamin K in CKD: is its supplementation advisable in CKD patients? Kidney Blood Press Res. 2021;46(5):523–30. https://doi.org/10.1159/000516611.
116. Nigwekar SU, Thadhani R, Brandenburg VM. Calciphylaxis. N Engl J Med. 2018;378(18):1704–14. https://doi.org/10.1056/NEJMra1505292.
117. Chen TY, Lehman JS, Gibson LE, Lohse CM, El-Azhary RA. Histopathology of calciphylaxis: cohort study with clinical correlations. Am J Dermatopathol. 2017;39:795–802.
118. Kramann R, Brandenburg VM, Schurgers LJ, et al. Novel insights into osteogenesis and matrix remodelling associated with calcific uraemic arteriolopathy. Nephrol Dial Transplant. 2013;28:856–68.
119. Moe SM, Chen NX. Calciphylaxis and vascular calcification: a continuum of extra-skeletal osteogenesis. Pediatr Nephrol. 2003;18:969–75.
120. Shroff R, Long DA, Shanahan C. Mechanistic insights into vascular calcification in CKD. J Am Soc Nephrol. 2013;24:179–89.
121. Chen NX, O'Neill K, Akl NK, Moe SM. Adipocyte induced arterial calcification is prevented with sodium thiosulfate. Biochem Biophys Res Commun. 2014;449:151–6.
122. Ghosh T, Winchester DS, Davis MDP, El-Azhary R, Comfere NI. Early clinical presentations and progression of calciphylaxis. Int J Dermatol. 2017;56:856–61.
123. Daudén E, Oñate MJ. Calciphylaxis. Dermatol Clin. 2008;26:557–68.
124. Polizzotto MN, Bryan T, Ashby MA, Martin P. Symptomatic management of calciphylaxis: a case series and review of the literature. J Pain Symptom Manag. 2006;32:186–90.
125. Nigwekar SU, Wolf M, Sterns RH, Hix JK. Calciphylaxis from nonuremic causes: a systematic review. Clin J Am Soc Nephrol. 2008;3:1139–43.
126. Weenig RH, Sewell LD, Davis MD, McCarthy JT, Pittelkow MR. Calciphylaxis: natural history, risk factor analysis, and outcome. J Am Acad Dermatol. 2007;56:569–79.
127. Bazari H. Case records of the Massachusetts General Hospital (Case 7-2007). N Engl J Med. 2007;356:1049–57.
128. Brandenburg VM, Evenepoel P, Floege J, et al. Lack of evidence does not justify neglect: how can we address unmet medical needs in calciphylaxis? Nephrol Dial Transplant. 2016;31:1211–9.
129. Baby D, Upadhyay M, Joseph MD, Asopa SJ, Choudhury BK, Rajguru JP, Gupta S. Calciphylaxis and its diagnosis: a review. J Fam Med Prim Care. 2019;8(9):2763–7. https://doi.org/10.4103/jfmpc.jfmpc_588_19.
130. Sato T, Ichioka S. How should we manage multiple skin ulcers associated with calciphylaxis? J Dermatol. 2012;39(11):966–8.
131. Zitt E, Konig M, Vychytil A, et al. Use of sodium thiosulphate in a multi-interventional setting for the treatment of calciphylaxis in dialysis patients. Nephrol Dial Transplant. 2013;28(5):1232–40.
132. Nigwekar SU, Kroshinsky D, Nazarian RM, Goverman J, Malhotra R, Jackson VA, Kamdar MM, Steele DJ, Thadhani RI. Calciphylaxis: risk factors, diagnosis, and treatment. Am J Kidney Dis. 2015;66(1):133–46. https://doi.org/10.1053/j.ajkd.2015.01.034.

133. An J, Devaney B, Ooi KY, Ford S, Frawley G, Menahem S. Hyperbaric oxygen in the treatment of calciphylaxis: a case series and literature review. Nephrology (Carlton). 2015;20:444–50.
134. Sowers KM, Hayden MR. Calcific uremic arteriolopathy: pathophysiology, reactive oxygen species and therapeutic approaches. Oxid Med Cell Longev. 2010;3:109–21.
135. Cicone JS, Petronis JB, Embert CD, Spector DA. Successful treatment of calciphylaxis with intravenous sodium thiosulfate. Am J Kidney Dis. 2004;43(6):1104–8.
136. Gupta DR, Sangha H, Khanna R. Chemical peritonitis after intraperitoneal sodium thiosulfate. Perit Dial Int. 2012;32(2):220–2.
137. Sherman C. Chemical peritonitis after intraperitoneal sodium thiosulfate. Perit Dial Int. 2013;33(1):104.
138. Strazzula L, Nigwekar SU, Steele D, et al. Intralesional sodium thiosulfate for the treatment of calciphylaxis. JAMA Dermatol. 2013;149(8):946–9.
139. Baldwin C, Farah M, Leung M, et al. Multi-intervention management of calciphylaxis: a report of 7 cases. Am J Kidney Dis. 2011;58:988–91.
140. Nordheim E, Dahle DO, Syse IM, Åsberg A, Reisæter AV, Hartmann A. Resolution of calciphylaxis after urgent kidney transplantation in 3 patients with end-stage kidney failure. Transplant Direct. 2016;2(11):e113.
141. Buckwalter JA, Glimcher MJ, Cooper RR, Recker R. Bone biology. I: structure, blood supply, cells, matrix, and mineralization. Instr Course Lect. 1996;45:371–86.
142. Downey PA, Siegel MI. Bone biology and the clinical implications for osteoporosis. Phys Ther. 2006;86(1):77–91.
143. Robling AG, Castillo AB, Turner CH. Biomechanical and molecular regulation of bone remodeling. Annu Rev Biomed Eng. 2006;8:455–98. https://doi.org/10.1146/annurev.bioeng.8.061505.095721.
144. Datta HK, Ng WF, Walker JA, Tuck SP, Varanasi SS. The cell biology of bone metabolism. J Clin Pathol. 2008;61(5):577–87. https://doi.org/10.1136/jcp.2007.048868.
145. Sims NA, Gooi JH. Bone remodeling: multiple cellular interactions required for coupling of bone formation and resorption. Semin Cell Dev Biol. 2008;19(5):444–51. https://doi.org/10.1016/j.semcdb.2008.07.016.
146. Matsuo K, Irie N. Osteoclast-osteoblast communication. Arch Biochem Biophys. 2008;473(2):201–9. https://doi.org/10.1016/j.abb.2008.03.027.
147. Dallas SL, Prideaux M, Bonewald LF. The osteocyte: an endocrine cell... and more. Endocr Rev. 2013;34(5):658–90. https://doi.org/10.1210/er.2012-1026.
148. Michigami T. Skeletal mineralization: mechanisms and diseases. Ann Pediatr Endocrinol Metab. 2019;24(4):213–9. https://doi.org/10.6065/apem.2019.24.4.213.
149. Murshed M. Mechanism of bone mineralization [Erratum in: Cold Spring Harb Perspect Med 2020 Aug 3;10(8)]. Cold Spring Harb Perspect Med. 2018;8(12):a031229. https://doi.org/10.1101/cshperspect.a031229.
150. Dardenne O, Prud'homme J, Arabian A, Glorieux FH, St-Arnaud R. Targeted inactivation of the 25-hydroxyvitamin D(3)-1(α)-hydroxylase gene (CYP27B1) creates an animal model of pseudovitamin D-deficiency rickets. Endocrinology. 2001;142:3135–41.
151. Panda DK, Miao D, Tremblay ML, Sirois J, Farookhi R, Hendy GN, Goltzman D. Targeted ablation of the 25-hydroxyvitamin D 1α-hydroxylase enzyme: evidence for skeletal, reproductive, and immune dysfunction. Proc Natl Acad Sci. 2001;98:7498–503.
152. Suda T, Takahashi N, Abe E. Role of vitamin D in bone resorption. J Cell Biochem. 1992;49:53–8.
153. Curtis EM, Harvey NC, Cooper C. The burden of osteoporosis. In: Harvey NC, Cooper C, editors. Osteoporosis: a life course epidemiology approach to skeletal health. Boca Raton: CRC Press; 2018. p. 1–20.
154. National Kidney Foundation. K/DOQI clinical practice guidelines for chronic kidney disease: evaluation, classification, and stratification. Am J Kidney Dis. 2002;39:S1–S266.
155. Jamal S. Fractures in men and women with dialysis-dependent renal failure. Endocrinol Rounds. 2003;3
156. Jamal SA, Gilbert J, Gordon C, Bauer DC. Cortical PQCT measures are associated with fractures in dialysis patients. J Bone Miner Res. 2006;21:543–8.

157. Jamal SA, Leiter RE, Jassal V, Hamilton CJ, Bauer DC. Impaired muscle strength is associated with fractures in hemodialysis patients. Osteoporosis Int. 2006;17(9):1390–7.
158. Malluche HH, Faugere MC. Renal osteodystrophy. New Engl J Med. 1989;321:317–8.
159. Lindberg JS, Moe SM. Osteoporosis in end-stage renal disease. Semin Nephrol. 1999;19:115–22.
160. Nickolas TL, McMahon DJ, Shane E. Relationship between moderate to severe kidney disease and hip fracture in the United States. J Am Soc Nephrol. 2006;17:3223–32.
161. Alem AM, Sherrard DJ, Gillen DL, et al. Increased risk of hip fracture among patients with end-stage renal disease. Kidney Int. 2000;58:396–9.
162. Kidney Disease: Improving Global Outcomes (KDIGO) CKD-MBD Work Group. KDIGO clinical practice guideline for the diagnosis, evaluation, prevention, and treatment of chronic kidney disease-mineral and bone disorder (CKD-MBD). Kidney Int. 2009;113:S1–130.
163. Jamal SA, West SL, Miller PD. Fracture risk assessment in patients with chronic kidney disease. Osteoporos Int. 2012;23:1191–8. https://doi.org/10.1007/s00198-011-1781-0.
164. Elkington JR. Hydrogen ion turnover in health and disease. Ann Intern Med. 1972;57:660–80.
165. Kraut JA. The role of metabolic acidosis in the pathogenesis of renal osteodystrophy. Adv Ren Replace Ther. 1995;2(1):40–51. https://doi.org/10.1016/s1073-4449(12)80070-7.
166. Moe S, Drüeke T, Cunningham J, Goodman W, Martin K, Olgaard K, Ott S, Sprague S, Lameire N, Eknoyan G, Kidney Disease: Improving Global Outcomes (KDIGO). Definition, evaluation, and classification of renal osteodystrophy: a position statement from Kidney Disease: Improving Global Outcomes (KDIGO). Kidney Int. 2006;69(11):1945–53. https://doi.org/10.1038/sj.ki.5000414.
167. Sharma S, Gupta A. Adynamic bone disease: revisited. Nefrologia (Engl Ed). 2021. https://doi.org/10.1016/j.nefro.2020.11.012.
168. Kurz P, Monier-Faugere MC, Bognar B, Werner E, Roth P, Vlachojannis J, Malluche HH. Evidence for abnormal calcium homeostasis in patients with adynamic bone disease. Kidney Int. 1994;46(3):855–61. https://doi.org/10.1038/ki.1994.342.
169. Coen G, Ballanti P, Bonucci E, Calabria S, Costantini S, Ferrannini M, Giustini M, Giordano R, Nicolai G, Manni M, Sardella D, Taggi F. Renal osteodystrophy in predialysis and hemodialysis patients: comparison of histologic patterns and diagnostic predictivity of intact PTH. Nephron. 2002;91(1):103–11. https://doi.org/10.1159/000057611.
170. Coco M, Rush H. Increased incidence of hip fractures in dialysis patients with low serum parathyroid hormone. Am J Kidney Dis. 2000;36:115–1121.
171. Atsumi K, Kushida K, Yamazaki K, Shimizu S, Ohmura A, Inoue T. Risk factors for vertebral fractures in renal osteodystrophy. Am J Kidney Dis. 1999;33(2):287–93. https://doi.org/10.1016/s0272-6386(99)70302-1.
172. Sherrard DJ, Hercz G, Pei Y, Maloney NA, Greenwood C, Manuel A, Saiphoo C, Fenton SS, Segre GV. The spectrum of bone disease in end-stage renal failure—an evolving disorder. Kidney Int. 1993;43(2):436–42. https://doi.org/10.1038/ki.1993.64.
173. Morelli MB, Santulli G, Gambardella J. Calcium supplements: good for the bone, bad for the heart? A systematic updated appraisal. Atherosclerosis. 2020;296:68–73. https://doi.org/10.1016/j.atherosclerosis.2020.01.008.
174. Torres PU, Bover J, Mazzaferro S, de Vernejoul MC, Cohen-Solal M. When, how, and why a bone biopsy should be performed in patients with chronic kidney disease. Semin Nephrol. 2014;34:612–25.
175. Jablonski G, Klem KH, Dnaielsen CC, Mosekilde L, Gordeladze JO. Aluminum-induced bone disease in uremic rats: effect of deferoxamine. Biosci Rep. 1996;16:49–63.
176. Bover J, Urena P, Brandenburg V, et al. Adynamic bone disease: from bone to vessels in chronic kidney disease. Semin Nephrol. 2014;34:626–40.
177. Cannata-Andia JB. Pathogenesis, prevention and management of low-bone turnover. Nephrol Dial Transplant. 2000;15:15–7.
178. Naji Rad S, Deluxe L. Osteitis fibrosa cystica. Treasure Island (FL): StatPearls Publishing; 2022.
179. Slatopolsky E, Gonzalez E, Martin K. Pathogenesis and treatment of renal osteodystrophy. Blood Purif. 2003;21(4–5):318–26.

Blood Clotting Complications in Dialysis

8

Stephen Z. Fadem

Introduction and Historical Perspective

Despite the discovery of dialysis in the 1800s by the Scottish chemist Thomas Graham, its use as a practical means of therapy remained unsuccessful, not just because of the lack of the right dialysis membrane but because of the inability to find a suitable anticoagulant.

The first attempted dialysis used hirudin, found in the saliva of blood-sucking leeches, and a direct inhibitor of thrombin. Georg Haas, a physician in the German town of Giessen, began experimenting with dialysis in 1914 and resumed his work after World War I with great disappointment because the hirudin he was using was too toxic. By 1924, a group at Johns Hopkins led by John Jacob Abel, Leonard Rowntree, and B. B. Turner was studying dialysis therapy in animals. Abel informed Haas of a purified leech extract, leading to an attempted treatment in a patient in 1924 that was successful for 15 min. This was the first human dialysis in history [1].

A leading John Hopkins physiologist and colleague of Abel, William H. Howell, was avidly studying blood clotting mechanisms, but it was his medical student, Jay McLean, who isolated heparin, a substance he found in the liver that inhibited coagulation. Howell also continued experiments with heparin [2], and by 1927, Haas was able to use it successfully in a follow-up dialysis procedure. The early work that led to its commercial availability by 1937 incorporated efforts by Charles Best, the Toronto physiologist who also contributed to the discovery and purification of insulin [3, 4].

S. Z. Fadem (✉)
Section of Nephrology, Department of Medicine, Baylor College of Medicine, Houston, TX, USA
e-mail: fadem@bcm.edu

S. Z. Fadem et al. (eds.), *Complications in Dialysis*,
https://doi.org/10.1007/978-3-031-44557-6_8

Before delving into how clotting, thrombosis, and bleeding disorders affect dialysis patients, we will first review how the clotting system works and how it is affected by chronic kidney disease [5].

The Clotting System

The two distinct pathways of clotting include the extrinsic system and the intrinsic system. They share mutual factors and a common pathway. The extrinsic pathway is exemplified by the crusty scab that forms over a nick or scrape. The intrinsic pathway protects us from the adverse consequence of internal bleeding but can sometimes malfunction, leading to venous thromboembolism. Intrinsic clotting can also be the effect of atrial fibrillation; blood pooling in the left atrium enables thrombus formation. As the thrombi break up, they shower emboli into the cerebral vessels, causing a stroke.

A major step in the clotting mechanism is the activation of thrombin, for it is thrombin that activates fibrinogen, leading to the cross-linked fibrin clot. This mechanism is fortunately balanced by antithrombin. Heparin is an activator of antithrombin and hence, an essential anticoagulant.

The Extrinsic Pathway

Injury to endothelial tissue exposes tissue factor (Factor III), which is also present in white blood cells. Once exposed, it activates Factor VII, which cascades to activate Factor X. The tissue factor also activates Factor VIII, which activates Factor X. The factors are serine proteases that cleave peptides at the serine locus, leading to their activation.

The Intrinsic Pathway

When damage to endothelial cells occurs, the exposure of phosphatidylserine binds circulating high molecular weight kininogen (HMWK). This cascades to activate Factor XII (Hageman Factor), activating Factor XI, then Factor IX (Christmas Factor). Tissue factor (Factor III) having bound to Factor VII and activating Factor X leads to the common pathway. Factor VII also activates Factor IX (Christmas Factor) [6].

Von Willebrand factor (VWF) is a glycoprotein with multiple binding sites. In addition to being present in the α-granules of platelets, it is in plasma and endothelial cells. With vascular injury, VWF leaks from damaged endothelial cells and is exposed to collagen. It also bridges with nearby platelets binding the glycoprotein Ib–IX receptor on their surface (GPIb-IX), leading to the activation of surface integrins that disrupt the α-granules and dense granules. The process is amplified as more VWF and thromboxane A2 are expressed from disturbed granules. The binding to collagen anchors the platelet to the exposed subendothelium and binds fibrinogen.

VWF is cleaved by the enzyme ADAMTS13; thus, high levels of ADAMTS13 distinguish the genetically determined ADAMTS13 deficiency-related thrombocytopenic purpura (TTP) from an acquired form of TTP results of a Shiga toxin produced by selected species of *Escherichia coli.* In this manifestation, diarrhea-associated hemolytic uremic syndrome, ADAMTS13 levels are not typically decreased. In atypical HUS, diarrhea is not present; it is the result of a disorder in the alternate complement pathway [7].

VWF is a carrier protein for Factor VIII. Factor VIII is activated through the thrombin activation of Factors XI and V. Activated Factor VIII stabilizes fibrin by creating cross-links.

GPIb-IX also interfaces with an integrin found on white blood cells and may also play a role in inflammation [8]. Inflammation and coagulation are correlated. Kallikreins play an active role in inflammation. They are activated from prekallikreins by Factor XI. When exposed to kallikrein, HMWK releases bradykinin, a proinflammatory vasodilator. The enzymatic breakdown of bradykinin is achieved through converting enzyme, the same enzyme that converts angiotensin 1 to angiotensin 2. Thus converting enzyme inhibitors increases bradykinin levels and can lead to a cough when bradykinin triggers airway sensor nerves [9]. Kallikrein inhibits the activation of Factor XII.

The Common Pathway

The activation of Factor X (Stuart-Prower Factor) by either activated Factor III (Tissue Factor) along with activated Factor VII through the extrinsic pathway or Factor IXa and Factor VIIIa from the intrinsic pathway, along with activated Factor V, converts prothrombin (Factor II) to Thrombin (IIa), the essential catalyst for the formation of fibrin (Ia) from fibrinogen (I). Platelets that have formed plugs on the cell wall can be stabilized by the cross-linking of fibrin. Calcium is essential for this reaction, explaining why citrate and oxalate, both binders of calcium, are able to inhibit coagulation. Both activated Factor XIII and Factor VIII are able to stabilize the cross-links. See Fig. 8.1.

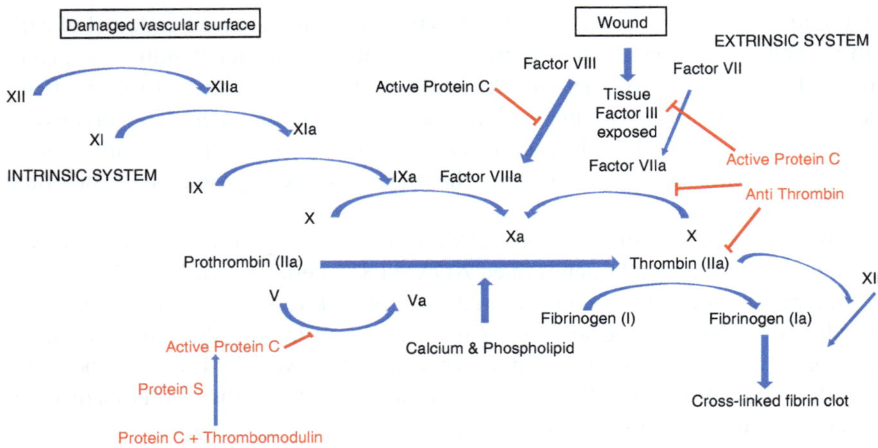

Fig. 8.1 Diagram of the clotting cascade

The Platelet System

Damage to a cell wall attracts platelets and stimulates them. Platelets are small particles in the blood that contain two types of granules and a series of canals. The α-granules contain several products essential to clotting, including fibrinogen, von Willebrand Factor (VWF), Factor V, and Factor VIII. The second type, dense granules, contains ADP, ATP, and serotonin. Once platelets have been stimulated, they release the contents of their granules into canals, leading to the generation of thrombin from thromboplastin and the deposition of fibrin from precursor fibrinogen. The platelet membrane contains arachidonic acid, which is converted first to an endoperoxide, and then to thromboxane A2, a powerful platelet aggregator. Arachidonic acid is also present in endothelial cell membranes, but here the conversion to endoperoxide leads to the formation of prostacyclin, a potent inhibitor of platelet aggregation. As long as the cell wall is intact, prostacyclin can work to prevent platelet aggregation and clot formation.

Serum Albumin

Albumin binding to thromboxane decreases its platelet aggregating ability. Thus, as one would expect, in low albumin states, thromboxane is more active. There is an inverse relationship between serum albumin and the risk of venous thromboembolism in hospitalized acutely ill patients [10]. That is also why nephrotic syndrome is associated with venous thromboembolism.

Inhibitors of Coagulation

The coagulation system must be in equilibrium. Either excessive and unchecked coagulation or inadequate coagulation can cause bleeding disorders. Anticlotting mechanisms can either be anti-Factor (or anticoagulant) or fibrinolytic. Clinical diseases such as hemophilia or VWF deficiency can lead to clotting disorders and excessive bleeding. Vitamin K is a cofactor affecting four clotting factors (Factor II, V, VII, and X). Warfarin, a vitamin K antagonist, interferes with these four proteases and is used as an anticoagulant. Subclinical vitamin K deficiency is commonly present in the dialysis population. Not only can this potentially lead to bleeding disorders, but the absence of vitamin K2 (MK-7) can promote vascular calcification [11], although a 2-year randomized controlled trial did not support MK-7 supplementation in dialysis patients to protect bone mineral density [12].

Antithrombin is a thrombin inhibitor that also blocks the activation of Factor X. Its activity increases 1000-fold in the presence of heparin. The endothelial glycosaminoglycan, heparan sulfate, has both antithrombin activity and induces prostacyclin production from endopeptidase.

The inhibition of activated Factor X blocks its stimulatory effects on releasing inflammatory cytokines, IL-6 and IL-8. The activation of protein C can be blocked by $\alpha 2$ macroglobulin and $\alpha 1$ antitrypsin. It is activated by thrombin and is anti-inflammatory. In addition, activated protein C (APC) degrades and thus prevents the activation of Factor V, Factor VIII, and Tissue Factor III. Protein S, synthesized by endothelial cells and hepatocytes in the presence of vitamin K, also augments Factors V and VIII deactivation. It also augments the blockage of Factor X and Factor VII by the Tissue Factor Pathway Inhibitor (TFPI), an extrinsic pathway inhibitor. Protein S is inactivated by inflammation through the complement system. When binding with thrombin, an endothelial cell membrane receptor, thrombomodulin, increases APC activity by 1000-fold. This is further augmented by the endothelial protein C receptor (EPCR) [13]. Protein S and Protein C deficiency are rarely seen in the dialysis population.

Anticoagulants

Heparin

The discovery of heparin was a milestone in the development of hemodialysis, and the routine use of unfractionated heparin is the mainstay of dialysis anticoagulation. It is a linear, highly sulfated glycosaminoglycan composed of repeating disaccharide units. Its molecular weight can vary from 2000 to 40,000 Daltons. Heparin is negatively charged and has a half-life that ranges between 0.5 and 2 h. In dialysis clinics, a bolus dose is generally followed by maintenance. Although it can be reversed with protamine, that practice is rarely required with current protocols.

The plastics that come into contact with blood as it passes through the dialyzer activate complement, white blood cells, and platelets, triggering thrombin and fibrin generation. Heparin augments antithrombin (AT) and also exerts its effect on activated Factor X. AT deficiency may be familial or acquired with an increase in intravascular coagulation, and this can lead to heparin resistance.

The heparin catastrophe of 2008 occurred because of African Swine Fever, a virus that deprecated the Chinese pig population. Heparin is made from pig intestines, and this infection led to a critical shortage in the availability of heparin for exportation. An unregulated manufacturer, Changzhou Scientific Protein Laboratories, based in the People's Republic of China, substituted over-sulfated chondroitin sulfate, an inexpensive product that mimicked the in vitro properties of heparin. The product entered the US market and was passed off as heparin. As a result, several patients died of anaphylactoid shock during dialysis care [14].

Low Molecular Weight Heparin (LMWH)

LMWH is cleared by the kidney but not by hemodialysis, and if used, the dose in kidney patients must be reduced. There is an increased risk of bleeding when used in dialysis patients. LMWH exerts its effect against the active Factor X, while unfiltered heparin (UFH) acts both on Factor II and Factor X.

Otherwise, LMWH is useful when other anticoagulants must be stopped in anticipation of surgery. Its prolonged activity allows for it to be injected subcutaneously rather than administered intravenously. A dosage adjustment is recommended when using LMWH products such as enoxaparin in patients with severe renal impairment <30 mL/min. Enoxaparin has also been associated with hyperkalemia in severe kidney disease. A systemic review has not established that it does lead to an increased bleeding risk in ESRD patients but fell short of recommending its use as an anticoagulant in dialysis patients [15].

The development of antibodies against platelets and heparin is a rare condition. HIT can be cautiously managed by using low molecular weight heparin rather than unfractionated heparin where otherwise indicated. LMWH is contraindicated when thrombocytopenia is associated with a positive in vitro test for antiplatelet antibodies in the presence of LMWH.

Warfarin

Warfarin is a vitamin K antagonist and thus impairs the activation of Factors II, VII, IX, and X. It has a risk of increased bleeding in patients on dialysis and, therefore, should be reserved for indications where other anticoagulants cannot be used. It is absorbed from the gastrointestinal tract, and its absorption, metabolism, and activity are related to diet and alcohol consumption. Patients who are on warfarin must be monitored closely. Its use has decreased with the development of newer anticoagulants, but it is still the only oral anticoagulant recommended for metal heart valves [16]. Newer agents are being evaluated that may be superior to warfarin for mechanical valve therapy [17].

Rivaroxaban

Rivaroxaban is a once-daily anticoagulant directed against Factor Xa. It is indicated for use in treating non-valvular atrial fibrillation and VTE. If used in the dialysis population, the dosage needs to be reduced. It should not be used with nonsteroidal anti-inflammatory drugs (NSAIDs) or amiodarone. In TOCKET AF, the pivotal trial comparing rivaroxaban with warfarin for noninferiority in use for atrial fibrillation, ESRD patients were excluded.

Apixaban

Apixaban is a Factor Xa inhibitor that, like rivaroxaban, can block thrombin formation. It has been used since 2012 to treat non-valvular atrial fibrillation and VTE. It has a low bleeding profile when compared with rivaroxaban and warfarin in CKD Stages 4 and 5 and the dialysis population [16]. In the general population, it reduced the risk of stroke when compared with aspirin [18].

When compared with warfarin for atrial fibrillation in the general population, the hazard ratio (HR) of systemic embolism or ischemic stroke was 0.79 (95% CI 0.66–0.95; $P < 0.001$ for noninferiority). Patients with a GFR <25 mL/min were excluded from the study [18].

Citrate

Citrate has been known to block blood clotting by reducing ionized calcium (iCa). Sodium citrate is used rarely in the dialysis population but may be suitable as a locking agent with dialysis catheter use [19]. It is used mainly with continuous renal replacement therapy (CRRT) in acute kidney injury. Its main side effect is hypocalcemia, and ionized calcium levels are monitored closely during the treatment.

Management of Clotting Disorders

In this section, we will discuss the management of venous thromboembolism (VTE), arteriovenous (AV) access, valvular disease, and atrial fibrillation in patients with end-stage kidney disease.

Venous Thromboembolism

Venous thromboembolism (VTE) is more common in patients with kidney disease. An 11.8-year study of 19,073 adults characterized by the level of kidney disease had an adjusted relative risk of 1.71 (95% CI 1.18–2.49) [20]. In other reviews, the HR for VTE is 4.5 (95% CI 4.1–4.9). VTE patients have a higher risk of bleeding because of anticoagulants (adjusted HR—AHR 2, 95% CI 1.3–2.9) and a higher mortality rate (aHR 2.4, 95% CI 2.0–2.8) [21].

A hypercoagulable state can be incited by inflammation and infection. This implicates endothelial cells, platelets and leukocytes, and coagulation factors. The release of polyphosphate, a potent proinflammatory signal, from the dense granules of platelets both activates factor V and decreases tissue factor pathway inhibitor activity. Protein C protects endothelial cells, and its decrease can potentiate their vulnerability. Leukocytes can extend fibers that, while designated to trap microorganisms, can also increase platelet adhesion and fibrin formation [22]. Plasminogen activator inhibitor (PAI)-I, a blocker of fibrinolysis, increases in response to the renin–angiotensin–aldosterone system (RAAS). RAAS is also associated with fibrinogen increases and D-dimer. The incidence of VTE is twice as high in AV grafts than in AV fistula patients [23].

A higher incidence of VTE was confirmed in phase 3 clinical trials of cancer patients treated with both recombinant erythropoietin and darbepoetin vs. placebo. The treated arms had a 7.5% incidence compared with the placebo arm of 4.9% [24]. This was not demonstrated in dialysis patients [25].

124 dialysis patients were retrospectively studied. 74 were in the apixaban and 50 in the warfarin group. The patients were studied for nearly 3 years. Bleeding events were 18% in the apixaban and 42% in the warfarin groups ($P = 0.01$). Major bleeding events were also significantly less 5.4 vs. 22%, respectively; $P = 0.01$) [26]. In a retrospective cohort review of USRDS data from 2013 to 2018, outcomes for patients treated with apixaban or warfarin were compared. In the 12,206 patients treated for VTE, apixaban was associated with a lower risk of VTE (HR 0.58; 95% CI 0.43–0.77), major bleeding (HR 0.78, 95% CI 0.62–0.98), and no difference in deaths [27].

A total of 203 patients in a retrospective cohort study from 2013 through 2021 were prescribed either 5 mg twice each day or 2.5 mg twice each day. The patients were either undergoing dialysis or were CKD Stages 4 and 5. The endpoints of the study were clinically relevant bleeding within 6 months of beginning therapy or VTE recurrence. The 125 patients treated with 5 mg had a significantly higher bleeding rate than the 78 patients treated with 2.5 mg (14.4% vs. 3.8%, $p = 0.02$). The rates of VTE recurrence were not significantly different between the two groups [28]. Evidence for using dabigatran or rivaroxaban in managing VTE in dialysis patients is lacking [29].

Thrombosing Arteriovenous (AV) Access

Vascular access narrowing can be a consequence of turbulence and can reduce blood flow leading to a clotted access. The narrowing that impairs flow also reduces dialysis clearance. Clotting in the dialyzer can lead to blood loss. The development of a clot in an AV fistula is responsible for 65–85% of access loss, while AV grafts have an even higher incidence of clotting. However, AV grafts are easier to declot than AV fistulas.

Early surveillance is needed to intervene before the thrombosis occurs. Outflow stenosis may cause prolonged bleeding or a change in the physical examination characterized by the appearance of a high-pitched bruit, increased pulse force, or aneurysmal enlargement. Inflow obstruction is characterized by the decreased thrill and bruit intensity. Any thrombosis may lead to downward trending Kt/*V* values. Accesses should be evaluated at least monthly. Thrombosis and stenosis result from a combination of vascular wall damage, stasis, and a hypercoagulable state. In the past, efforts at systemic anticoagulation with warfarin [30], the use of fish oil, and antiplatelet medications have been attempted [31, 32]. Antiplatelet therapy was shown to be improved prolonged access patency [33].

Multiple disorders in the clotting system can be associated with AV access thrombosis. Increased levels of fibrinogen, Tissue Factor III, Factor VII, XII, VIII, APC, thrombin-AT complexes, D dimers, antiphospholipid antibodies, anticardiolipin antibodies, decreased vitamin K, decreased VWF, as well as lowered AT and endothelial and access wall dysfunction, coupled with altered flow dynamics set a stage for clotting, and support the need for regular vigilance [5, 8].

Antiphospholipid antibody syndrome (APS) can cause increased clotting. It may occur in patients with systemic lupus erythematosus, or it may be idiopathic. There have been several studies that have looked at antiphospholipid antibodies, lupus anticoagulants (LA), and IgG anticardiolipin antibodies (ACL) in ESKD patients. Data from these studies were pooled by Ames et al. [34]. They were unable to conclude that antiphospholipid antibodies caused fistula occlusions. Fistula occlusion and LA are associated, however.

Atrial Fibrillation

Atrial fibrillation is associated with venous stasis and clot formation in the atria. Clots can embolize from the atrium to the cerebral vasculature and cause strokes. Antithrombotic therapy, particularly with warfarin, apixaban, and rivaroxaban, is standard therapy in the general population [35]. The ideal anticoagulant for atrial fibrillation will minimize the incidence of embolic stroke by avoiding clots associated with status and also remove the protection the clotting system affords patients in the event of injury. The risk of anticoagulation is a major bleed, particularly a stroke. Chronic kidney disease patients have an increased risk of developing atrial fibrillation, and this risk rises once dialysis has been started. It is conservatively estimated that 10% of dialysis patients have atrial fibrillation. Direct oral anticoagulants (DOACs), also referred to as nonvitamin K anticoagulants (NOACs), directly block active Factor Xa. They do not require monitoring and have been shown to be safer in the non-dialysis population [36]. Controversy exists as to whether there is conclusive evidence to recommend anticoagulation with DOACs in patients who have atrial fibrillation. DOACs are eliminated by the kidney and may accumulate with severe kidney disease. Large trials that established the safety of DOACs in treating atrial fibrillation excluded patients with severe CKD.

A 2-year analysis of 244 patients on rivaroxaban, either 20 mg or 15 mg each day, from the Fresenius Medical Care North America (FMCNA) database was evaluated. Thirty-nine had a stroke, 10 had a major bleeding episode, and 36 had an embolic CVA. These values did not significantly differ from those of patients being treated with warfarin [37].

The Valkyrie Study randomized 132 patients to a vitamin K antagonist (VKA), rivaroxaban 10 mg daily, or rivaroxaban and vitamin K2 (RVK2) group. The study continued for 36 months, but premature discontinuation occurred in 255 of the patients. The endpoint was cardiovascular events, and the risk-adjusted hazard ratio (aHR), when adjusted for the competing risk of death, was 0.39 (95% CI 0.17–0.90; $P < 0.03$) in the rivaroxaban group, 0.48 (95% CI 0.22–1.08; $P < 0.08$) in the RVK2 group. The risk of stroke, all-cause mortality, and cardiac mortality did not differ between the treatment groups [38]. Pooled studies compared 3744 DOAC with 26,973 warfarin patients. DOACs and warfarin were similarly effective. The Factor Xa inhibitors did not reduce the incidence of major or intracranial bleeding but did reduce the risk of gastrointestinal bleeding [39].

A retrospective USRDS data review from 2010 to 2015 compared atrial fibrillation patients who were anticoagulated with either warfarin ($n = 25{,}523$) or apixaban ($n = 2351$) and found no differences in the incidence of stroke or systemic embolism. Major bleeding events were lower with apixaban. However, the incidence of stroke, systemic embolism, or death with the 5 mg twice a day dose of apixaban was lower compared with the 2.5 mg twice a day or with warfarin. These observations required confirmation in randomized trials [40]. When apixaban was compared with warfarin in a USRDS data review from 2013 to 2018, it was confirmed that there were no differences in the risk of stroke or systemic embolism in patients treated with apixaban and warfarin. Apixaban 5 mg twice daily was associated with a lower risk of bleeding than either lower dose apixaban or warfarin. The 5 mg twice daily apixaban dose was associated with a lower risk of mortality than warfarin (HR 0.85; 95% CI 0.78–0.92). There is no survival advantage of using warfarin and the lowered dosage of apixaban [41].

In a 3-year retrospective review of USRDS data, Mavrakanas and Charytan analyzed 2082 patients. Four hundred seventy-three patients were on P2Y12 inhibitors such as clopidogrel, and 117 of them received a P2Y12 inhibitor and apixaban. Three hundred fifty-six patients did not receive an anticoagulant. 1609 patients did not receive a P2Y12 inhibitor, but 404 of them received apixaban. The data review demonstrated no effect on preventing stroke with either anticoagulant. When compared with using no anticoagulant, the use of apixaban and a P2Y12 together significantly increased the risk of fatal or intracranial bleeding (HR 8.82, 95% CI 2.06–37.76; $p = 0.003$) [35].

The Renal Hemodialysis Patients Allocated Apixaban Versus Warfarin in Atrial Fibrillation (RENAL-AF) trial was a randomized trial that was inconclusive and stopped prematurely because of enrollment difficulties. With 2.5 mg or 5 mg of apixaban administered twice a day, the incidence of stroke and bleeding events was similar to warfarin. The study demonstrated a tenfold incidence of stroke or systemic embolism in the group treated with either anticoagulant [42], which contrasts with the ARISTOTLE trial for non-dialysis patients [18].

Although other clinical trials with research with Factor XI antagonists in the dialysis population are underway, there is currently no solid evidence for recommending anticoagulation for atrial fibrillation in patients receiving dialysis [43]. In dialysis patients who are anticoagulated, retrospective studies demonstrate that there are no risk differences in preventing strokes or systemic emboli between warfarin and apixaban but that apixaban at the 5 mg twice daily dose offers a survival advantage over warfarin or the lower apixaban dose [41]. Despite variable results, current guidelines recommend the use of DOACs in atrial fibrillation patients on hemodialysis [44].

Bleeding

Bleeding in dialysis patients accounts for increased morbidity, hospitalization rates, and death. It has been estimated that CKD-associated bleeding risks are tenfold that of the general population. It has long been recognized that platelet function is abnormal in uremia [45], but the exact mechanisms associated with increased bleeding in CKD patient has yet to be clarified. Decreased calcium availability, α-granule abnormalities, decreased serotonin, and diminished ADP availability have all been described.

Abnormal arachidonic acid metabolism reduces thromboxanes. Increased fibrin fragment binding to glycoprotein (GP) IIb/IIIa receptors on the platelet wall decreases adhesion and aggregation. Uremic toxins impair ADP-induced platelet aggregation.

All of these factors contribute to the observation that bleeding disorders are more prevalent in kidney patients. At the chairside, it is difficult to separate inflammation or coagulation abnormalities related to the uremic environment from those pertaining to the anticoagulants and other medications required during dialysis. Heparin strongly increases antithrombin activity. Dialyzer membranes can activate platelets. Paradoxically, dialysis can improve coagulation and reduces the risk of bleeding [5].

Head Trauma in Dialysis Patients

A subdural hematoma (SDH) occurs when blood collects between the dura and arachnoid membranes as a result of a tear in the veins bridging the cerebral cortex and dural sinus. It is associated with damage to the cerebral cortex but can also increase intracranial pressure and lead to death. In the elderly, falls are the most common cause of an SDH. The incidence of trauma-related SDH in the general population climbs with age. In a Japanese epidemiological analysis of a national database, only 2.6% were using warfarin. 20.3% required burr hole procedure [46].

The risks of SDH in hemodialysis patients can be related to age, the use of anticoagulants, or injuries such as falls. SDH in dialysis patients independent of trauma and the use of oral anticoagulants has been well described since the early days of therapy [47]. The occurrence of nontraumatic SDH is also seen in the dialysis population; the incidence in one study was 3.37% independent of atrial fibrillation and the use of anticoagulants [19].

The use of warfarin was also associated with intracranial hemorrhage in the general population and also in patients undergoing hemodialysis. An analysis of 2793 SDH occurrences in the USRDS registry demonstrated that 68% were patients >65 years old. The mortality rate at <30 days was 39%. The increase in SDH was discordant between hemodialysis and peritoneal dialysis [48]. Other analyses have shown an increased incidence of SDH in hemodialysis when compared with peritoneal dialysis independent of warfarin use. Its cause may be related to the routine use of heparin required for hemodialysis [49]. Falls are common in the dialysis population, particularly in aged or frail patients. Any unwitnessed fall necessitates brain imaging to exclude an acute intracranial bleeding episode.

Gastrointestinal Bleeding in Dialysis Patients

Abnormalities in the gastrointestinal tract lead to increased episodes of gastrointestinal bleeding. The reasons are multifactorial and include the bleeding disorders inherent in ESRD patients, including abnormal platelet activation by dialyzer membranes, the need for anticoagulation during dialysis, and medications such as NSAIDs or aspirin. The dialysis procedure is characterized by subclinical blood loss [50]. The evaluation of GI bleeding should include a complete blood count and platelet count. The reticulocyte count will help separate blood loss from chronic anemia. Stools for blood and an endoscopy or colonoscopy may be required. The incidence of a lower gastrointestinal blooding episode requiring hospitalization ranges from 20 to 30 per 100,000 persons per year. Vascular ectasias can cause recurrent bleeding and may instigate 19–32% of colon bleeding episodes. Local coagulation measures can be attempted in cases where they do not spontaneously resolve. Other sources of bleeding include diverticular disease, especially in polycystic kidney disease patients and the elderly. Ischemic colitis, malignancies, and hemorrhoids may also occur [51].

Conclusion

This chapter began with a review of the coagulation and fibrinolytic systems. Take-home points are that patients undergoing dialysis have abnormal clotting functions that may result in excessive bleeding or clotting. Hemodialysis patients are unique because they require anticoagulation and can have vitamin K production or calcium metabolism disorders. They may have dialyzer-induced platelet aggregation. VTE is nearly twice as common in the dialysis population. The AV access is particularly vulnerable to thrombosing, and regular surveillance is necessary. Everyday disorders like atrial fibrillation react differently to standard therapy, as was recently demonstrated in a randomized clinical trial that did not support the use of DOACs in dialysis-based atrial fibrillation. Head trauma can occur in dialysis patients, particularly if they are a fall risk and especially if they are anticoagulated. Any unwitnessed fall should lead to the suspicion of a potential intracranial bleeding episode.

References

1. Benedum J. The early history of the artificial kidney. Anasthesiol Intensivmed Notfallmed Schmerzther. 2003;38(11):681–8. https://doi.org/10.1055/s-2003-43386.
2. Howell WH. The purification of heparin and its presence in blood. Am J Phys. 1925;71(3):553–62. https://doi.org/10.1152/ajplegacy.1925.71.3.553.
3. Ong CS, Marcum JA, Zehr KJ, Cameron DE. A century of heparin. Ann Thorac Surg. 2019;108(3):955–8. https://doi.org/10.1016/j.athoracsur.2019.03.104.
4. Murray GD, Best CH. The use of heparin in thrombosis. Ann Surg. 1938;108(2):163–77. https://doi.org/10.1097/00000658-193808000-00002.
5. Lutz J, Menke J, Sollinger D, Schinzel H, Thürmel K. Haemostasis in chronic kidney disease. Nephrol Dial Transplant. 2013;29(1):29–40. https://doi.org/10.1093/ndt/gft209.
6. Osterud B, Rapaport SI. Activation of factor IX by the reaction product of tissue factor and factor VII: additional pathway for initiating blood coagulation. Proc Natl Acad Sci U S A. 1977;74(12):5260–4. https://doi.org/10.1073/pnas.74.12.5260.
7. Sadler JE. Von Willebrand factor, ADAMTS13, and thrombotic thrombocytopenic purpura. Blood. 2008;112(1):11–8. https://doi.org/10.1182/blood-2008-02-078170.
8. Jain N, Corken A, Kumar A, Davis C, Ware J, Arthur J. Role of platelets in chronic kidney disease. J Am Soc Nephrol. 2021;32(7):1551–8. https://doi.org/10.1681/asn.2020121806.
9. Fox AJ, Lalloo UG, Belvisi MG, Bernareggi M, Chung KF, Barnes PJ. Bradykinin-evoked sensitization of airway sensory nerves: a mechanism for ACE-inhibitor cough. Nat Med. 1996;2(7):814–7. https://doi.org/10.1038/nm0796-814.
10. Chi G, Gibson CM, Liu Y, Hernandez AF, Hull RD, Cohen AT, et al. Inverse relationship of serum albumin to the risk of venous thromboembolism among acutely ill hospitalized patients: analysis from the APEX trial. Am J Hematol. 2019;94(1):21–8. https://doi.org/10.1002/ajh.25296.
11. McCabe KM, Adams MA, Holden RM. Vitamin K status in chronic kidney disease. Nutrients. 2013;5(11):4390–8. https://doi.org/10.3390/nu5114390.
12. Levy-Schousboe K, Marckmann P, Frimodt-Møller M, Peters CD, Kjærgaard KD, Jensen JD, et al. Vitamin K supplementation and bone mineral density in dialysis: results of the double-blind, randomised, placebo-controlled RenaKvit trial. Nephrol Dial Transplant. 2022;2022:gfac315. https://doi.org/10.1093/ndt/gfac315.

13. Ezihe-Ejiofor JA, Hutchinson N. Anticlotting mechanisms 1: physiology and pathology. Contin Educ Anaesth Crit Care Pain. 2013;13(3):87–92. https://doi.org/10.1093/bjaceaccp/mks061.
14. Blossom DB, Kallen AJ, Patel PR, Elward A, Robinson L, Gao G, et al. Outbreak of adverse reactions associated with contaminated heparin. N Engl J Med. 2008;359(25):2674–84. https://doi.org/10.1056/NEJMoa0806450.
15. Lim W, Cook DJ, Crowther MA. Safety and efficacy of low molecular weight heparins for hemodialysis in patients with end-stage renal failure: a meta-analysis of randomized trials. J Am Soc Nephrol. 2004;15(12):3192–206. https://doi.org/10.1097/01.Asn.0000145014.80714.35.
16. Fatima H, Nwankwo I, Anam M, Maharjan S, Amjad Z, Abaza A, et al. Safety and efficacy of apixaban vs warfarin in patients with stage 4 and 5 chronic kidney disease: a systematic review. Cureus. 2022;14(10):e30230. https://doi.org/10.7759/cureus.30230.
17. Kluge KE, Seljeflot I, Arnesen H, Jensen T, Halvorsen S, Helseth R. Coagulation factors XI and XII as possible targets for anticoagulant therapy. Thromb Res. 2022;214:53–62. https://doi.org/10.1016/j.thromres.2022.04.013.
18. Granger CB, Alexander JH, McMurray JJ, Lopes RD, Hylek EM, Hanna M, et al. Apixaban versus warfarin in patients with atrial fibrillation. N Engl J Med. 2011;365(11):981–92. https://doi.org/10.1056/NEJMoa1107039.
19. Fayed A, Tarek A, Refaat MI, Abouzeid S, Salim SA, Zsom L, et al. Retrospective analysis of nontraumatic subdural hematoma incidence and outcomes in Egyptian patients with end-stage renal disease on hemodialysis. Ren Fail. 2021;43(1):1322–8. https://doi.org/10.1080/0886022x.2021.1979038.
20. Wattanakit K, Cushman M, Stehman-Breen C, Heckbert SR, Folsom AR. Chronic kidney disease increases risk for venous thromboembolism. J Am Soc Nephrol. 2008;19(1):135–40. https://doi.org/10.1681/asn.2007030308.
21. Molnar AO, Bota SE, McArthur E, Lam NN, Garg AX, Wald R, et al. Risk and complications of venous thromboembolism in dialysis patients. Nephrol Dial Transplant. 2018;33(5):874–80. https://doi.org/10.1093/ndt/gfx212.
22. Branchford BR, Carpenter SL. The role of inflammation in venous thromboembolism. Front Pediatr. 2018;6:142. https://doi.org/10.3389/fped.2018.00142.
23. Roetker NS, Guo H, Ramey DR, McMullan CJ, Atkins GB, Wetmore JB. Hemodialysis vascular access and risk of major bleeding, thrombosis, and cardiovascular events: a cohort study. Kidney Med. 2022;4(6):100456. https://doi.org/10.1016/j.xkme.2022.100456.
24. Bennett CL, Silver SM, Djulbegovic B, Samaras AT, Blau CA, Gleason KJ, et al. Venous thromboembolism and mortality associated with recombinant erythropoietin and darbepoetin administration for the treatment of cancer-associated anemia. JAMA. 2008;299(8):914–24. https://doi.org/10.1001/jama.299.8.914.
25. Suttorp MM, Hoekstra T, Ocak G, van Diepen AT, Ott I, Mittelman M, et al. Erythropoiesis-stimulating agents and thrombotic events in dialysis patients. Thromb Res. 2014;134(5):1081–6. https://doi.org/10.1016/j.thromres.2014.07.030.
26. Reed D, Palkimas S, Hockman R, Abraham S, Le T, Maitland H. Safety and effectiveness of apixaban compared to warfarin in dialysis patients. Res Pract Thromb Haemost. 2018;2(2):291–8. https://doi.org/10.1002/rth2.12083.
27. Wetmore JB, Herzog CA, Yan H, Reyes JL, Weinhandl ED, Roetker NS. Apixaban versus warfarin for treatment of venous thromboembolism in patients receiving long-term dialysis. Clin J Am Soc Nephrol. 2022;17(5):693–702. https://doi.org/10.2215/cjn.14021021.
28. Knueppel P, Bang SH, Troyer C, Barriga A, Shin J, Cadiz CL, et al. Evaluation of standard versus reduced dose apixaban for the treatment of venous thromboembolism in patients with severe renal disease (ESRD-VTE). Thromb Res. 2022;220:91–6. https://doi.org/10.1016/j.thromres.2022.10.014.
29. Cheung CYS, Parikh J, Farrell A, Lefebvre M, Summa-Sorgini C, Battistella M. Direct oral anticoagulant use in chronic kidney disease and dialysis patients with venous thromboembolism: a systematic review of thrombosis and bleeding outcomes. Ann Pharmacother. 2021;55(6):711–22. https://doi.org/10.1177/1060028020967635.

30. Bennett WM. Should dialysis patients ever receive warfarin and for what reasons? Clin J Am Soc Nephrol. 2006;1(6):1357–9. https://doi.org/10.2215/cjn.01700506.
31. Quencer KB, Oklu R. Hemodialysis access thrombosis. Cardiovasc Diagn Ther. 2017;7(Suppl 3):S299–s308. https://doi.org/10.21037/cdt.2017.09.08.
32. Kumpfbeck A, Rockman CB, Jacobowitz GR, Lugo JZ, Barfield ME, Scher LA, et al. Anticoagulation therapy is associated with increased access-related wound infections after hemodialysis access creation. Ann Vasc Surg. 2022;80:136–42. https://doi.org/10.1016/j.avsg.2021.08.032.
33. Mizuno T, Nakamura M, Satoh N, Tsukada H, Matsumoto A, Hamasaki Y, et al. Patency with antiplatelet treatment after vascular access intervention therapy: a retrospective observational study. Ren Replace Ther. 2018;4(1):43. https://doi.org/10.1186/s41100-018-0184-5.
34. Ames PRJ, Merashli M, Bucci T, Pastori D, Pignatelli P, Violi F, et al. Antiphospholipid antibodies in end-stage renal disease: a systematic review and meta-analysis. Hemodial Int. 2020;24(3):383–96. https://doi.org/10.1111/hdi.12847.
35. Mavrakanas TA, Charytan DM. Apixaban versus no anticoagulation by P2Y12 inhibitor prescription status in dialysis patients with atrial fibrillation. Kidney360. 2022;3(10):1769–71. https://doi.org/10.34067/kid.0003002022.
36. Ktenopoulos N, Sagris M, Theofilis P, Lionaki S, Rallidis LS. Direct oral anticoagulants in patients on chronic dialysis and concomitant atrial fibrillation: a common clinical impasse. Front Biosci (Schol Ed). 2022;14(3):21. https://doi.org/10.31083/j.fbs1403021.
37. Chan KE, Edelman ER, Wenger JB, Thadhani RI, Maddux FW. Dabigatran and rivaroxaban use in atrial fibrillation patients on hemodialysis. Circulation. 2015;131(11):972–9. https://doi.org/10.1161/CIRCULATIONAHA.114.014113.
38. De Vriese AS, Caluwé R, Van Der Meersch H, De Boeck K, De Bacquer D. Safety and efficacy of vitamin K antagonists versus rivaroxaban in hemodialysis patients with atrial fibrillation: a multicenter randomized controlled trial. J Am Soc Nephrol. 2021;32(6):1474–83. https://doi.org/10.1681/asn.2020111566.
39. Li W, Zhou Y, Chen S, Zeng D, Zhang H. Use of non-vitamin K antagonists oral anticoagulants in atrial fibrillation patients on dialysis. Front Cardiovasc Med. 2022;9:1005742. https://doi.org/10.3389/fcvm.2022.1005742.
40. Siontis KC, Zhang X, Eckard A, Bhave N, Schaubel DE, He K, et al. Outcomes associated with apixaban use in patients with end-stage kidney disease and atrial fibrillation in the United States. Circulation. 2018;138(15):1519–29. https://doi.org/10.1161/CIRCULATIONAHA.118.035418.
41. Wetmore JB, Weinhandl ED, Yan H, Reyes JL, Herzog CA, Roetker NS. Apixaban dosing patterns versus warfarin in patients with nonvalvular atrial fibrillation receiving dialysis: a retrospective cohort study. Am J Kidney Dis. 2022;80(5):569–79.e1. https://doi.org/10.1053/j.ajkd.2022.03.007.
42. Pokorney SD, Chertow GM, Al-Khalidi HR, Gallup D, Dignacco P, Mussina K, et al. Apixaban for patients with atrial fibrillation on hemodialysis: a multicenter randomized controlled trial. Circulation. 2022;146(23):1735–45. https://doi.org/10.1161/circulationaha.121.054990.
43. Benz AP, Eikelboom JW. Apixaban compared with warfarin in patients with atrial fibrillation and end-stage renal disease: lessons learned. Circulation. 2022;146(23):1746–8. https://doi.org/10.1161/circulationaha.122.061647.
44. Faisaluddin M, Alwifati N, Naeem N, Balasubramanian S, Narasimhan B, Iqbal U, Dani SS. Safety and efficacy of direct oral anticoagulants versus warfarin for atrial fibrillation in end-stage renal disease on hemodialysis: A meta-analysis of randomized control trials. Am J Cardiol. 2023;206:309–311. https://doi.org/10.1016/j.amjcard.2023.08.116.
45. Boccardo P, Remuzzi G, Galbusera M. Platelet dysfunction in renal failure. Semin Thromb Hemost. 2004;30(5):579–89. https://doi.org/10.1055/s-2004-835678.

46. Toi H, Kinoshita K, Hirai S, Takai H, Hara K, Matsushita N, et al. Present epidemiology of chronic subdural hematoma in Japan: analysis of 63,358 cases recorded in a national administrative database. J Neurosurg. 2018;128(1):222–8. https://doi.org/10.3171/2016.9.Jns16623.
47. Talalla A, Halbrook H, Barbour BH, Kurze T. Subdural hematoma associated with long-term hemodialysis for chronic renal disease. JAMA. 1970;212(11):1847–9. https://doi.org/10.1001/jama.1970.03170240051007.
48. Sood P, Sinson GP, Cohen EP. Subdural hematomas in chronic dialysis patients: significant and increasing. Clin J Am Soc Nephrol. 2007;2(5):956–9. https://doi.org/10.2215/cjn.03781106.
49. Wang IK, Cheng YK, Lin CL, Peng CL, Chou CY, Chang CT, et al. Comparison of subdural hematoma risk between hemodialysis and peritoneal dialysis patients with ESRD. Clin J Am Soc Nephrol. 2015;10(6):994–1001. https://doi.org/10.2215/cjn.08140814.
50. Rosenblatt SG, Drake S, Fadem S, Welch R, Lifschitz MD. Gastrointestinal blood loss in patients with chronic renal failure. Am J Kidney Dis. 1982;1(4):232–6. https://doi.org/10.1016/s0272-6386(82)80059-0.
51. Saeed F, Agrawal N, Greenberg E, Holley JL. Lower gastrointestinal bleeding in chronic hemodialysis patients. Int J Nephrol. 2011;2011:272535. https://doi.org/10.4061/2011/272535.

Strategies to Avoid and Treat Peritoneal Dialysis Catheter Complications

9

Anjali Bhatt Saxena

Strategies to Avoid and Treat Peritoneal Dialysis Catheter Complications

Successful PD therapy depends upon permanent and safe access to the peritoneal cavity. A good catheter provides obstruction-free access and should not be a source of infection. Mechanical catheter problems cause the transfer to HD in nearly 20% of PD patients. Peritoneal infections, which are often catheter-related, are responsible for another 30–50% of PD technique failures [1, 2]. Therefore, proper catheter placement and management are imperative.

Types of Peritoneal Dialysis Catheters

Globally, the most widely used catheter is the standard Tenckhoff, followed by the swan-neck [3]. PD catheters have essentially three segments: intraperitoneal, tunneled, and extraperitoneal. The intraperitoneal segment is the portion of the catheter that resides inside the peritoneal cavity; side holes along the length of the intraperitoneal portion deliver and drain dialysate. The extraperitoneal segment passes through a subcutaneous tunnel within the abdominal wall (intramural), exits through the skin, and has an external (outside the body) segment. The catheter may contain one or two polyester cuffs, typically 1 cm long, referred to as the internal (preperitoneal) and external (subcutaneous) cuffs.

A. B. Saxena (✉)
Division of Nephrology, Stanford University, Stanford, CA, USA

Santa Clara Valley Medical Center, San Jose, CA, USA

S. Z. Fadem et al. (eds.), *Complications in Dialysis*,
https://doi.org/10.1007/978-3-031-44557-6_9

The Tenckhoff catheter is available with straight or coiled intraperitoneal segments; a meta-analysis was unable to find any benefit of the coiled over the straight catheter, and one randomized control trial (RCT) found that straight catheters required less surgical intervention due to catheter dysfunction than coiled catheters [4]. The swan-neck catheter, a modified Tenckhoff catheter, features a pre-formed 180° bend between the two cuff shield [3, 5]. These catheters can be placed in an arcuate tunnel so that both external and internal segments of the tunnel can easily be directed downwards, which is the optimal direction of the external catheter to reduce exit site infection risk. Additionally, the pre-formed angle between cuffs eliminates the risk of the catheter straightening over time due to rubber "shape memory," thus potentially reducing the risk of internal catheter tip migration and external cuff extrusion [6]. Pre-sternal catheters, another modification of catheter design, enter the peritoneum in the traditional location and are then tunneled subcutaneously and ipsilaterally up to the chest wall, where they finally exit the skin. The unique design of the pre-sternal catheter offers several benefits in certain settings: it is easily visible even in the obese patient with a large pannus, it allows patients with abdominal ostomies and pediatric patients in diapers to utilize PD without risk of exit site cross-contamination, and it may reduce the risk of catheter trauma (a risk factor for exit site infection) because the chest is a rather rigid structure with minimal wall motion. A long catheter tunnel, combined with three cuffs, may reduce peri-catheter bacterial contamination of the peritoneal cavity and reduce the incidence of peritonitis [7].

Embedded PD catheters are inserted into the peritoneum weeks to months before expected use, with the extraperitoneal segment "buried" in the subcutaneous fat until use is required. As with standard catheter placement, the intraperitoneal segment is implanted into the peritoneum; the extraperitoneal segment passes through a subcutaneous tunnel within the abdominal wall (intramural) but is then "buried" subcutaneously in the lower abdominal region where it remains until purposefully exteriorized weeks to months later for initiation of PD, usually in an ambulatory setting. Benefits of embedded catheters include (1) allowing the catheter to heal in a sterile environment and (2) avoiding delays in the initiation of PD since the catheter is already healed and ready to use as soon as it is exteriorized. Published reports suggest a 10–12% futility rate (catheter never used due to patient death, transplantation, initiation on HD, renal recovery). Of 306 embedded catheters, 85% had primary function, and 56% of those without initial function were successfully secondarily salvaged [8]. One study of 66 embedded catheters reported a 4.3% increased odds of non-function for each week's increase in embedment. Others opine that embedded catheter complication rates do not have a linear association with time and suggest that embedment duration between 6 and 21 weeks minimizes both futility and complication rates [8, 9].

Catheter-Related Complications

The most common PD catheter complications include exit site (ES) and tunnel infection, impaired flow, external cuff extrusion, dialysate leaks, and infusion pain. Catheter-related infections can result from improper catheter placement, poor wound healing at the ES, external catheter trauma, interference with the normal healing process during and after catheter placement, and inadequate routine ES care. ES infections have been shown to be a result of sinus tract bacterial colonization. Therefore, it is imperative for a new ES to heal in a sterile environment. One way to achieve this is by keeping the original post-surgical dressing in place for 5–7 days after catheter placement, removing it only in the case of frank bleeding or drainage. Trained PD personnel should be the first to uncover the original catheter dressing, and they should always wear masks while inspecting the ES in this perioperative period. After the ES is well healed, trauma to the external segment of the catheter predisposes to infection by allowing bacterial colonization of the sinus tract and exit site and impairing normal tissue regeneration [10].

Effective and successful PD requires excellent catheter function. Therefore, it is imperative to maintain optimal catheter flow and address problems immediately. Most flow problems are due to one of four causes: (1) constipation, (2) fibrin plugging or occlusion of the internal catheter lumen by fibrin, (3) catheter migration, and (4) omental wrapping.

Constipation is the most common cause of catheter flow problems and clinically presents with slow or incomplete emptying during the drain phase of the exchange and little to no difficulty filling the peritoneum; occasionally, it can manifest as a complete inability to drain. When impaired catheter drainage is associated with constipation, stool-filled bowel loops either obstruct catheter side holes or cause loculated fluid collections that are not readily accessible for drainage. Constipation is commonly encountered in PD patients and can often be corrected with simple measures. When initially confronted with a poorly draining catheter, assume constipation is the cause and treat it accordingly. Osmotic laxatives such as polyethylene glycol 3350 or lactulose can be given initially. If ineffective, a stimulant laxative can be added, but caution is advised because these can cause cramping or diarrhea. Enemas should be avoided in PD patients to reduce the risk of translocation of bowel wall bacteria from the intestine into the peritoneum. Any phosphate-containing laxatives or enemas must be completely avoided. If laxatives are ineffective in improving catheter flow despite a good cathartic response, proceed to a flat-plate radiograph which will provide information regarding both bowel stool content and PD catheter tip location (see below). When the radiograph shows a large stool burden, continue efforts to relieve constipation. Prevention of constipation is important and should consist of education regarding healthy bowel habits, high fiber diet, regular physical activity to promote bowel motility, and regular use of emollient laxatives such as docusate in patients who do not have daily bowel movements (or who have persistently hard stool).

When a successful laxative regimen fails to restore proper drainage, an abdominal radiograph can both confirm relief of constipation and evaluate for catheter tip migration. The catheter coil or tip (for straight catheters) should be situated in the true pelvis for best flow. Catheter position is optimized at the time of placement, but over time displacement can occur. When a catheter is incidentally seen to be displaced but continues to function appropriately, it is not necessary to reposition it. On the other hand, a poorly draining and displaced PD catheter will require repositioning. An initial approach is a trial of laxatives to stimulate peristalsis and encourage the movement of the catheter toward the lower pelvis. If the catheter fails to function after simple maneuvers are implemented (e.g., laxatives, forced flushing), guidewire manipulation under fluoroscopy may be attempted. Two Canadian centers reported a 63% and 77% success rate with this technique [11, 12]. If these maneuvers are unsuccessful, laparoscopic repositioning of the catheter tip back to the true pelvis and anchoring is necessary.

Prolonged catheter drain times, or the complete inability to drain or fill the peritoneum via the PD catheter, may be caused by fibrin plugging or omental wrapping. Fibrin plugging is a condition in which the PD catheter lumen becomes obstructed with fibrin clots. Fibrin and fibrin clots form normally within the peritoneal fluid, and when they lodge within the catheter lumen, dysfunction ensues. When faced with the inability to drain or fill, and constipation has been eliminated, evaluate for fibrin plugging. Two first steps are recommended: (1) manual compression of the PD fluid fill-bag to cause increased inflow pressure in an attempt to dislodge the clot and/or (2) in the clinic, an experienced PD provider attaches a sterile syringe to the catheter and attempts vigorous flushes with heparinized saline. If this is unsuccessful, fibrinolysis can be attempted by injecting a thrombolytic (tissue-type plasminogen activator, t-PA, or urokinase)m 1 mg/mL to fill the volume of the catheter and transfer set, followed by a 1-h dwell [13]. Afterwards, draining is reattempted using a manual PD solution twin-bag; if draining is slow, a 60 mL syringe can be used to withdraw fluid manually, and if successful, then the twin-bag drain procedure is reattempted. If the obstruction persists, fluoroscopic guidewire manipulation can be attempted to clear a fibrin sheath [13]. Ultimately, minimally invasive laparoscopic exploration of the peritoneum and catheter may be required to evaluate and treat the cause of catheter dysfunction. It can be performed with little disruption to PD therapy by performing low-volume, supine PD post-operatively.

Catheter entrapment or “wrapping” is another reason for flow dysfunction and is caused by the direct obstruction of catheter drain holes by the omentum. Omental wrapping is not detectable by plain abdominal radiographs. It often requires laparoscopic surgery to diagnose and remove the obstruction; its presence may be suggested by an abnormal pattern of contrast distribution when iodinated contrast is injected directly into the catheter under fluoroscopic visualization (catheter-gram). Under unobstructed conditions, injected contrast should quickly emit from the catheter and cause rapid pelvic opacification. Catheter obstructions will cause contrast to pool in certain areas where the catheter drain holes remain patent rather than distribute evenly within the peritoneum. With or without imaging suggestive of omental wrapping, when faced with a poorly draining or nonfunctional but properly placed PD catheter without constipation, often laparoscopic exploration will quickly identify and allow treatment of omental wrapping. The risk of future omental wrapping can be decreased by omentopexy of low-hanging omentum—either at the time of omental de-wrapping surgery or, preferably, at the time of catheter placement.

References

1. Mujais S, Story K. Peritoneal dialysis in the US: evaluation of outcomes in contemporary cohorts. Kidney Int Suppl. 2006;103:S21–6.
2. Flanigan M, Gokal R. Peritoneal catheters and exit-site practices toward optimum peritoneal access: a review of current developments. Perit Dial Int. 2005;25(2):132–9.

3. Negoi D, Prowant BF, Twardowski ZJ. Current trends in the use of peritoneal dialysis catheters. Adv Dial Int. 2006;22:147–52.
4. Chow KM, Wong SSM, Ng JKC, Cheng YL, Leung CB, Pang WF, et al. Straight versus coiled peritoneal dialysis catheters: a randomized controlled trial. Am J Kidney Dis. 2020;75(1):39–44.
5. Twardowski ZJ, Nolph KD, Khanna R, Prowant BF, Ryan LR, Nichols KW. The need for a "swan neck" permanently bent, arcuate peritoneal dialysis catheter. Perit Dial Bull. 1985;5:219–23.
6. Gadallah M. The role of peritoneal dialysis catheter configuration in preventing catheter tip migration. Adv Perit Dial. 2000;16:47–50.
7. Twardowski ZJ, Prowant BF, Pickett B, Nichols WK, Nolph KD, Khanna R. Four-year experience with swan neck presternal peritoneal dialysis catheter. Am J Kidney Dis. 1996;27(1):99–105.
8. Brown PA, McCormick BB, Knoll G, Su Y, Doucette S, Fergusson D, et al. Complications and catheter survival with prolonged embedding of peritoneal dialysis catheters. Nephrol Dial Transplant. 2008;23(7):2299–303.
9. Sinha S, Fok M, Davenport A, Banga N, Lindsey B, Fernando B, et al. Use of the embedded peritoneal dialysis catheter. Ann R Coll Surg Engl. 2018;100(7):534–44.
10. Crabtree JH, Fishman A, Siddiqi RA, Hadnott LL. The risk of infection and peritoneal catheter loss from implant procedure exit-site trauma. Perit Dial Int. 1999;19(4):366–71.
11. Miller M, McCormick B, Lavoie S, Biyani M, Zimmerman D. Fluoroscopic manipulation of peritoneal dialysis catheters: outcomes and factors associated with successful manipulation. Clin J Am Soc Nephrol. 2012;7(5):795–800.
12. Li P, Choo D, Deved V, Shah N, Shurraw S, Zuidema S, et al. Salvage of malfunctioning peritoneal dialysis catheters: an algorithm for recanalization and repositioning. J Vasc Interv Radiol. 2021;32(6):902–6.
13. Sahani MM, Mukhtar KN, Boorgu R, Leehey DJ, Popli S, Ing TS. Tissue plasminogen activator can effectively declot peritoneal dialysis catheters. Am J Kidney Dis. 2000;36(3):675.

Cycler Issues, Overfill, Inflow, and Drain Pain

10

Rafia Chaudhry

Introduction

The early peritoneal dialysis cycler was developed in Seattle in 1962 [1, 2], and the institution of the peritoneal dialysis cycler allowed Continuous Cycling Peritoneal Dialysis (CCPD) or Automated PD (APD) to be implemented. In CCPD, individualized patient-specific peritoneal dialysis parameters are programmed into the cycler, which then automatically carries out peritoneal dialysis exchanges for the patient. As the peritoneal dialysis cycler technology has advanced, worldwide trends in the use of peritoneal dialysis demonstrate an increasing number of patients on peritoneal dialysis, with the use of automated peritoneal dialysis (APD) in 130 countries increasing by 14.5% in developing countries, and by 30.3% in developed countries between 1997 and 2008 [3].

Cycler-Related Issues in CCPD

The parameters that are programmed into the cycler include fill volume, dwell time, number of exchanges, duration of the fill, dwell and drain times, number of pauses, and optional modifications including tidal volume, last fill volume. The clinician's understanding of the mechanics of the cycler and the actual delivery of the programmed dialysate prescription to the patient is crucial in addressing and resolving some of the cycler-related complications discussed below. A lack of timely resolution of any of these PD cycler-related issues will have a significant impact on patients' quality of life and may result in patients switching from CCPD to CAPD and even HD.

R. Chaudhry (✉)
University of California, San Francisco, San Francisco, CA, USA
e-mail: rafia.chaudhry@ucsf.edu

S. Z. Fadem et al. (eds.), *Complications in Dialysis*,
https://doi.org/10.1007/978-3-031-44557-6_10

Inflow Pain

Inflow pain is described as sharp or burning pain during at the beginning of a dwell or dialysate infusion. This is attributed to a number of possible causes which include dialysate pH, catheter position (where the tip may be next to bowel or bladder), constipation, or intra-abdominal adhesions.

Inflow pain can be addressed by reducing the dialysate infusion rate and using a slightly increased bicarbonate or bicarbonate-lactate dialysate solution. If these steps do not resolve the discomfort, consider imaging (abdominal X-ray and then CT abdomen) to rule out adhesions and evaluate for optimizing the position of the PD catheter, recognizing that the PD catheter tip can migrate after initial placement, with physiologic activities including peristalsis and constipation.

Drain Pain

There is an overall impression that drain pain is now more common than a few decades ago, although data on this is lacking. This may be potentially due to increased use of the PD cycler. Drain pain occurs due to a siphoning effect of draining fluid where the hydraulic forces applied to drain dialysate from the patient's peritoneal cavity can pull sensitive visceral organs or parietal peritoneum toward the PD catheter resulting in referred pain (usually pelvic) (Fig. 10.1). In the event of no-flow (dialysate flow rate of less than 12 mL/min) or slow-flow state (dialysate flow rate of less than 50 mL/min), the cycler can increase the pneumatic forces up to 15 kPa or 113 mmHg for up to 10 seconds resulting in further discomfort.

Other potential factors contributing to drain pain include PD catheter placement (either the length or position of the catheter can be the culprit), and some

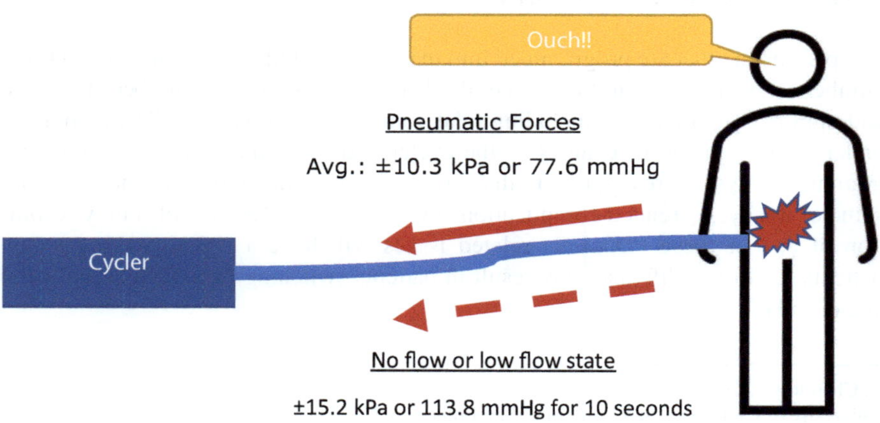

Fig. 10.1 Pneumatic forces generated by the cycler are increased in "low flow" or "no flow" states and cause a suctioning effect against visceral organs or parietal peritoneum resulting in drain pain

observational data suggest obesity or high BMI may also predispose to increased drain pain.

The recommended interventions for drain pain start with the basics, ensuring an effective bowel regimen, including laxatives, to address constipation and potentially moving PD catheter tip away from the parietal peritoneum or visceral organs. If the drain pain persists, consider imaging (starting with an abdominal and pelvic X-ray) to assess the catheter position, especially if there is an associated slow flow in the PD catheter.

Role of Tidal PD (TPD) in Addressing Drain Pain

TPD is when a fixed volume of residual dialysate solution is programmed to remain in the peritoneal cavity to act as a buffer between the patient's peritoneum and intra-abdominal tissue, thus dispersing hydraulic forces (Fig. 10.2).

In a large cross-sectional survey at 6 large PD units with a total of 293 patients on APD, 4–37% of APD patients were on Tidal Peritoneal Dialysis (TPD) at individual centers. Drain pain was the most common indication for TPD (86% of patients [$n = 72$] were on TPD due to drain pain). Other indications for TPD included "low transport status" [8 patients] and frequent disruptive low-drain-volume alarms [4 patients] [4].

Overfill or Increased Intra Peritoneal Volume (IIPV) IIPV or "overfill" occurs when excessive dialysate solution, i.e., effluent accumulates in the peritoneal cavity, beyond the target volume, or PD prescription fill volume. IIPV is an underrecognized complication of TPD.

Some of the culprit reasons for IIPV in TPD include inadequate estimation of total ultrafiltration (UF) volume, while catheter malfunction (resulting in slow flow during drain phase), and bypassing of the complete initial drain (I-Drain) without reaching target drain volumes can lead to IIPV events in non-TPD as well. The I-Drain is programmed at 70–85% of the last fill volume, or if there is a manual

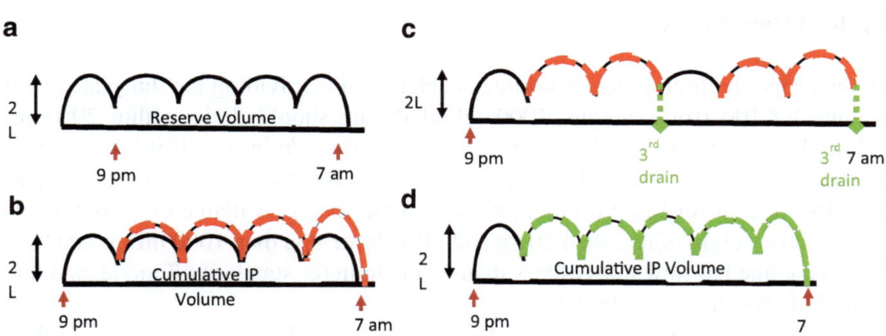

Fig. 10.2 (**a**) Tidal PD; (**b**) risk of cumulative IP volume with tidal PD; Strategies to avoid overfill: (**c**) Tidal full drain every "*n*" cycle (in this case every 3rd) or (**d**) tidal total expected UF drain. *PD* peritoneal dialysis, *IP* intraperitoneal, *UF* ultrafiltration

daytime exchange programmed into the prescription, the cycler will prompt the patient to enter the exchange volume to calculate I-drain.

IIPV leads to Increased Intraperitoneal Pressure (IPP), and PD patients with pre-existing cardiac or pulmonary conditions may be more susceptible to the physiologic effects of IIPV or IPP. The clinical signs and symptom severity varies from mild symptoms to potentially life-threatening events and may include abdominal or back pain, dialysate leakage into the abdominal wall, genital tissues, or pleural cavity, dialysate leakage around PD catheter site, cardiac complications including heart failure exacerbation, pericardial effusions, and pulmonary complications including shortness of breath, severe respiratory distress, and hydrothorax.

IIPV is associated with a high drain volume which is equivalent to the end-dwell volume (DV) to fill volume (FV) ratio (DV/FV). The FV is programmed dialysate solution volume per exchange. DV/FV >1.6 can be used as the threshold value for an increased risk of an IIPV event, while DV/FV >2 is associated with increased severity of IIPV events [5].

IIPV can be avoided by educating patients about signs and symptoms of IIPV, and steps to implement in the event that the patient experiences any of them. The patient should be instructed to do a stat drain on the cycler and hold further PD exchanges, including manual exchanges, and then notify the PD RN as soon as possible.

For patients on tidal PD, IIPV can be avoided by the PD team (decision in collaboration with nephrologist and PD RNs) by programming either, or both options below, into cycler (Fig. 10.2):

- Tidal full drain: Complete drainage of peritoneal cavity at pre-specified drain cycle intervals, for example, every third cycle drain.
- Tidal total ultrafiltration: Clinician specifies expected total ultrafiltration volume per night, and the cycler drains a percentage of this total expected UF volume (based on number of exchanges) + tidal volume with each cycle.

Cycler Flow Issues

The appropriate drain time per minute is calculated by dividing the dialysate or fill volume by 100 (for example, 2000 mL dialysate should drain within 20 min). "Slow-flow" is defined as flow rate of less than 50 mL/min, i.e., if it takes greater than 20 min to fill or drain 2 L of dialysate solution for standard fill modes, and less than 15 mL/min for low fill mode, with the latter being available only to patients with a body weight of less than 20 kg and fill volume less than 1000 mL, while "no-flow" is defined as flow rates of less than 12 mL/min for standard fill mode, and less than 3 mL/min for low fill mode.

The most common reason for inadequate drain speed, i.e., slow-flow or no-flow are mechanical issues, including obstruction secondary to kinks, fibrin, constipation, and catheter malfunction. Patients should be advised to attempt initial repositioning, i.e., turning sides, sitting up to resolve these issues, in an attempt to mobilize the catheter tip from potentially obstructing intra-abdominal tissue. However, if the slow drain alarm persists, patients should contact their PD RN to investigate potential kinks, fibrin, and catheter malfunction.

References

1. Nolph D. Peritoneal dialysis. 3rd ed. Dordrecht: Kluwer Academic Publishers; 1989.
2. Oreopoulos DG, Thodis E. The history of peritoneal dialysis: early years at Toronto Western Hospital. Dial Transplant. 2010;39(8):338–43.
3. Jain AK, Blake P, Cordy P, Garg AX. Global trends in rates of peritoneal dialysis. J Am Soc Nephrol. 2012;23(3):533–44. https://doi.org/10.1681/ASN.2011060607.
4. Blake PG, Sloand JA, McMurray S, Jain AK, Matthews S. A multicenter survey of why and how tidal peritoneal dialysis (TPD) is being used. Perit Dial Int. 2014;34(4):458–60.
5. Blake P. Drain pain, overfill, and how they are connected. Perit Dial Int. 2014;34(4):342–4. https://doi.org/10.3747/Pdi.2014.00104.

Infections in Peritoneal Dialysis

11

Megha Salani

Introduction

This chapter will focus on infections related to peritoneal dialysis (PD), including exit site infections, tunnel infections, and peritonitis.

Exit site infections (ESIs) present as erythema around the exit site (ES) with possible purulent drainage. Tunnel infections lead to erythema, edema, and tenderness over the catheter tract and may cause discharge, particularly with pressure on the cuff.

Peritonitis often presents as abdominal pain and fever and sometimes with nausea or diarrhea. Patients should be instructed to monitor the dialysis effluent and call their unit for cloudy fluid as this could be an early sign of peritonitis. A decline in ultrafiltration may precede overt symptoms.

Diagnosis

ESIs are diagnosed by visual inspection. If purulent drainage can be expressed from the sinus tract, it should be cultured. Swabbing the skin around the exit site can yield contaminants. If a tunnel infection is suspected, an ultrasound can be valuable to assess for fluid collections [1].

When peritonitis is suspected, it is important to obtain an effluent cell count, Gram stain, and culture with antibiotic susceptibilities. Blood cultures are only needed if systemic symptoms are present. To obtain a reliable effluent sample, the dialysate fluid should dwell for 2–4 h and, after centrifugation, be incubated in aerobic and anaerobic blood culture bottles.

M. Salani (✉)
Vanderbilt University Medical Center, Nashville, TN, USA
e-mail: Megha.salani@vumc.org

S. Z. Fadem et al. (eds.), *Complications in Dialysis*,
https://doi.org/10.1007/978-3-031-44557-6_11

Table 11.1 Differential diagnosis

Cloudy fluid	Abdominal pain
Infectious peritonitis	Infectious peritonitis
Pancreatitis	Pancreatitis
Chemical peritonitis	Ischemic bowel
Malignant ascites	Cholecystitis
Eosinophilic peritonitis	Diverticulitis
Encapsulating peritoneal sclerosis	Appendicitis
Chylous ascites	Constipation
Fibrin	Incarcerated hernia
Blood	Ruptured viscus
Catheter-associated trauma	Pyelonephritis
Drugs	Nephrolithiasis

A diagnosis of peritonitis is made if two of the three criteria are met: abdominal pain and/or cloudy effluent, a cell count of more than 100 white blood cells (WBCs) with at least 50% polymorphonuclear cells (PMNs), or a positive culture. The differential diagnosis for cloudy fluid and abdominal pain can be found in Table 11.1.

In addition to infectious peritonitis, pancreatitis and chemical peritonitis may also have greater than 100 WBC with over 50% PMN. Fluid that has been dwelling for more than a day can be cloudy with WBC over 100; typically, it has a mononuclear cell predominance.

With eosinophilic peritonitis, greater than 10% of eosinophils are observed. About half of these episodes are due to infection, and the other half are idiopathic. A higher absolute cell count could indicate infectious peritonitis, while a higher eosinophil count is associated with idiopathic etiology. Eosinophilic peritonitis should be treated as infectious until culture data return. When idiopathic, it may be associated with a new catheter or the recent initiation of PD. Eosinophilic peritonitis typically resolves in 2–6 weeks without intervention. Steroids and/or antihistamines can be helpful [2].

Some causes of abdominal pain can lead to secondary peritonitis, such as cholecystitis, diverticulitis, appendicitis, incarcerated hernia, or ruptured viscus. There have been rare cases of aseptic peritonitis with icodextrin use that is thought to be due to a peptidoglycan contaminant. This is a diagnosis of exclusion, presenting with a cell count of 350–3000 with sterile culture, improving when icodextrin has been stopped, and recurring if icodextrin from the same or similar lot is reintroduced.

Preventative Measures

Prevention of ES infections (ESIs) and tunnel infections focus on local care and topical antibiotics. Very tight clothing or taut anchoring of the catheter can traumatize the ES.

The nasal carriage of *S. aureus* is a risk factor for *S. aureus* PD infections, but no differences were seen in the total number of ESIs when nasal mupirocin was used. Therefore, the nasal carriage is not routinely checked [3, 4].

Mupirocin and/or gentamicin cream at the exit site reduces the risk of ESI [5, 6]. When compared with one another, variations in outcomes with mupirocin and gentamicin cream have not been reproduced in other studies. There is a theoretical risk of antibiotic resistance or fungal growth, but this is outweighed by the benefits seen in clinical outcomes with fewer ESIs.

Preventing peritonitis begins even prior to PD catheter placement. Parenteral antibiotics at the time of insertion reduce early peritonitis [7]. Several reviews have demonstrated no differences with the catheter type or the surgical technique; experts recommend that the catheter naturally lie laterally or downward from the exit site with avoidance of the belt line and skin folds [8, 9]. Patients should be instructed to avoid heavy lifting and showering/bathing after catheter insertion surgery until cleared by their dialysis team. The catheter should remain untouched until the first dressing change—1 week after surgery unless being used for urgent start protocols. Training should be done one-on-one with a qualified nurse. Patients trained by less experienced nurses may have fewer infections, highlighting the importance of continuous education for trainers [10]. Double bag or Y-set connectology can reduce peritonitis rates for patients on continuous ambulatory peritoneal dialysis (CAPD), and the "flush before fill" technique has been demonstrated to reduce peritonitis with CAPD and with cyclers that have this option [11].

Patients on PD may need stool softeners and/or laxatives to avoid constipation. Empty the peritoneal cavity prior to undergoing any medical procedure. Dental work can cause transient bacteremia with hematogenous spread causing peritonitis. Therefore, prophylaxis with a single dose of 2 g of amoxicillin is recommended [12]. Colonoscopy and colposcopy are associated with a translocation of enteric and vaginal microbes, respectively [13]. Prophylaxis with cefazolin and gentamicin should be given prior to endoscopy and GU instrumentation.

Aseptic Technique

- Keep windows and doors shut during exchanges.
- Keep room off limits to pets and toddlers.
- Wear mask.
- Wash hands with soap and water.
- Dry hands completely before exchange.

Educating patients on aseptic techniques and on protocols for wet and dry contamination and providing prophylaxis for wet contamination are important to reduce peritonitis risk (Table 11.2).

Table 11.2 Contamination

Types of contamination	Dry contamination	Wet contamination
Definition	Outside closed system	Open system
Examples	Leak or disconnection distal to closed clamp	Leak during instillation Leak or break in tubing proximal to a clamp Touch contamination during an exchange
Patient education	Keep clamp on transfer set closed, stop dialysis, call unit	Close clamp on transfer set, stop dialysis, call unit
Management	Change sterile tubing	Change sterile tubing and give prophylaxis

Apart from prophylaxis, bacterial antibiotic use should prompt concurrent antifungal use due to the risk of fungal peritonitis from fungal overgrowth in the gut. This can be accomplished with oral nystatin 500,000 units four times daily or fluconazole 200 mg every 48 h [14, 15].

Repeat training routinely after peritonitis, catheter infection, hospitalization, or a change in medical status, mental acuity, dexterity, or vision. Use connection assist devices when indicated [16]. Units should audit infection rates and outcomes to compare to national and international data and develop continuous quality improvement programs. The infection rate should be fewer than 0.5 episodes per patient year. Monitoring of specific organisms and susceptibilities can help to guide unit-specific empiric therapy. If the culture-negative rate is greater than 15–20%, the unit should reassess culture techniques.

Causes

For every episode of peritonitis, a root cause analysis must be performed. Peritonitis prior to training is usually due to *S. aureus*. Bacteria can gain access to the peritoneal cavity intraluminally from touch contamination or periluminally via the ES and tunnel. The former is most commonly *S. epidermidis*, diphtheroids, and Gram-negative rods (GNRs); the latter *S. aureus, Pseudomonas*, and also GNRs. Enteric organisms, including GNRs, Candida, and anaerobes, can enter the cavity across the bowel wall and warrant evaluation for primary pathology. Hematogenous seeding is a less common cause. Risk factors include dental work or intravascular device infection. PD-associated peritonitis rarely causes bacteremia. Transvaginal spread can lead to bacterial or fungal infections, particularly after instrumentation or if there is a communication to the peritoneal space.

PD-related peritonitis culture data shows a predominance of Gram-positive organisms, accounting for approximately 60% of cases. Coagulase-negative Staphylococcus (CoNS) was the most common of these at about 30%. Gram-negative infections comprised 15–20% of cases and fungi 3–4% [17].

Management of Exit Site and Tunnel Infections

Exit sites can be either perfect or good (Figs. 11.1 and 11.2). When the appearance of the ES is equivocal (Fig. 11.3), continue local care and topical antibiotics. The choice of antibiotic can be tailored to the Gram stain. The patient should be

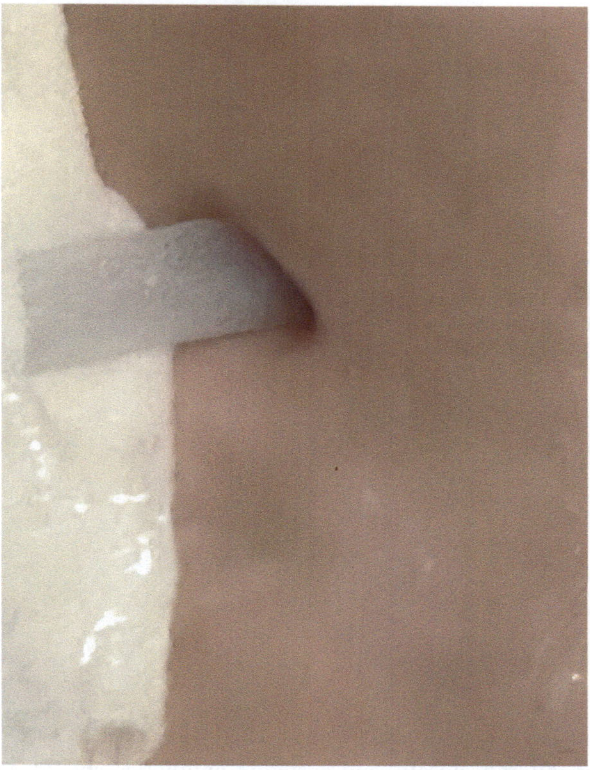

Fig. 11.1 Perfect cuff. (*Photo by Stephen Z. Fadem*)

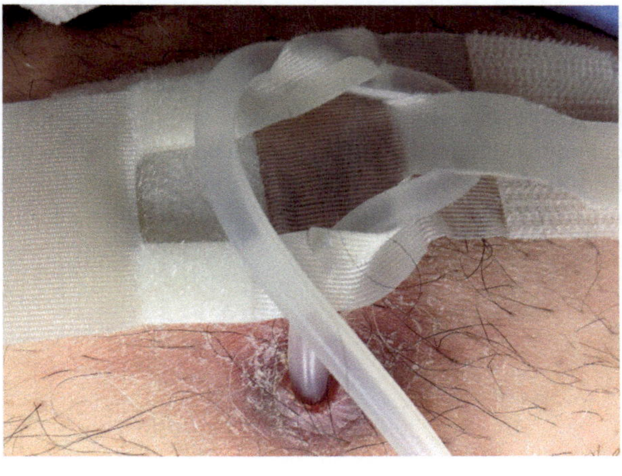

Fig. 11.2 Good cuff with scale. (*Photo by Thomas Golper*)

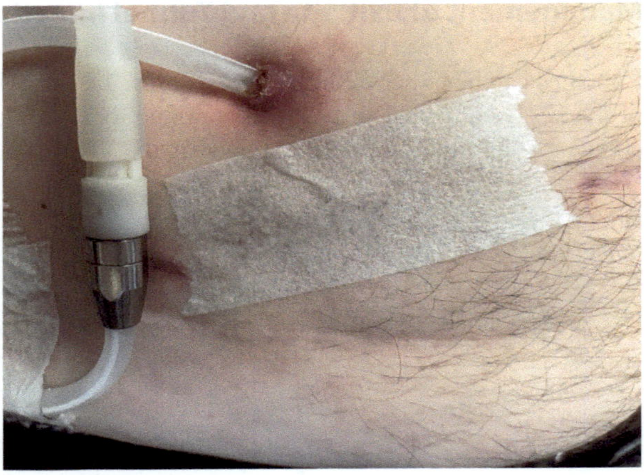

Fig. 11.3 Equivocal cuff. (*Photo by Thomas Golper*)

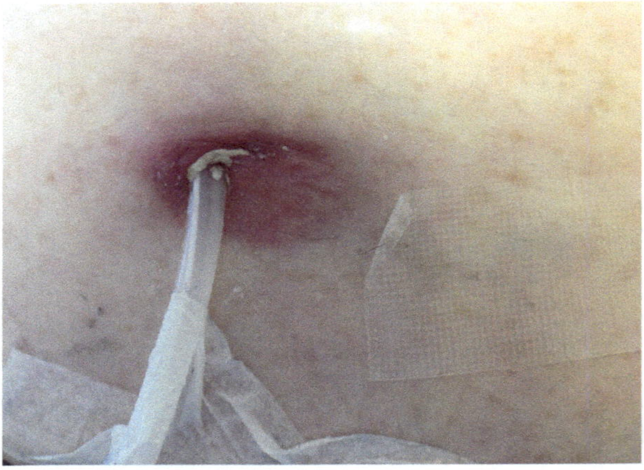

Fig. 11.4 Acute exit site infection. (*Photo by Thomas Golper*)

monitored closely, and systemic antibiotics should be added if the condition is worsening or if there is no improvement by 2 weeks [18]. For most ESIs (Fig. 11.4), a first-generation cephalosporin is the first line. Change to a quinolone for GNRs and to vancomycin for methicillin-resistant *S. aureus* (MRSA). If there is no improvement over 1–2 weeks, consider adding a second antibiotic. For Staphylococcal infections, adding rifampin can help penetrate biofilms. After clinical improvement, antibiotics should be continued for one additional week. An infection lasting for over 4 weeks is considered chronic (Fig. 11.5), even if initially improved with antibiotics. Re-culture and adjust antibiotics as needed. Evaluate the

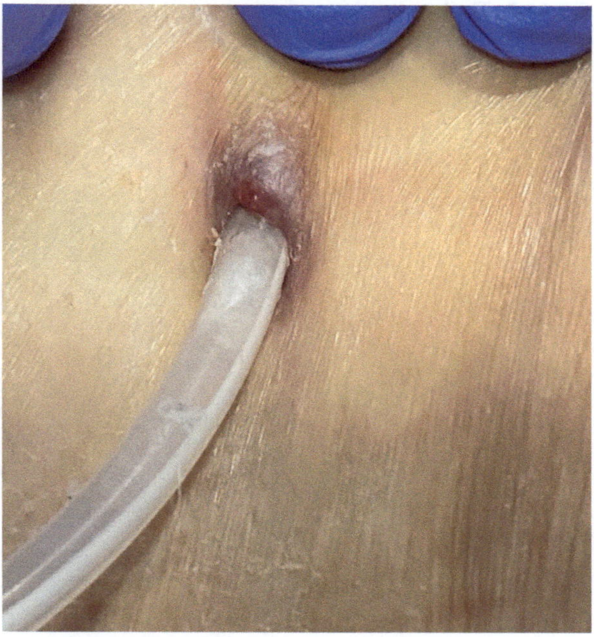

Fig. 11.5 Chronic exit site infection. (*Photo by Stephen Z. Fadem*)

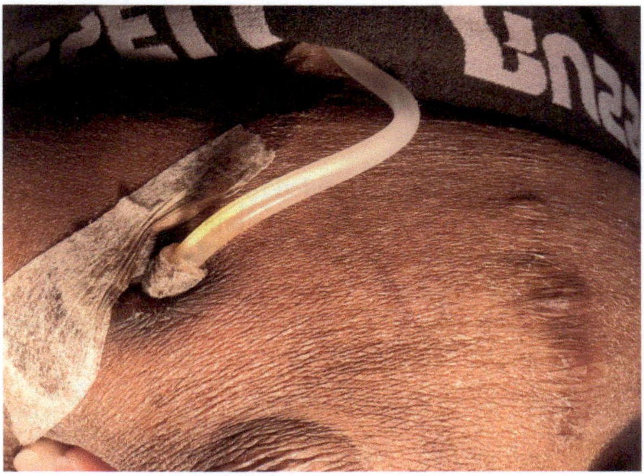

Fig. 11.6 Cuff extrusion. (*Photo by Thomas Golper*)

need for debridement of granulation tissue or removing an exposed cuff. An exposed cuff is more safely removed by an abrasive rather than by a sharp blade (Fig. 11.6). An eschar can be associated with a chronic exit site infection (Fig. 11.7). A

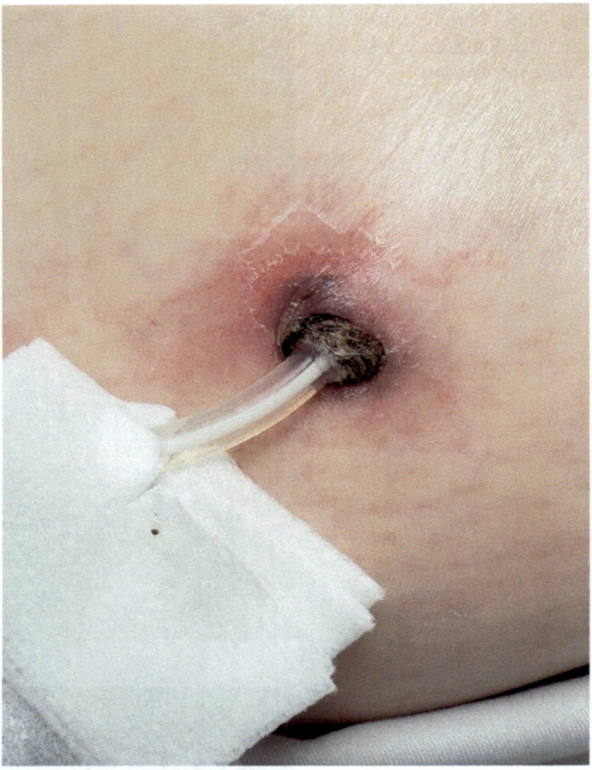

Fig. 11.7 Thick eschar. (*Photo by Thomas Golper*)

traumatized cuff can be avoided by relieving any tension on the catheter (Fig. 11.8). A cuff infection may require prolonged antibiotic use. Consider catheter removal with concurrent catheter placement. For acute or chronic ESIs with concurrent peritonitis, consider catheter removal and wait 2–4 weeks before replacing the catheter.

Figures 11.1, 11.2, 11.3, 11.4, 11.5, 11.6, 11.7 and 11.8 various depictions of exit sites.

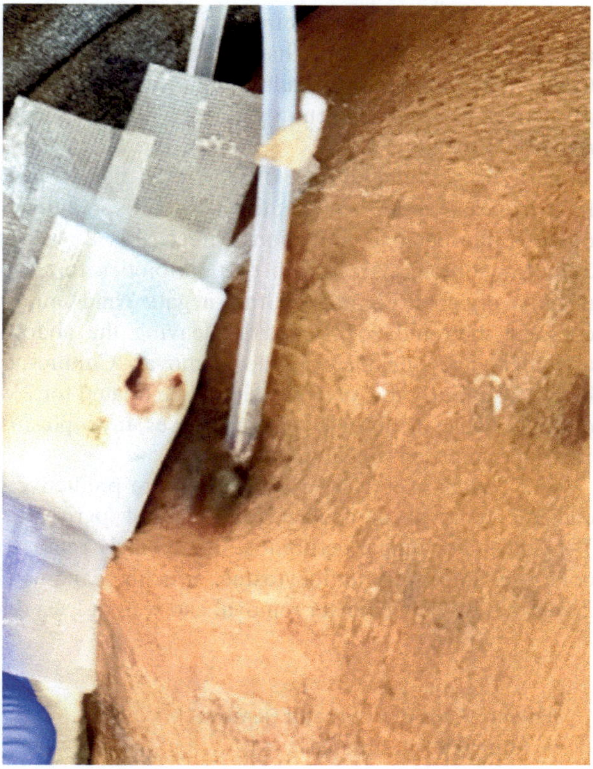

Fig. 11.8 Traumatized exit site. (*Photo by Stephen Z. Fadem*)

Management of Peritonitis

The mainstay of peritonitis treatment is to begin antibiotics quickly, ideally right after the culture is collected. In addition to antibiotics, manage pain with rapid in and out flushes and monitor for ultrafiltration problems. Use intraperitoneal heparin for drainage problems or fibrin.

The PROMPT study showed an increased risk of PD failure with delay of initiating antibiotics [19]. Intraperitoneal antibiotics are preferred but an IV dose may be necessary to prevent treatment delays. Initial treatment includes Gram-positive and Gram-negative coverage with adjustments once culture and susceptibility are obtained. Antibiotics can be given continuously, in each dialysate bag, or intermittently, with a larger dose that dwells for at least 6 h [20]. Possible empiric therapy includes cefazolin 500 mg/L load then 125 mg/L or 15–20 mg/kg daily and ceftazidime 500 mg/L load then 125 mg/L or 1000–1500 mg daily.

Empiric use of vancomycin can increase resistance but is still preferred if the patient is an MRSA carrier, has a history of MRSA infection, or has a history of a CoNS infection that is difficult to treat. Avoid prolonged or repeated use of aminoglycosides if possible, even in patients without residual kidney function, due to the risk of ototoxicity.

Peritonitis should improve over 36–48 h of appropriate antibiotics. For *S. aureus*, Enterococcus, and Gram-negative peritonitis, continue treatment for 3 weeks. For other Gram-positive infections, treat for 2 weeks. For Pseudomonas and Stenotrophomonas, treat with two antibiotics for 3–4 weeks. If multiple Gram-negative organisms or mixed Gram-negative and Gram-positive organisms are present, add metronidazole. Consider leaving the abdomen dry, evaluate for acute abdomen, and consider catheter removal. Culture-negative peritonitis typically behaves similarly to CoNS and should be treated for 2 weeks. If it is not improving, consider unusual etiologies such as viruses, mycoplasma, mycobacteria, Legionella, or a superimposed fungal infection.

Cell counts over 1090/mL on day 3 are predictive of treatment failure [21]. If catheter removal is needed for bacterial peritonitis, continue antibiotics for 7–14 days. For fungal peritonitis, immediately remove the catheter. Treat with fluconazole, amphotericin/flucytosine, or echinocandins [22]. Continue treatment for 2 weeks following catheter removal and wait at least 4–6 weeks before reinsertion.

When to Consider Catheter Removal

- Fungal peritonitis*.
- Bowel perforation*.
- Refractory peritonitis.
- Mycobacterial peritonitis.
- Pseudomonas or Stenotrophomonas peritonitis with concurrent ESI and/or tunnel infection.
- Unresolving peritonitis with concurrent ESI and/or tunnel infection.
- Relapsing or recurrent peritonitis.
- Ongoing ESI.

*Remove catheter immediately

Outcomes

In general, peritonitis resolves with treatment in 69–78% of cases, leads to catheter removal in 18–19%, and mortality in 2.5–9% [17, 23, 24]. The best outcomes are seen with CoNS, Streptococci, and culture-negative peritonitis. Corynebacteria, Enterococci, *S. aureus*, and non-pseudomonal GNRs pose a moderate risk. Polymicrobial, pseudomonal, and fungal infections have the poorest prognosis [17, 25]. Despite having a good response, relapse and recurrence are often caused by CoNS (see Table 11.3 for definitions). This is likely due to repeated touch

Table 11.3 Definitions in peritonitis

Refractory peritonitis	Not improving after 5 days of appropriate antibiotics
Recurrent peritonitis	2 episodes in <4 weeks with different organisms
Relapsing peritonitis	2 episodes in <4 weeks with same organism
Repeat peritonitis	2 episodes in >4 weeks with same organism

contaminations, shorter duration of antibiotics, fewer catheter removals, the formation of a biofilm, and a less robust immune response [26, 27]. Retraining is key. For a first relapse, treat with a longer course of antibiotics. For a second relapse, consider simultaneous catheter removal and placement.

Approximately 25% of hospitalizations of patients on PD are due to peritonitis, and it is the reason for about 30% of transfers to HD [28]. After severe infection, about 50% of patients resume PD, and the 2-year technique survival is about 30% [23, 29]. Stopping PD can be by patient or physician's choice, or related to permanent damage to the peritoneal membrane. This will be further addressed in the chapter on membrane dysfunction.

The mortality rate of fungal peritonitis is 5–53%. Lower mortality rates are seen with *Candida albicans* than with other fungi. Higher mortality is associated with bowel obstruction, lower residual kidney function, and when the catheter is not removed [22].

Conclusion

PD-related infections include ESIs, tunnel infections, and peritonitis. The key to good outcomes is with continuous training of patients and staff, ensuring preventative measures, expeditious treatment of infections with close follow-up, and tracking of data to modify strategies. Follow-up includes monitoring for improvement and adjusting antibiotics as more data is obtained. This is important to ensure adequate treatment but also for appropriate antibiotic stewardship. If patients are not improving despite appropriate antibiotics, catheter removal should be considered. Removing the catheter in a timely manner to allow for eradication of the infection can lead to fewer complications and enhance long-term technique survival.

References

1. Plum J, Sudkamp S, Grabensee B. Results of ultrasound-assisted diagnosis of tunnel infections in continuous ambulatory peritoneal dialysis. Am J Kidney Dis. 1994;23(1):99–104. https://doi.org/10.1016/s0272-6386(12)80818-3.

2. Fontán MP, Rodríguez-Carmona A, Galed I, Iglesias P, Villaverde P, García-Ureta E. Incidence and significance of peritoneal eosinophilia during peritoneal dialysis-related peritonitis. Perit Dial Intern. 2003;23(5):460–4. https://doi.org/10.1177/089686080302300510.
3. Mupirocin Study Group. Nasal mupirocin prevents *Staphylococcus aureus* exit-site infection during peritoneal dialysis. Mupirocin Study Group. J Am Soc Nephrol. 1996;7(11):2403–8. https://doi.org/10.1681/ASN.V7112403.
4. Luzar MA, Coles GA, Faller B, et al. *Staphylococcus aureus* nasal carriage and infection in patients on continuous ambulatory peritoneal dialysis. NEJM. 1990;322(8):505–9. https://doi.org/10.1056/NEJM199002223220804.
5. Htay H, Johnson DW, Wu SY, Oei EL, Foo MWY, Choo JCJ. Comparison of topical chlorhexidine and mupirocin for the prevention of exit-site infection in incident peritoneal dialysis patients. Perit Dial Intern. 2017;37(3):266–72. https://doi.org/10.3747/pdi.2016.00257.
6. Bernardini J, Bender F, Florio T, et al. Randomized, double-blind trial of antibiotic exit site cream for prevention of exit site infection in peritoneal dialysis patients. J Am Soc Nephrol. 2005;16(2):539–45. https://doi.org/10.1681/ASN.2004090773.
7. Gadallah MF, Ramdeen G, Mignone J, Patel D, Mitchell L, Tatro S. Role of preoperative antibiotic prophylaxis in preventing postoperative peritonitis in newly placed peritoneal dialysis catheters. Am J Kidney Dis. 2000;36(5):1014–9. https://doi.org/10.1053/ajkd.2000.19104.
8. Strippoli G, Tong A, Johnson D, Schena F, Craig J. Catheter-related interventions to prevent peritonitis in peritoneal dialysis: a systematic review of randomized, controlled trials. J Am Soc Nephrol. 2004;15(10):2735–46. https://doi.org/10.1097/01.ASN.0000141463.95561.79.
9. Nessim SJ. Optimising PD peritonitis prevention and treatment: an infectious goal. Perit Dial Intern. 2022;42(2):108–9. https://doi.org/10.1177/08968608221082838.
10. Chow KM, Szeto CC, Law MC, Fung JSF, Li PKT. Influence of peritoneal dialysis training nurses' experience on peritonitis rates. Clin J Am Soc Nephrol. 2007;2(4):647–52. https://doi.org/10.2215/CJN.03981206.
11. Smith CA. Reduced incidence of peritonitis by utilizing "flush before fill" in APD. Adv Perit Dial. 1997;13:224–6.
12. Limeres Posse J, Alvarez Fernandez M, Fernandez Feijoo J, et al. Intravenous amoxicillin/clavulanate for the prevention of bacteraemia following dental procedures: a randomized clinical trial. J Antimicrob Chemother. 2016;71(7):2022–30. https://doi.org/10.1093/jac/dkw081.
13. Chaudhry RI, Chopra T, Fissell R, Golper TA. Strategies to prevent peritonitis after procedures: our opinions. Perit Dial Intern. 2019;39(4):315–9. https://doi.org/10.3747/pdi.2018.00148.
14. Lo WK, Chan CY, Cheng SW, Poon JFM, Chan DTM, Cheng IKP. A prospective randomized control study of oral nystatin prophylaxis for candida peritonitis complicating continuous ambulatory peritoneal dialysis. Am J Kidney Dis. 1996;28(4):549–52. https://doi.org/10.1016/S0272-6386(96)90466-7.
15. Restrepo C, Chacon J, Manjarres G. Fungal peritonitis in peritoneal dialysis patients: successful prophylaxis with fluconazole, as demonstrated by prospective randomized control trial. Perit Dial Intern. 2010;30(6):619–25. https://doi.org/10.3747/pdi.2008.00189.
16. Piraino B. Can we reduce rates of *Staphylococcus aureus* and other peritonitis in peritoneal dialysis patients? Perit Dial Intern. 2010;30(3):277–9. https://doi.org/10.3747/pdi.2010.00052.
17. Mujais S. Microbiology and outcomes of peritonitis in North America. Kidney Intern. 2006;70(S103):S55–62. https://doi.org/10.1038/sj.ki.5001916.
18. Twardowski ZJ. Exit-site care in peritoneal dialysis patients. Perit Dial Intern. 1994;14(3_suppl):S39–42. https://doi.org/10.1177/089686089401403S08.
19. Muthucumarana K, Howson P, Crawford D, Burrows S, Swaminathan R, Irish A. The relationship between presentation and the time of initial administration of antibiotics with outcomes of peritonitis in peritoneal dialysis patients: the PROMPT study. Kidney Intern Rep. 2016;1(2):65–72. https://doi.org/10.1016/j.ekir.2016.05.003.
20. Szeto CC, Li PKT. Peritoneal dialysis-associated peritonitis. Clin J Am Soc Nephrol. 2019;14(7):1100–5. https://doi.org/10.2215/CJN.14631218.

21. Chow KM, Szeto CC, Cheung KKT, et al. Predictive value of dialysate cell counts in peritonitis complicating peritoneal dialysis. Clin J Am Soc Nephrol. 2006;1(4):768–73. https://doi.org/10.2215/CJN.01010306.
22. Chang TI, Kim HW, Park JT, et al. Early catheter removal improves patient survival in peritoneal dialysis patients with fungal peritonitis: results of 94 episodes of fungal peritonitis at a single center. Perit Dial Intern. 2011;31(1):60–6. https://doi.org/10.3747/pdi.2009.00057.
23. Bunke CM, Brier ME, Golper TA. Outcomes of single organism peritonitis in peritoneal dialysis: Gram negatives versus gram positives in the Network 9 Peritonitis Study. Kidney Intern. 1997;52(2):524–9. https://doi.org/10.1038/ki.1997.363.
24. Kavanagh D, Prescott GJ, Mactier RA. Peritoneal dialysis-associated peritonitis in Scotland (1999–2002). Nephrol Dial Transplant. 2004;19(10):2584–91. https://doi.org/10.1093/ndt/gfh386.
25. Perez Fontan M, Rodriguez-Carmona A, Garcia-Naveiro R, Rosales M, Villaverde P, Valdes F. Peritonitis-related mortality in patients undergoing chronic peritoneal dialysis. Perit Dial Intern. 2005;25(3):274–84. https://doi.org/10.1177/089686080502500311.
26. Dasgupta MK. Biofilms and infection in dialysis patients. Semin Dial. 2002;15(5):338–46. https://doi.org/10.1046/j.1525-139X.2002.00084.x.
27. Jung K, Luthje P, Lundahl J, Brauner A. Low immunogenicity allows *Staphylococcus epidermidis* to cause PD peritonitis. Perit Dial Intern. 2011;31(6):672–8. https://doi.org/10.3747/pdi.2009.00150.
28. Mujais S, Story K. Peritoneal dialysis in the US: evaluation of outcomes in contemporary cohorts. Kidney Intern. 2006;70(S103):S21–6. https://doi.org/10.1038/sj.ki.5001912.
29. Prasad KN, Singh K, Rizwan A, et al. Microbiology and outcomes of peritonitis in Northern India. Perit Dial Intern. 2014;34(2):188–94. https://doi.org/10.3747/pdi.2012.00233.

Peritoneal Membrane Dysfunction

12

Shweta Bansal

Introduction

As an established alternative to hemodialysis (HD), the adequacy of peritoneal dialysis (PD) is dependent on patient compliance and the performance of the peritoneal membrane. Owing to improved technology and the decline in peritonitis rates, membrane dysfunction (inadequate solute transport or inadequate water removal) has become an emerging factor leading to PD transfer to HD. In the latest Peritoneal Dialysis Outcomes and Practice Patterns Study, inadequate solute clearance and water removal led to approximately 13%–16% and 4%–10% of patients transferring to HD, respectively [1]. This chapter discusses the pathophysiology of membrane dysfunction and describes the methodology of functional assessment, the clinical presentation of abnormalities, and the diagnostic and management strategies to treat membrane dysfunction.

Peritoneal Membrane

The peritoneal membrane consists of a complex capillary wall endothelium and a single layer of mesothelial cells. Between these layers lies a submesothelial, interstitial tissue. This is a gel-like matrix containing fibroblasts, adipocytes, and collagen fibers. The permeability of this membrane is determined by the resistances created by each component. Based on the three-pore model initially derived from a computer simulation for peritoneal transport mechanisms, solute and water

S. Bansal (✉)
Division of Nephrology, Department of Medicine, University of Texas Health San Antonio, San Antonio, TX, USA
e-mail: bansals3@uthscsa.edu

S. Z. Fadem et al. (eds.), *Complications in Dialysis*,
https://doi.org/10.1007/978-3-031-44557-6_12

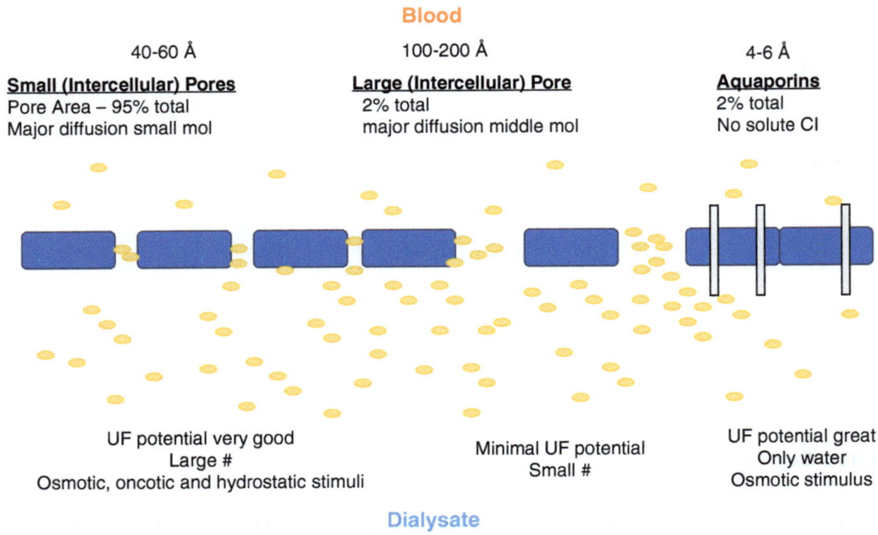

Fig. 12.1 Pores, glucose, ultrafiltration, and osmotic forces, "3 Pore Model"*. *Courtesy of Thomas Golper and John Burkart

transport occurs through three-pore types located in the capillary endothelium [2] (Fig. 12.1).

Large intercellular pores (radius 12–15 nm) are believed to be intercellular gaps and account for less than 1% of the effective total pore area for small solute diffusion. They play a minor role in ultrafiltration (UF). "Small intercellular pores" (radius 4 nm) account for approximately 90% of total pore area and are the primary route for solute diffusion and for over 50% of glucose-induced ultrafiltration. The third pore type is made up of aquaporin-1 (AQP-1) channels. These channels comprise only 1–2% of the total pore area but contribute up to 40% of ultrafiltration. The newer pore-matrix model also considers the fact that capillaries with three types of pores are distributed throughout the interstitial matrix, resulting in varying distances between capillary lumens and the peritoneal cavity.

Evaluation of Peritoneal Membrane Permeability

Peritoneal Equilibration Test (PET): This test semi-quantitatively measures the peritoneal membrane transfer rates for solutes (usually urea and creatinine) based on the ratio of their concentration in dialysate(D)/plasma(P) ratio at hour 0, 2, and 4 (t) during the dialysate dwell; and for glucose, based on the ratio of dialysate glucose at dwell times $t2$ or $t4$ to dialysate glucose at 0 dwell time (D_t/D_0). The PET provides a valuable tool for categorizing and monitoring changes in the peritoneal membrane transport/function [3].

Fast PET: This allows an assessment of net ultrafiltration and categorization of solute transport status using only the 4-h $D/P_{creatinine}$ ratio and glucose concentration. The only disadvantage is the unavailability of a ratio from intermediate time points. This may pose a problem if planning continuous cyclic peritoneal dialysis (CCPD) regimens with shorter dwell times and increases the possibility of error.

Modified PET: 4.25% exchange instead of 2.5% is used to create a maximal osmotic gradient to evaluate the ultrafiltration failure [4]. Some experienced programs only use this modified PET as the initial PET.

Mini-PET: It is a simple and fast method to assess transcellular free water transport reflecting AQP-1 deficiency/dysfunction. For this test, standardized PET is shortened to 1 h using 4.25% exchange, and dialysate sodium [Na] at hour 1 is also measured [5].

Membrane Dysfunction

Membrane dysfunction is not well-defined but usually implies impaired transport of water and solutes. It presents clinically as either increasing edema and hypertension due to impaired water removal and/or inadequate solute clearance resulting in high blood urea, creatinine, uremic symptoms, and worsening anemia. Before membrane dysfunction is deemed as the cause of impaired water removal and solute clearance, common non-membrane issues such as non-adherence with prescribed dialysis treatments and dietary restrictions, catheter malfunction, or PD fluid leaks need to be considered and evaluated. After ruling out these problems, an initial evaluation for membrane dysfunction consists of performing a PET with 4.25% exchange to assess both solute and water transport. Ultrafiltration Failure (UFF) is defined as UF of <400 mL after 4 h of 4.25% exchange (the "rule of 4s"). The PET allows a logical approach to the differential diagnosis and treatment of UFF.

1. *High transporter (PET $D/P_{creatinine}$ >0.81):* This is the largest group of patients with membrane dysfunction. They have good low molecular weight solute diffusive transport but have poor UF due to rapid absorption of glucose and dissipation of the osmotic gradient during standard PD using glucose-containing dialysate. This clinical picture, called Type I Ultrafiltration Failure (UFF), may develop over the course of months to years, may be transient subsequent to recent peritonitis, or may be intrinsic to a particular patient's peritoneal membrane.
   (a) *Type I UFF:* The development of slowly increasing solute permeability is a typical feature of chronic PD. The pathomorphological attribution of type I UFF is probably both fibrosis and angiogenesis, resulting in an increased effective capillary surface area. The avascular submesothelial fibrotic layer results in decreased osmotic pressure (possibly due to glucose uptake by interstitial myofibroblast) and increased diffusive resistance toward the endothelial exchange area of the capillaries. Additionally, by angiogenesis, an increased number of perfused capillaries under the fibrotic matrix rapidly

dissipate the glucose-driven osmotic pressure gradient between plasma water and dialysate. The factors contributing to morphologic and functional alterations have been uremia, peritonitis, and the non-physiologic nature of dialysis fluids (low pH, high lactate and glucose concentrations) leading to significantly increased circulating nitric oxide (NO), advanced glycation end products, vascular endothelial growth factor (VEGF), endothelial nitric oxide synthase, and inflammatory cytokines [interleukin (IL-1β), tumor necrosis factor-alpha (TNF-α), and IL-6]. The increase in effective peritoneal surface area is strongly related to VEGF and NO [6].

Accurate longitudinal measurements of peritoneal transport showed a marked decline in small-pore fluid transport which cannot be explained just by the rapid disappearance of an osmotic pressure gradient. A reasonable yet unproven theory of this pore dysfunction is that the decreased microcirculatory hydrostatic pressure gradient is caused by vasculopathy characterized by wall thickening and duplication of the capillary basement membrane, leading to the narrowing of the microvascular lumina [7]. High glucose-induced pseudohypoxia as a result of a high NADH-NAD^+ ratio causing upregulation of hypoxia-inducible factor-1 gene and microinflammation might be involved in the development of fibrosis and vasculopathy [8].

(b) *Recent peritonitis:* Acute peritonitis is associated with an enormous intraperitoneal network of pro- and anti-inflammatory cytokines and a complex interaction of peritoneal cell lines [9]. A rapid and reversible increase in the effective peritoneal surface area occurs most likely under the influence of NO, proinflammatory cytokines (IL-1β, TNF-α, IL-6), and prostaglandins [10]. This results in an increase in the $D/P_{creatinine}$, a proportionate decrease in the D_t/D_0glucose, and a significant reduction in net UF as compared with baseline [11]. Fortunately, these changes are generally transient. However, hyperpermeability of the membrane and morphologic changes such as submesothelial fibrosis and angiogenesis are typical and important results of recurrent infectious episodes and may lead to type I UFF [1].

2. Average transport (PET $D/P_{creatinine}$ 0.5–0.8): Membrane dysfunction in this category represents a selective defect in peritoneal free water transport through the AQP-1 channel (ultrasmall pore). Normally functioning AQP-1 channels lead to a rapid dilution of dialysate [Na] in the early part of the dwell. AQP-1-mediated UF is responsible for 40–50% of the effective transcapillary UF in glucose-containing dialysate and is thought to decline with vintage on PD, causing this selective defect in water transport (Type II UFF). Functional alteration of AQP-1 channels, rather than a decrease in their expression, is responsible for less free water removal in long-term PD. The underlying mechanism, while not clear, is likely a glycation- or NO-mediated process. Mini-PET or dialysate [Na] at 1 h can be used to assist in diagnosing defective transport through AQP-1 channels. The dip in dialysate [Na] is abnormally small.

Patients with mechanical problems (catheter malfunction or dialysate leak) or an increase in the rate of absorption of dialysate via lymphatics (type IV UFF) present in a similar fashion to true membrane failure, although peritoneal membrane function is intact [12].

3. Low transport (PET $D/P_{creatinine} < 0.5$): This category represents the least number of patients with membrane dysfunction and often stems from conditions leading to a severe reduction in effective peritoneal membrane contact surface area rather than a change in the intrinsic transport capacity (type III UFF) [13, 14]. Therefore, signs and symptoms of both fluid overload and inadequate solute removal may be present.
   (a) Abdominal adhesions: Adhesions are a common cause of decreased surface area. Adhesions are a consequence of blood, inflammation, and/or infection, often related to repeated episodes of frequent or severe peritonitis or abdominal surgery, particularly in the setting of bowel pathology.
   (b) Encapsulating peritoneal sclerosis (EPS): It is a rare complication associated with significant morbidity and mortality, characterized by intraperitoneal inflammation and fibrosis, which at times results in the encasement of bowel loops. EPS causes impairment of both solute and volume clearance and bowel obstruction. EPS is a slowly progressive, frequently asymptomatic disorder that occurs after generally >5 years of PD and multiple episodes of peritonitis. It develops in a stepwise fashion; in the early inflammation stage, patients present with non-specific symptoms of anorexia, nausea, diarrhea, and intermittent abdominal pain. The later ileus stage is characterized by intermittent bowel obstruction from bowl encapsulation. Bowel tethering and peritoneal calcification in the presence of characteristic symptoms are highly suggestive [15].
   (c) Compromised peritoneal blood flow: It is an extremely rare cause of membrane failure. A significant decrease in the peritoneal clearance of urea and creatinine has been observed in a few patients with systemic vascular disease (e.g., systemic lupus erythematosus, vasculitis, scleroderma, or malignant hypertension), but this was not associated with UFF [16, 17]

Prevention of Membrane Dysfunction

Avoidance and prompt treatment of PD-related infections are the key steps to prevent membrane dysfunction of all types [18]. The use of glucose-sparing dialysates fluids such as icodextrin has been associated with stable peritoneal permeability and better volume control in long-term PD patients [19]. In pre-clinic studies, phloretin, a non-selective blocker of facilitative glucose channels, reduced glucose absorption by >30% and resulted in a >50% higher UF rate compared to control animals [20]. Analysis of the balANZ trial revealed that compared to a progressive increase in peritoneal membrane permeability with conventional solutions, patients who performed PD with the neutral pH, lactate-buffered and low GDP dialysate had a stable rate of membrane transport over the 2 years of observation [21]. Long-term histomorphological and functional data are lacking, and these solutions are currently not commercially available in the US. Upregulation of the RAAS system in response to acute inflammation and chronic exposure to a bioincompatible PD solution plays an important role in the morphologic alteration of the peritoneal membrane. Few retrospective trials of patients on PD treated with 2 years of angiotensin-converting enzyme inhibitors have shown beneficial effects on the development of these alterations [22, 23]. Emphasizing lower dietary sodium intake and the regular use of high-dose diuretics can reduce reliance on hypertonic dialysate for fluid removal, and thus spare the membrane from glucose-induced inflammation and fibrosis, as explained above. Additionally, given the high prevalence of constipation in the ESRD population, one should regularly prescribe laxatives. This can help avoid catheter malfunction from contributing to poor fluid removal.

Management of Membrane Dysfunction

Treatment of high transport related problems involves shortening dwell times by switching continuous ambulatory PD patients to continuous cyclic PD (CCPD), shortening the dwell times if already on CCPD, and using icodextrin for any very long dwells (Table 12.1). Dietary sodium reduction, high-dose and combination diuretics, and laxative use are important adjuncts. Combination therapy with furosemide and a thiazide-like diuretic is effective [24].

Discontinuing PD and resting the peritoneum for at least 4 weeks by a temporary transfer to HD have been associated with significant improvement in UF capacity and normalization of solute transport characteristics in more than 81% of patients [25, 26]. Peritoneal rest enabled patients with UFF to continue PD for a median period of 23 months (range, 13–46 months). If this rest strategy is applied late in the course of UFF, e.g., > 6 months after development of UFF, it may not be effective to reverse the higher transport characteristics and UF capacity [27].

Membrane dysfunction in low transporters is more difficult to treat. Increasing dialysate volume to engage more surface area and utilizing every available hour for

Table 12.1 Preventive and management strategies for peritoneal membrane dysfunction

Goal		Strategy
Prevention	From the onset	Low sodium diet
		High-dose loop diuretic
		RAAS Blocker
		Regular laxatives
		Biocompatible dialysate (if available)
Treatment	High transporter	Switch CAPD patients to CCPD to shorten dwell time
		Shorten dwell times in CCPD
		Icodextrin for long dwell
	Low transporter	Increase dialysate volume
	General	Peritoneal dialysis rest in selected patients
		Continue the preventative strategies

RAAS renin angiotensin aldosterone system, *CAPD* continuous ambulatory peritoneal dialysis, *CCPD* continuous cyclical peritoneal dialysis dwelling may be helpful. Surgical restoration of surface area can be selectively helpful. In EPS, Tamoxifen and prednisone have been associated with improved survival in several retrospective studies, but overall, the prognosis is poor [28, 29].

Conclusion

The potential for membrane dysfunction increases as patients are successfully maintained on PD for longer periods of time. Therefore, an astute management approach avoiding peritonitis and high glucose exposure is the key to prevention. The modified PET is an essential tool to assist in the workup and formulating a logical therapeutic approach to manage these patients.

References

1. Lambie M, Zhao J, McCullough K, Davies SJ, Kawanishi H, Johnson DW, et al. Variation in peritoneal dialysis time on therapy by country: results from the peritoneal dialysis outcomes and practice patterns study. Clin J Am Soc Nephrol. 2022;17(6):861–71. https://doi.org/10.2215/CJN.16341221.
2. Rippe B, Stelin G, Haraldsson B. Computer simulations of peritoneal fluid transport in CAPD. Kidney Int. 1991;40(2):315–25. https://doi.org/10.1038/ki.1991.216.
3. Misra M, Khanna R. The clinical interpretation of peritoneal equilibration test. Semin Dial. 2014;27(6):598–602. https://doi.org/10.1111/sdi.12285.
4. La Milia V, Pozzoni P, Virga G, Crepaldi M, Del Vecchio L, Andrulli S, et al. Peritoneal transport assessment by peritoneal equilibration test with 3.86% glucose: a long-term prospective evaluation. Kidney Int. 2006;69(5):927–33. https://doi.org/10.1038/sj.ki.5000183.
5. La Milia V, Di Filippo S, Crepaldi M, Del Vecchio L, Dell'Oro C, Andrulli S, et al. Mini-peritoneal equilibration test: a simple and fast method to assess free water and small solute transport across the peritoneal membrane. Kidney Int. 2005;68(2):840–6. https://doi.org/10.1111/j.1523-1755.2005.00465.x.
6. Mortier S, De Vriese AS, Lameire N. Recent concepts in the molecular biology of the peritoneal membrane—implications for more biocompatible dialysis solutions. Blood Purif. 2003;21(1):14–23. https://doi.org/10.1159/000067867.
7. Krediet RT. Acquired decline in ultrafiltration in peritoneal dialysis: the role of glucose. J Am Soc Nephrol. 2021;32(10):2408–15. https://doi.org/10.1681/ASN.2021010080.
8. Krediet RT, Parikova A. Relative contributions of pseudohypoxia and inflammation to peritoneal alterations with long-term peritoneal dialysis patients. Clin J Am Soc Nephrol. 2022;17(8):1259–66. https://doi.org/10.2215/CJN.15371121.
9. Horton JK, Davies M, Topley N, Thomas D, Williams JD. Activation of the inflammatory response of neutrophils by Tamm-Horsfall glycoprotein. Kidney Int. 1990;37(2):717–26. https://doi.org/10.1038/ki.1990.38.
10. Albrektsen GE, Wideroe TE, Nilsen TI, Romundstad P, Radtke M, Hallan S, et al. Transperitoneal water transport before, during, and after episodes with infectious peritonitis in patients treated with CAPD. Am J Kidney Dis. 2004;43(3):485–91. https://doi.org/10.1053/j.ajkd.2003.10.043.
11. Szeto CC, Chow KM, Wong TY, Leung CB, Wang AY, Lui SF, et al. Feasibility of resuming peritoneal dialysis after severe peritonitis and Tenckhoff catheter removal. J Am Soc Nephrol. 2002;13(4):1040–5. https://doi.org/10.1681/ASN.V1341040.

12. Teitelbaum I. Ultrafiltration failure in peritoneal dialysis: a pathophysiologic approach. Blood Purif. 2015;39(1–3):70–3. https://doi.org/10.1159/000368972.
13. Pannekeet MM, Imholz AL, Struijk DG, Koomen GC, Langedijk MJ, Schouten N, et al. The standard peritoneal permeability analysis: a tool for the assessment of peritoneal permeability characteristics in CAPD patients. Kidney Int. 1995;48(3):866–75. https://doi.org/10.1038/ki.1995.363.
14. Struijk DG, Krediet RT, Koomen GC, Boeschoten EW, Hoek FJ, Arisz L. A prospective study of peritoneal transport in CAPD patients. Kidney Int. 1994;45(6):1739–44. https://doi.org/10.1038/ki.1994.226.
15. Moriles KE, Hashmi MF. Encapsulating peritoneal sclerosis. Treasure Island: StatPearls; 2022.
16. Nolph KD, Stoltz ML, Maher JF. Altered peritoneal permeability in patients with systemic vasculitis. Ann Intern Med. 1971;75(5):753–5. https://doi.org/10.7326/0003-4819-75-5-753.
17. Brown ST, Ahearn DJ, Nolph KD. Reduced peritoneal clearances in scleroderma increased by intraperitoneal isoproterenol. Ann Intern Med. 1973;78(6):891–4. https://doi.org/10.7326/0003-4819-78-6-891.
18. Muthucumarana K, Howson P, Crawford D, Burrows S, Swaminathan R, Irish A. The relationship between presentation and the time of initial administration of antibiotics with outcomes of peritonitis in peritoneal dialysis patients: the PROMPT study. Kidney Int Rep. 2016;1(2):65–72. https://doi.org/10.1016/j.ekir.2016.05.003.
19. Cho Y, Johnson DW, Badve S, Craig JC, Strippoli GF, Wiggins KJ. Impact of icodextrin on clinical outcomes in peritoneal dialysis: a systematic review of randomized controlled trials. Nephrol Dial Transplant. 2013;28(7):1899–907. https://doi.org/10.1093/ndt/gft050.
20. Bergling K, Martus G, Oberg C. Phloretin improves ultrafiltration and reduces glucose absorption during peritoneal dialysis in rats. J Am Soc Nephrol. 2022;33:1857–63. https://doi.org/10.1681/ASN.2022040474.
21. Johnson DW, Brown FG, Clarke M, Boudville N, Elias TJ, Foo MW, et al. The effect of low glucose degradation product, neutral pH versus standard peritoneal dialysis solutions on peritoneal membrane function: the balANZ trial. Nephrol Dial Transplant. 2012;27(12):4445–53. https://doi.org/10.1093/ndt/gfs314.
22. Kolesnyk I, Dekker FW, Noordzij M, le Cessie S, Struijk DG, Krediet RT. Impact of ACE inhibitors and AII receptor blockers on peritoneal membrane transport characteristics in long-term peritoneal dialysis patients. Perit Dial Int. 2007;27(4):446–53.
23. Kolesnyk I, Noordzij M, Dekker FW, Boeschoten EW, Krediet RT. A positive effect of AII inhibitors on peritoneal membrane function in long-term PD patients. Nephrol Dial Transplant. 2009;24(1):272–7. https://doi.org/10.1093/ndt/gfn421.
24. Tzamaloukas AH. Avoiding the use of hypertonic dextrose dialysate in peritoneal dialysis. Semin Dial. 2000;13(3):156–9. https://doi.org/10.1046/j.1525-139x.2000.00041.x.
25. de Alvaro F, Castro MJ, Dapena F, Bajo MA, Fernandez-Reyes MJ, Romero JR, et al. Peritoneal resting is beneficial in peritoneal hyperpermeability and ultrafiltration failure. Adv Perit Dial. 1993;9:56–61.
26. Miranda B, Selgas R, Celadilla O, Munoz J, Sanchez Sicilia L. Peritoneal resting and heparinization as an effective treatment for ultrafiltration failure in patients on CAPD. Contrib Nephrol. 1991;89:199–204. https://doi.org/10.1159/000419767.
27. De Sousa E, Del Peso G, Alvarez L, Ros S, Mateus A, Aguilar A, et al. Peritoneal resting with heparinized lavage reverses peritoneal type I membrane failure. A comparative study of the resting effects on normal membranes. Perit Dial Int. 2014;34(7):698–705. https://doi.org/10.3747/pdi.2013.00286.
28. Summers AM, Clancy MJ, Syed F, Harwood N, Brenchley PE, Augustine T, et al. Single-center experience of encapsulating peritoneal sclerosis in patients on peritoneal dialysis for end-stage renal failure. Kidney Int. 2005;68(5):2381–8. https://doi.org/10.1111/j.1523-1755.2005.00701.x.
29. Kawanishi H, Kawaguchi Y, Fukui H, Hara S, Imada A, Kubo H, et al. Encapsulating peritoneal sclerosis in Japan: a prospective, controlled, multicenter study. Am J Kidney Dis. 2004;44(4):729–37.

Metabolic Complications of Peritoneal Dialysis

13

Osama El Shamy

Hyperglycemia

Given that the majority of peritoneal dialysis solutions utilized are dextrose-based, concerns about potential hyperglycemia are warranted. Goldstein et al. [1] estimated daily glucose absorption for patients on continuous ambulatory peritoneal dialysis (CAPD) in the range of 100–300 g. However, most PD patients in the United States are on automated peritoneal dialysis (APD). A pilot study [2] to determine glucose absorption in patients on APD using peritoneal equilibration test (PET) results and effluent glucose concentrations estimated the mean daily glucose absorption to be 89.7 g. Does this amount of glucose absorption significantly affect glycemic control in PD patients?

A meta-analysis [3] of under 14,000 incident PD patients set out to assess rates of new-onset diabetes mellitus (NODM), new-onset impaired glucose tolerance, and new-onset impaired fasting glucose. The study found that approximately 55% of PD patients may develop at least one kind of glucose metabolism disturbance. However, there was no significant difference in NODM rates between PD and HD patients, perhaps because insulin resistance is common in both.

The mainstay of hyperglycemia treatment in PD patients is insulin, administered either intraperitoneally (IP) or subcutaneously (SC). While IP administration is more convenient for patients and has been shown to result in better glycemic control [4, 5], it does require a 30% greater amount of insulin compared to the SC route [6].

Given the intermittent nature of thrice weekly HD, one would expect greater fluctuations in blood glucose levels when compared to PD, especially CAPD, and this was corroborated by Chen et al. [7] Patients on thrice weekly HD had higher

O. El Shamy (✉)
Division of Nephrology and Hypertension, Vanderbilt University Medical Center, Nashville, TN, USA

S. Z. Fadem et al. (eds.), *Complications in Dialysis*,
https://doi.org/10.1007/978-3-031-44557-6_13

rates of both hypo- and hyperglycemia and higher mean amplitude of glycemic excursion, as well as the largest amplitude of glycemic excursion compared to CAPD. It is owing to these fluctuations in blood glucose levels and the effect of anemia and hypoproteinemia on hemoglobin A1c that makes it an unreliable determinant of glycemic control. KDIGO recommends targeting hemoglobin A1c levels of <8% for patients on dialysis [8]. The most accurate way to determine these fluctuations in dialysis patients is through continuous glucose monitoring systems.

Icodextrin use may cause an overestimation of blood glucose levels measured using finger-stick meters. Icodextrin is systemically hydrolyzed to maltose, maltotriose, and maltotetraose [9], all of which contribute to osmolality and contribute to the mild hyponatremia sometimes observed. It is believed that maltose interferes with glucose assays that utilize glucose dehydrogenase (such as glucose dehydrogenase/coenzyme PQQ) based devices [9, 10]. Glucometers using other assays, such as glucose oxidase, have been preferred.

Hyperlipidemia

When compared to the general population, ESKD patients have higher rates of cardiovascular disease (CVD). CVD-associated mortality is one of the leadings causes of death in the ESKD population [11]. Abnormal lipid metabolism predisposes to the development of CVD. Mechanisms of abnormal lipid metabolism in dialysis patients [12] include increased production of and decreased clearance of very low-density lipoprotein triglycerides (VLDL-TG) [13–16] and increased peritoneal losses of glycosaminoglycans, alpha-acid glycoprotein, HDL-C, and other regulatory macro molecules [17].

Studies in HD patients demonstrate that low serum total cholesterol levels are associated with a higher mortality rate [18, 19]. Dyslipidemias seen in PD patients are different in that they tend to have high total cholesterol, LDL, and triglyceride levels and low HDL and apolipoprotein A1 levels [20]. A prospective study of PD patients from the United States Renal Data System (USRDS) examined the association between serum total cholesterol and triglyceride with morbidity and mortality [21]. Reference ranges used for total cholesterol and triglycerides were 176–225 mg/dL and 201–300 mg/dL, respectively. A significant mortality hazard ratio (HR) was demonstrated in the lowest total cholesterol category (≤125 mg/dL, HR 1.94), with the remaining categories demonstrating a reverse J-shaped curve association. Similar findings were also seen in patients regardless of whether they were taking lipid-modifying medications and in patients with serum albumin levels ≤3.0 g/dL. Patients with serum albumin >3.0 g/dL and total cholesterol levels >275 mg/dL were found to have increased all-cause mortality. Low-to-normal triglyceride levels were protective, regardless of lipid-modifying medication administration.

These findings challenge the utility of lipid-modifying medications in the PD patient population, consistent with a prior finding that dialysis patients, especially patients on PD and those with atherosclerotic cardiovascular disease, are less likely to be treated for their hyperlipidemia [22]. The use of these medications was associated with decreased all-cause and cardiovascular mortality in patients with total cholesterol levels >226 mg/dL, diabetics, and patients with a Charlson Comorbidity Index score > 2 [23].

The use of statins is the standard of care for treating elevated LDL levels in PD patients. Yet, like the general population, these patients have the potential to develop statin therapy side effects such as myalgia and asthenia. The use of combined ezetimibe-simvastatin in PD patients demonstrated effective dyslipidemia treatment with neither of these side effects [24].

Weight Gain

The caloric load of dextrose-based PD solutions is significant. The greater the mass of dextrose instilled, the greater the caloric load (for example, 1.5 L of 1.5% dextrose contain 83 kcal, whereas 2.5 L of 4.25% dextrose contain 393 kcal). Rates of obesity in PD patients tend to correlate with other risk factors such as muscle wasting, dynapenia, and sarcopenia. A study assessing obesity rates in PD patients found 81.8% and 100% obesity rates in patients with moderate and severely reduced muscle mass, respectively [25].

The evolution of body fat mass in incident PD patients is of interest. Visceral fat mass is associated with insulin resistance, hyperglycemia, and dyslipidemia in the general population. It is a predictor of cardiovascular disease in PD patients [26]. Using serial assessments of body composition, nutrition status, and adipokine levels, Choi et al. [27] determined changes in fat composition and adipokines in incident PD patients during the first 24 months of dialysis, finding a continuous rise in leptin, body weight, and visceral and subcutaneous fat mass. However, the adjusted model did not demonstrate a correlation between body weight or fat mass and patient outcomes. A similar study [28] of incident PD patients found that after 1 year on PD, 50.6% and 65.9% of patients had an increase in their dry weight and fat mass, respectively. Interestingly, non-fast transporters had greater weight gain than fast transporters.

Demonstrating the variation of weight gain among PD patients, a retrospective analysis [29] of 114 prevalent PD patients over a 2-year period found that only 8 patients gained >10 kg. These patients were non-diabetic, had little residual kidney function (RKF), mostly normal cardiac function, and were high average transporters.

The effect of excessive fat accumulation (EFA) may have on the long-term outcomes of PD patients is important. Defining EFA as a change in percentage of body fat by 5.0% in men and 5.4% in women, Kim et al. [30] found the greatest body weight increase and EFA occurred within 2 years of PD treatment. There were increased mortality and PD failure rates in this subset of patients. Other studies had demonstrated no effect on mortality.

In conclusion, while there is verified weight gain in patients on PD, its rate and effect on long-term modality and patient survival are yet to be fully determined.

Hyponatremia

Mild, clinically insignificant hyponatremia in PD patients is common and likely multifactorial. Sodium sieving in the initial stages of the PD cycle may increase serum sodium concentrations and stimulate thirst. This can result in increased water consumption. Patients with chronic kidney disease are also more likely to be anorexic. Anorexia in PD patients can be exacerbated by abdominal discomfort (fullness), peritoneal protein losses, inflammation, and resultant malnutrition culminating in decreased solute intake. This may mislead the clinician into thinking the patient is well dialyzed. Another possible contributing factor is the subclinical hypokalemia often observed in PD patients. To maintain volume and tonicity, the deficit of cellular potassium triggers cells to gain sodium from the extracellular fluid. Given that the majority of PD solutions used are dextrose-based, patients can develop hyperglycemia which results in hyperosmolality and a subsequent shift of water from the intracellular to the extracellular space. Similarly, patients with little to no RKF may use icodextrin-based solutions as part of their daily exchanges. As mentioned above, icodextrin is metabolized to maltose, and it accumulates in extracellular fluid, creating an osmotic gradient with a resultant shift of free water to the extracellular space. Finally, inadequate ultrafiltration, a cause of PD technique failure, can result in hyponatremia due to increased extracellular free water and low serum sodium concentrations.

In an observational study of over 4000 incident US PD patients, sodium levels <140 mEq/L were associated with higher mortality [31]. This effect was attenuated but remained significant when factoring in APD versus CAPD, laboratory characteristics, RKF, and nutritional status for sodium levels <136 mEq/L. These observations support the findings of a previous study that demonstrated higher all-cause mortality in patients with serum sodium <137 mEq/L. In the previous study, a 1 mEq/L increase in sodium was associated with 21% lower all-cause mortality [32].

Hypokalemia

Hypokalemia prevalence ranges from 10 to 36% in PD patients [33, 34]. This is likely due to the absence of potassium in dialysate, the lingering effect of pre-ESKD potassium dietary restriction, and anorexia. Furthermore, absorbed glucose stimulates insulin release, which causes potassium movement into the cells.

The correlation between serum potassium levels and mortality in PD patients is U-shaped [35]. Potassium levels <3.5 and ≥5.5 mEq/L were associated with increased all-cause mortality. In addition, there is a correlation between hypokalemia and peritonitis. Hypokalemia can cause dysmotility, constipation, and intestinal bacterial overgrowth, with subsequent transmural migration potentially resulting in the development of peritonitis [36]. Hypokalemia can contribute to muscle weakness which might detrimentally affect connection skills.

Thus, the treatment of hypokalemia is important. Potassium supplementation and/or liberalizing dietary intake are the mainstays. Achieving potassium levels of 4–5 mEq/L in PD patients using a protocol-based potassium supplementation regimen resulted in lower peritonitis rates compared to conventional reactive potassium supplementation in PD patients with serum potassium <3.5 mEq/L. [37]

Protein Losses

Peritoneal protein losses (PPL) range from 4.8 to 10 g per day [38, 39]. While some studies have correlated PPL with mortality, malnutrition, inflammation, and cardiovascular events, these findings are not universal. A multivariable regression model adjusting for age, gender, serum IL-6 and albumin levels, RKF, amongst other things found increased all-cause mortality with higher Charlson Comorbidity Index scores, extracellular water excess, and lower PPL [38]. The latter finding is puzzling; overhydration was the strongest predictor of PPL, consistent with prior studies that found central venous congestion to be a major determinant of PPL, owing to elevated venous pressures in the peritoneal microcirculation [40].

Sarcopenia is one of the causes of mortality in patients on dialysis, owing to age-related loss of skeletal muscle mass and strength. Unexpectedly, a cross-sectional study of 100 PD patients found no correlation between PPL and muscle mass, strength, or sarcopenia [41].

Knowing that hypoalbuminemia is associated with mortality in ESKD patients, some clinicians may be hesitant to start hypoalbuminemia patients on PD due to PPL. An analysis of USRDS data found that while patients with hypoalbuminemia were less likely to be initiated on PD, those on PD had lower mortality compared to their HD counterparts (HR 0.88, $p < 0.05$) [42].

Gastroesophageal Reflux

Gastrointestinal (GI) symptoms such as discomfort, pain, and vomiting are common in uremic patients. Rates of gastroesophageal reflux (GERD) are significantly higher amongst CKD patients compared to the general population (77.5% vs 38.6%). Aside from increased gastrin levels, decreased gastrointestinal motility, and amyloid deposition, Helicobacter pylori (HP) plays a pivotal role in the development of GI symptoms in HD and PD patients [43, 44]. However, HP rates in CKD patients are lower than in the general population (40% vs 75%). It is recommended that ESKD patients with GI symptoms undergo endoscopic evaluation, especially as part of kidney transplant evaluation.

The prevalence of GERD in the PD population is thought to be due to the effect of intraperitoneal pressures (which are directly correlated with fill volumes, body habitus, and positioning) resulting in decreased basal tone of the lower esophageal sphincter [45, 46]. However, manometric assessment of lower esophageal sphincter pressures in CAPD patients during filling, emptying, and refilling did not demonstrate any differences in mean distal esophageal amplitude, duration, or velocity of peristalsis [47, 48].

Comparing endoscopic and pathological findings in HD and PD patients, HP rates were significantly higher in PD patients [49]. However, rates of GERD, [48, 49] erosive reflux esophagitis, and non-erosive reflux disease were similar between the two groups [49].

Conclusion

In conclusion, PD patients suffer from the same metabolic issues as the general population and the hemodialysis population, except that glucose loading and peritoneal protein losses magnify and alter these common complications.

References

1. Grodstein GP, Blumenkrantz MJ, Kopple JD, Moran JK, Coburn JW. Glucose absorption during continuous ambulatory peritoneal dialysis. Kidney Int. 1981;19(4):564–7. https://doi.org/10.1038/ki.1981.53. PMID: 7241890.
2. Kotla SK, Saxena A, Saxena R. A model to estimate glucose absorption in peritoneal dialysis: a pilot study. Kidney360. 2020;1(12):1373–9. https://doi.org/10.34067/KID.0004722020. PMID: 35372892; PMCID: PMC8815531.
3. Xue C, Gu YY, Cui CJ, Zhou CC, Wang XD, Ruan MN, Huang LX, Chen SX, Yang B, Chen XJ, Qian YX, Wu J, Zhao XZ, Zhang YQ, Mei CL, Zhang SL, Xu J, Mao ZG. New-onset glucose disorders in peritoneal dialysis patients: a meta-analysis and systematic review. Nephrol Dial Transplant. 2020;35(8):1412–9. https://doi.org/10.1093/ndt/gfz116. PMID: 31236586.
4. Blaine E, Tumlinson R, Colvin M, Haynes T, Whitley HP. Systematic literature review of insulin dose adjustments when initiating hemodialysis or peritoneal dialysis. Pharmacotherapy. 2022;42(2):177–87. https://doi.org/10.1002/phar.2659. Epub 2022 Jan 17. PMID: 35000222.
5. Quellhorst E. Insulin therapy during peritoneal dialysis: pros and cons of various forms of administration. J Am Soc Nephrol. 2002;13(Suppl 1):S92–6.
6. Almalki MH, Altuwaijri MA, Almehthel MS, Sirrs SM, Singh RS. Subcutaneous versus intraperitoneal insulin for patients with diabetes mellitus on continuous ambulatory peritoneal dialysis: meta-analysis of non-randomized clinical trials. Clin Invest Med. 2012;35(3):E132–43. https://doi.org/10.25011/cim.v35i3.16589.
7. Chen XX, Duan Y, Zhou Y. Effects of hemodialysis and peritoneal dialysis on glycometabolism in patients with end-stage diabetic nephropathy. Blood Purif. 2021;50(4–5):506–12. https://doi.org/10.1159/000511722. Epub 2020 Dec 10. PMID: 33302273.
8. de Boer IH, Caramori ML, Chan JCN, et al. Executive summary of the 2020 KDIGO diabetes management in CKD guideline: evidence-based advances in monitoring and treatment. Kidney Int. 2020;98(4):839–48. https://doi.org/10.1016/j.kint.2020.06.024.
9. Ramos R, González T, Fulladosa X, Castelao AM, Grinyó JM. False hyperglycemies in diabetic patients using icodextrin in peritoneal dialysis. Dial Transplant. 2008;37:323–7.
10. Janssen W, Harff G, Caers M, Schellekens A. Positive interference of icodextrin metabolites in some enzymatic glucose methods. Clin Chem. 1998;44:2379–80.
11. Foley RN, Parfrey PS, Sarnak MJ. The clinical epidemiology of cardiovascular disease in chronic renal disease. Am J Kidney Dis. 1998;32(Suppl 3):S112–9.
12. Lal SM. Hyperlipidemia in continuous ambulatory peritoneal dialysis patients. ASAIO J. 1993;39(2):87–8. PMID: 8324266.

13. Turgan C, Feehally J, Bennet S, et al. Accelerated hypertriglyceridemia in patients on CAPD: a preventable abnormality. Int J Artif Organs. 1981;4:158–60.
14. Ramos JM, Heaton A, McGurk JG, et al. Sequential changes in serum lipids and their subfractions in patients receiving CAPD. Nephron. 1983;35:20–3.
15. Mordasini R, Frey F, Flury W, et al. Selective deficiency of hepatic triglyceride lipase in uremic patients. N Engl J Med. 1977;297:1362–6.
16. Rapoport J, Aviram M, Chaimovitz C, et al. Defective high density lipoprotein composition in patients on chronic hemodialysis. N Engl J Med. 1978;299:1326–9.
17. Lindholm B, Norbeck HE. Serum lipids and lipoproteins during CAPD. Acta Med Scand. 1986;220:143–51.
18. Lowrie EG, Lew NL. Death risk in hemodialysis patients: the predictive value of commonly measured variables and an evaluation of death rate differences between facilities. Am J Kidney Dis. 1990;15:458–82.
19. Iseki K, Yamazato M, Tozawa M, Takishita S. Hypocholesterolemia is a significant predictor of death in a cohort of chronic hemodialysis patients. Kidney Int. 2002;61:1887–93.
20. Prichard S, Sniderman A, Cianflone K, Marpole D. Cardiovascular disease in peritoneal dialysis. Perit Dial Int. 1996;16(Suppl 1):S19–22.
21. Habib AN, Baird BC, Leypoldt JK, Cheung AK, Goldfarb-Rumyantzev AS. The association of lipid levels with mortality in patients on chronic peritoneal dialysis. Nephrol Dial Transplant. 2006;21:2881–92.
22. Fox CS, Longenecker JC, Powe NR, et al. Undertreatment of hyperlipidemia in a cohort of United States kidney dialysis patients. Clin Nephrol. 2004;61:299–307.
23. Goldfarb-Rumyantzev AS, Habib AN, Baird BC, Barenbaum LL, Cheung AK. The association of lipid modifying medications with mortality in patients on long-term peritoneal dialysis. Am J Kidney Dis. 2007;50:791–802.
24. Suzuki H, Inoue T, Watanabe Y, Kikuta T, Sato T, Tsuda M. Efficacy and safety of ezetimibe and low-dose simvastatin as primary treatment for dyslipidemia in peritoneal dialysis patients. Adv Perit Dial. 2010;26:53–7. PMID: 21348380.
25. Guida B, Trio R, Di Maro M, Memoli A, Di Lauro T, Belfiore A, Santillo M, Cataldi M. Prevalence of obesity and obesity-associated muscle wasting in patients on peritoneal dialysis. Nutr Metab Cardiovasc Dis. 2019;29(12):1390–9. https://doi.org/10.1016/j.numecd.2019.05.057. Epub 2019 May 16. PMID: 31668791.
26. Lu Q, Cheng LT, Wang T, Wan J, Liao LL, Zeng J, et al. Visceral fat, arterial stiffness, and endothelial function in peritoneal dialysis patients. J Ren Nutr. 2008;18:495–502.
27. Choi SJ, Park MY, Kim JK, Hwang SD. The 24-month changes in body fat mass and adipokines in patients starting peritoneal dialysis. Perit Dial Int. 2017;37(3):290–7. https://doi.org/10.3747/pdi.2016.00053. Epub 2017 Jan 17. PMID: 28096439.
28. Caron-Lienert RS, Poli-de-Figueiredo CE, Figueiredo AEPL, da Costa BEP, Crepaldi C, Pizzato AC, Ferrari F, Giuliani A, Ronco C. The influence of glucose exposure load and peritoneal membrane transport on body composition and nutritional status changes after 1 year on peritoneal dialysis. Perit Dial Int. 2017;37(4):458–63. https://doi.org/10.3747/pdi.2016.00265. Epub 2017 Apr 13. PMID: 28408713.
29. Jolly S, Chatatalsingh C, Bargman J, Vas S, Chu M, Oreopoulos DG. Excessive weight gain during peritoneal dialysis. Int J Artif Organs. 2001;24(4):197–202. PMID: 11394699.
30. Kim JK, Park HC, Song YR, Kim HJ, Moon SJ, Kim SG. Effects of excessive body fat accumulation on long-term outcomes during peritoneal dialysis. Perit Dial Int. 2019;39(3):268–75. https://doi.org/10.3747/pdi.2018.00164. Epub 2019 Mar 6. PMID: 30846607.
31. Ravel VA, Streja E, Mehrotra R, Sim JJ, Harley K, Ayus JC, Amin AN, Brunelli SM, Kovesdy CP, Kalantar-Zadeh K, Rhee CM. Serum sodium and mortality in a national peritoneal dialysis cohort. Nephrol Dial Transplant. 2017;32(7):1224–33. https://doi.org/10.1093/ndt/gfw254. PMID: 27358272; PMCID: PMC5837718.
32. Chang TI, Kim YL, Kim H, et al. Hyponatremia as a predictor of mortality in peritoneal dialysis patients. PLoS One. 2014;9:e111373.

33. Yu HL, Lu XH, Su CY, Tang W, Wang T. Potassium metabolism in continuous ambulatory peritoneal dialysis patients. Ren Fail. 2014;36(5):748–54. https://doi.org/10.3109/0886022X.2014.884379. Epub 2014 Feb 11. PMID: 24512377.
34. Khan AN, Bernardini J, Johnston JR, Piraino B. Hypokalemia in peritoneal dialysis patients. Perit Dial Int. 1996;16(6):652. PMID: 8981546.
35. Torlén K, et al. Serum potassium and cause-specific mortality in a large peritoneal dialysis cohort. Clin J Am Soc Nephrol. 2012;7(8):1272–84. https://doi.org/10.2215/CJN.00960112.
36. Ribeiro SC, Figueiredo AE, Barretti P, Pecoits-Filho R, de Moraes TP, all centers that contributed to BRAZPD II study. Low serum potassium levels increase the infectious-caused mortality in peritoneal dialysis patients: a propensity-matched score study. PLoS One. 2015;10(6):e0127453. https://doi.org/10.1371/journal.pone.0127453. PMID: 26091005; PMCID: PMC4474697.
37. Pichitporn W, Kanjanabuch T, Phannajit J, Puapatanakul P, Chuengsaman P, Parapiboon W, Treamtrakanpon W, Boonyakrai C, Matayart S, Katavetin P, Perl J, Praditpornilpa K, Eiam-Ong S, Tungsanga K, Johnson DW. Efficacy of potassium supplementation in hypokalemic patients receiving peritoneal dialysis: a randomized controlled trial. Am J Kidney Dis. 2022;80(5):580–588.e1. https://doi.org/10.1053/j.ajkd.2022.03.013. Epub ahead of print. PMID: 35597332.
38. Malho Guedes A, Calças Marques R, Ribeiro B, Fernandes MT, Faísca M, Silva AP, Bragança J, Rodrigues A. Peritoneal protein loss, inflammation, and nutrition: refuting myths. Front Med (Lausanne). 2022;9:884061. https://doi.org/10.3389/fmed.2022.884061. PMID: 35692552; PMCID: PMC9178188.
39. Young GA, Brownjohn AM, Parsons FM. Protein losses in patients receiving continuous ambulatory peritoneal dialysis. Nephron. 1987;45(3):196–201. https://doi.org/10.1159/000184116. PMID: 3574568.
40. Krediet RT, Yoowannakul S, Harris LS, Davenport A. Relationships between peritoneal protein clearance and parameters of fluid status agree with clinical observations in other diseases that venous congestion increases microvascular protein escape. Perit Dial Int. 2019;39(2):155–62. https://doi.org/10.3747/pdi.2018.00016. Epub 2019 Jan 18. PMID: 30661003.
41. Do JY, Kim AY, Kang SH. Peritoneal protein loss is not associated with sarcopenia in peritoneal dialysis patients. Front Med (Lausanne). 2021;8:653807. https://doi.org/10.3389/fmed.2021.653807. PMID: 34336874; PMCID: PMC8316630.
42. Singh T, Astor BC, Waheed S. End-stage renal disease patients with low serum albumin: is peritoneal dialysis an option? Perit Dial Int. 2019;39(6):562–7. https://doi.org/10.3747/pdi.2018.00204. Epub 2019 Mar 9. PMID: 30852522.
43. Sugimoto M, Sakai K, Kita M, Imanishi J, Yamaoka Y. Prevalence of Helicobacter pylori infection in long-term hemodialysis patients. Kidney Int. 2009;75(1):96–103. https://doi.org/10.1038/ki.2008.508. Epub 2008 Oct 8. PMID: 18843261; PMCID: PMC3126916.
44. Khedmat H, Ahmadzad-Asl M, Amini M, Lessan-Pezeshki M, Einollahi B, Pourfarziani V, Naseri MH, Davoudi F. Gastro-duodenal lesions and Helicobacter pylori infection in uremic patients and renal transplant recipients. Transplant Proc. 2007;39(4):1003–7. https://doi.org/10.1016/j.transproceed.2007.03.034. PMID: 17524875.
45. Anderson JE, Yim KB, Crowell MD. Prevalence of gastroesophageal reflux disease in peritoneal dialysis and hemodialysis patients. Adv Perit Dial. 1999;15:75–8. PMID: 10682075.
46. Twardowski ZJ, Khanna R, Nolph KD, Scalamogna A, Metzler MH, Schneider TW, Prowant BF, Ryan LP. Intraabdominal pressures during natural activities in patients treated with continuous ambulatory peritoneal dialysis. Nephron. 1986;44(2):129–35. https://doi.org/10.1159/000184217. PMID: 3774076.
47. Hylander BI, Dalton CB, Castell DO, Burkart J, Rössner S. Effect of intraperitoneal fluid volume changes on esophageal pressures: studies in patients on continuous ambulatory peritoneal dialysis. Am J Kidney Dis. 1991;17(3):307–10. https://doi.org/10.1016/s0272-6386(12)80479-3. PMID: 1996574.
48. Song HJ, Kim SM, Lee YM, Hwang JA, Moon KM, Moon CG, Koo HS, Song KH, Kim YS, Lee TH, Huh KC, Choi YW, Kang YW, Hwang WM, Yun SR. Is there a difference in

the prevalence of gastroesophageal reflux disease between peritoneal dialysis and hemodialysis patients? Korean J Gastroenterol. 2013;62(4):206–12. https://doi.org/10.4166/kjg.2013.62.4.206. PMID: 24162707.
49. Usta M, Ersoy A, Ayar Y, Ocakoğlu G, Yuzbasioglu B, Erdem ED, Erdogan O. Comparison of endoscopic and pathological findings of the upper gastrointestinal tract in transplant candidate patients undergoing hemodialysis or peritoneal dialysis treatment: a review of literature. BMC Nephrol. 2020;21(1):444. https://doi.org/10.1186/s12882-020-02108-w. PMID: 33092560; PMCID: PMC7583226.

Miscellaneous Non-infectious Complications of Peritoneal Dialysis

14

Nupur Gupta

Introduction

There are complications related to infections and those unrelated to infection. Non-infectious complications can be annoying and bothersome and must be appreciated as they can lead to PD technique failure.

Hemoperitoneum (Fig. 14.1)

Hemoperitoneum is recognized by as little as 10 mL of blood in 2 L of effluent. The origin of the blood could be from the peritoneal membrane, intraperitoneal organs, or gynecological structures. Table 14.1 lists possible etiologies [1].

Laboratory testing includes culturing the PD effluent, coagulation studies, a complete blood count (CBC), effluent hematocrit, and serum amylase level. To determine its severity, both the effluent and systemic hematocrit level should also be assessed serially. An effluent hematocrit greater than 2% suggests severe bleeding. Heavy recurrent bleeding associated with pain and fever should prompt an urgent and aggressive evaluation that includes abdominal imaging studies, such as a computerized tomography (CT) scan, abdominal ultrasound, magnetic resonance imaging (MRI), or angiography.

In the presence of visible blood, the prevention of clotting should be attempted using intraperitoneal heparin (500–1000 units/L). Rapid exchanges can help clear the blood and clots. Dialysate temperatures cooler than body temperature can vasoconstrict bleeding blood vessels. Aspirin and other systemic anticoagulants should

N. Gupta (✉)
Indiana University School of Medicine, Indianapolis, IN, USA
e-mail: nugupta@iu.edu

S. Z. Fadem et al. (eds.), *Complications in Dialysis*,
https://doi.org/10.1007/978-3-031-44557-6_14

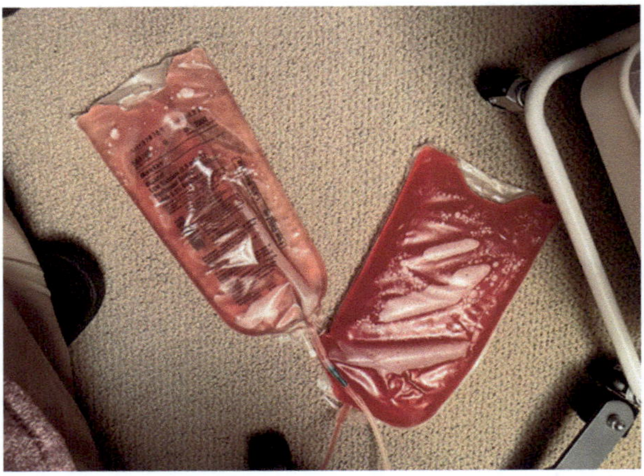

Fig. 14.1 Hemoperitoneum in peritoneal dialysis

Table 14.1 Etiologies for hemoperitoneum

Urological—cyst rupture
Gynecological—mensuration, endometriosis
Post-procedure—immediately after PD catheter placement
Gastrointestinal—intestinal wall injury, cholecystitis, pancreatitis, hepatic cysts
Trauma
Infection
Encapsulating peritoneal sclerosis

be stopped, if possible. In women of childbearing age, the use of oral contraceptives may prevent ovulation and control bleeding [2]. If bleeding persists, surgical exploration may be required [3].

Infusion Pain

Abdominal discomfort in PD could be experienced during inflow or outflow [4]. The inflow pain could be due to mechanical issues, dialysate temperature, or the acidic pH of the dialysate. Constipation causing bowel expansion and a forceful stream of infusing dialysate against sensitive tissue can be painful. Although the pain usually subsides after complete filling, it can disturb the quality of sleep in APD.

The first step to control abdominal discomfort is to decrease the infusion rate by adjusting the transfer set clamp. Changing the body position, for example, from sitting to standing, may move the catheter tip and decrease the pain. Malposition should be ruled out by abdominal over-penetrated (high kilovoltage) X-ray. If positioning is not the problem, the next step is to add 2–5 mEq of $NaHCO_3$ (25 mmol/L) to the dialysate just before infusion [5]. Note that care must be taken for any dialysate additives risk contamination, causing peritonitis. Higher pH (pH 7–7.4) dialysate has been shown to reduce infusion pain more than standard lactate-containing dialysate [6]. If the pain is not resolved, catheter flow studies should be considered. The catheter flow studies are performed by radiologically distilling contrast through the catheter and visualizing the flow into the peritoneal space under fluoroscopic guidance. This maneuver can show the location of the tip or demonstrate any obstruction to flow with greater accuracy than the flat plate X-ray.

Outflow Pain or Also Called Drain Pain

Drain pain is experienced due to the Bernoulli effect of the catheter as it siphons against abdominal structures. Its incidence is 13–25%. The problem may occur less often by preoperative planning for the position of the exit site. Various techniques have been explained. In one, the home dialysis nurse pre-marks the catheter location based on body habitus, using the catheter itself if the stencil is not available.

Pain can improve simply with time on therapy. Pain generally worsens during the later phase of the drain time on CAPD, the initial drain, and at the end of APD. This is due to a dry abdomen. If the patient has a dry day, the initial drain can cause drain pain due to catheter approximation against organs. The incidence is more frequently observed during APD due to the hydraulic suction by the cycler, especially if the tip of the catheter wedges near the walls of the rectum, uterus, or bladder. Tidal APD is an option which leaves 10–25% of the fluid in the abdomen at the end of each exchange. Tidal APD may not be helpful if the catheter wedges. If this is the case and the pain persists, relocation of the catheter must be considered.

The evaluation of drain pain should first exclude peritonitis, then obtain an abdominal X-ray to locate the catheter tip. Intensive catharsis with osmotic agents like lactulose can aid peristalsis and stimulate tip relocation. The patient should be referred for repositioning or replacement if malposition and drain pain persist.

Hydrothorax

Hydrothorax could occur due to the migration of peritoneal dialysate from the peritoneal cavity to the pleural cavity via pleuroperitoneal fistulas. Symptoms may include shortness of breath, chest tightness, or pleuritic chest pain. Most defects are congenital and right-sided, although some could develop after surgical procedure. The incidence is 1.6%, and many develop within 30 days of initiating PD. [7] In patients presenting with pleural effusions, hydrothorax should be considered. The evaluation must exclude other etiologies like congestive heart failure, infection, and malignancy. Unexplained weight gain, decreased ultrafiltration, and reabsorption of dialysate might be dominant features. Increased Intrabdominal pressure may be a minor contributing factor [8].

Diagnosis involves radiography and the biochemical analysis of thoracentesis-derived fluid. The PD-associated hydrothorax fluid is a transudate with a fluid glucose concentration that is higher than the serum glucose concentration. Pleural fluid glucose is influenced by previous dialysate composition, blood glucose, the rate of pleuroperitoneal leakage, and the duration of the pleural fluid presence in the normally absorptive pleura. Interpretation in a diabetic is complicated because of the equilibration of the pleural fluid with systemic glycemia. In patients with small diaphragmatic defects, glucose absorption from the pleural cavity may be greater than in patients with a larger defect. The pleural fluid glucose concentration cannot be used as the sole criterion for diagnosis, but it is generally accepted that pleural fluid with a glucose concentration greater than that of the serum concentration is consistent with hydrothorax [9].

The imaging of choice depends on the local expertise and availability. Peritoneal scintigraphy has a sensitivity of approximately 50%. Technetium 99m is instilled into the PD fluid, after which a series of images is obtained. Tracer uptake detected in the thoracic cavity confirms a communication between the peritoneum and the pleural space [10]. Alternative techniques that are used less frequently are CT and magnetic resonance peritoneography.

The treatment could be conservative or invasive. The conservative treatments are reducing intraabdominal pressure by smaller fill volumes and performing the dwell when positioned to minimize pressure, i.e., supine or standing [11]. Many patients have a recurrence with this conservative approach [12]. The persistence and recurrence of hydrothorax require permanent obliteration of the pleuroperitoneal communication with pleurodesis using autologous blood, talc, tetracycline, surgical or thoracoscopic correction, or video-assisted thoracoscopic (VATS) talc pleurodesis [13]. The VATS along with chemical pleurodesis has better outcomes. The VATS allows the defects to be visualized while chemical pleurodesis does not [14]. Chemical agents used in pleurodesis include talc or tetracycline. Both have disadvantages; talc can cause emboli while tetracycline can be painful [15]. If the patient is not asleep, anesthesia may be required when using tetracycline, although it is effective with no long-term complications. The choice of agent should depend on clinical conditions, local expertise, and availability of the agent. Hydrothorax is also discussed in Chap. 15.

Pneumoperitoneum (Fig. 14.2)

Pneumoperitoneum is usually characterized and diagnosed as subdiaphragmatic air on imaging. Although it is most likely an incidental finding, it could indicate a perforated viscus. The relevance of an asymptomatic pneumoperitoneum remains controversial; the reported incidence is 16–34% [16, 17]. The presence of a large pneumoperitoneum is significant, indicating either peritonitis or visceral perforation [17]. The initial evaluation should include a physical examination and thorough history. If the patient has abdominal pain, nausea, and vomiting, one should suspect peritonitis and viscus perforation.

The possible etiologies in an asymptomatic patient include recent laparoscopic procedures or air entry during the exchange. If PD exchanges are performed

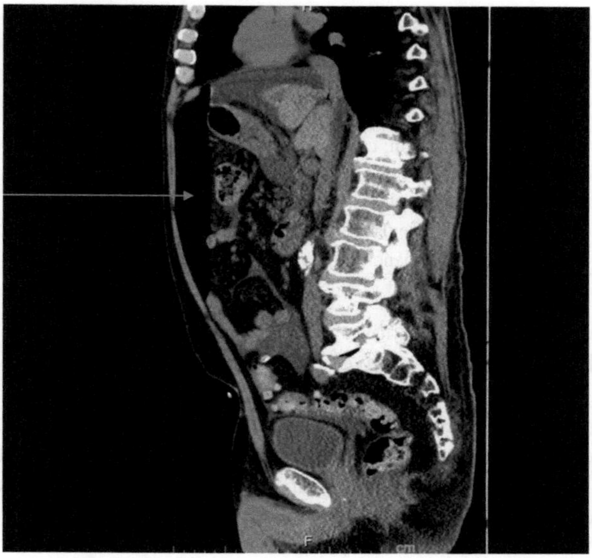

Fig. 14.2 Pneumoperitoneum in peritoneal dialysis

appropriately, there should be no air entry. Recurrent pneumoperitoneum suggests an inappropriate technique, predisposing to peritonitis. After ruling out peritonitis, diverticular disease and colonic micro perforations (inflammatory bowel disease, ischemic colitis) should be considered in patients with milder symptoms [18]. If the clinical examination and peritoneal fluid analysis are inconclusive, the next step is a CT scan with oral contrast media [19].

The air instilled during the exchange could present symptoms such as abdominal fullness and the inability to tolerate daytime exchange. The patient may present with abdominal fullness in one or all four quadrants. It is important to review the exchange technique with the patient to correct faulty practices. In most cases, the free air is reabsorbed in the abdominal cavity.

Intraperitoneal air can be a cause of systemic and PD effluent eosinophilia.

After a perforated viscus and peritonitis are ruled out, we recommend pneumoaspiration to help with symptomatic improvement. The pneumoaspiration is performed by connecting an empty drain bag and placing the patient in the Trendelenburg position. The air passes into the drainage bag, and the bag is seen inflating with air. A repeat X-ray can confirm a reduction in the pneumoperitoneum [19].

Chyloperitoneum

Chyloperitoneum is the presence of triglyceride-rich chylomicrons that results in a milky appearing effluent. The source of the chylomicrons is interruption of lymphatic drainage from the intestine to the main lymphatic duct. A high fatty meal increases lymph flow and can result in the milky white appearance of dialysate

Table 14.2 Etiologies of chyloperitoneum

1. Obstruction to lymphatic flow
2. Lymphatic cell proliferation: lymphoma, lymph node extension of a cancer of an abdominal or a pelvic organ, lymphangioleiomyomatosis
3. Venous congestion: constrictive pericarditis, CHF, SVC syndrome
4. Trauma/Post-surgical: blunt or penetrating abdominal trauma, abdominal surgery (including dialysis catheter placement), thoracic surgery (including lung and heart transplants)
5. Infections: tuberculosis, lymphatic filariasis
6. Miscellaneous: pancreatitis, drugs

effluent. The diagnosis is based on a triglyceride level in the peritoneal effluent higher than plasma levels [20].

Multiple etiologies are listed in Table 14.2.

The treatment of the chyloperitoneum mainly involves managing the underlying etiology, bowel rest, and changing to enteral nutrition without triglycerides. Temporarily transitioning from PD to hemodialysis accelerates the healing process [21].

Icodextrin Skin Rash

Icodextrin is an iso-osmotic high molecular weight polymer of starch that is extensively used for long dwells in CAPD and APD [22]. The skin lesions associated with icodextrin can vary from maculopapular exfoliative skin rash, itching, or leukocytoclastic vasculitis [23, 24]. The rash could be generalized or limited to the palm and soles. The lesions typically start within a few days but could appear after weeks of exposure. In the majority of cases, the lesions are limited to the palm and soles and do not warrant discontinuation. Rarely, exposure to icodextrin could accompany widespread exfoliative dermatitis, acute generalized exanthematous pustulosis, maculopapular rash, or chronic lymphocytic vasculitis. These severe episodes of skin hypersensitivity necessitate the permanent discontinuation of icodextrin [25, 26].

The incidence of this rash can vary from 2.3 to 18.9% [27, 28]. The patient that presents with a rash or itching within weeks or days of initiating icodextrin raises suspicion for an allergic reaction. Any other etiology for the allergic reaction (e.g., modification in the orally administered drugs and changes in the patient's diet or lifestyle habits) should be excluded. If no exact etiology is identified, the resolution of skin lesions after stopping the dialysate is proof of concept. Skin testing with the icodextrin patch is less sensitive and specific. The exact allergenic epitope for the hypersensitive reaction is unknown. It is absorbed from the peritoneal lymphatic to circulation [29]. The alpha-amylase metabolizes it to maltose and glucose polymer. The biopsy specimen shows peritoneal monocyte infiltration suggesting a type IV hypersensitivity reaction mediated through dendritic cells [30].The sensitization by the metabolites may be associated with a skin rash. The clinician should have heightened suspicion for any rash or itching developing while the patient is on icodextrin.

Conclusion

While we have not mentioned every known non-infectious complication, we have described the common and unique ones with the goal to provoke the reader to read in more detail as described in the references.

References

1. Greenberg A, Bernardini J, Piraino BM, Johnston JR, Perlmutter JA. Hemoperitoneum complicating chronic peritoneal dialysis: single-center experience and literature review. Am J Kidney Dis. 1992;19(3):252–6.
2. Dimitriadis CA, Bargman JM. Gynecologic issues in peritoneal dialysis. Adv Perit Dial. 2011;27:101–5.
3. Lew SQ. Hemoperitoneum: bloody peritoneal dialysate in ESRD patients receiving peritoneal dialysis. Perit Dial Int. 2007;27(3):226–33.
4. Prakash J, Tripathi K, Singh M. Complications of intermittent peritoneal dialysis. J Assoc Physicians India. 1990;38(12):906–8.
5. Bunchman TE, Ballal SH. Treatment of inflow pain by pH adjustment of dialysate in peritoneal dialysis. Perit Dial Int. 1991;11(2):179–80.
6. Mactier RA, Sprosen TS, Gokal R, et al. Bicarbonate and bicarbonate/lactate peritoneal dialysis solutions for the treatment of infusion pain. Kidney Int. 1998;53(4):1061–7.
7. Kawaguchi AL, Dunn JC, Fonkalsrud EW. Management of peritoneal dialysis-induced hydrothorax in children. Am Surg. 1996;62(10):820–4.
8. Mahale AS, Katyal A, Khanna R. Complications of peritoneal dialysis related to increased intra-abdominal pressure. Adv Perit Dial. 2003;19:130–5.
9. Chow KM, Szeto CC, Wong TY, Li PK. Hydrothorax complicating peritoneal dialysis: diagnostic value of glucose concentration in pleural fluid aspirate. Perit Dial Int. 2002;22(4):525–8.
10. Spadaro JJ, Thakur V, Nolph KD. Technetium-99m-labelled macroaggregated albumin in demonstration of trans-diaphragmatic leakage of dialysate in peritoneal dialysis. Am J Nephrol. 1982;2(1):36–8.
11. Bargman JM. Complications of peritoneal dialysis related to increased intraabdominal pressure. Kidney Int Suppl. 1993;40:S75–80.
12. Singh S, Vaidya P, Dale A, Morgan B. Massive hydrothorax complicating continuous ambulatory peritoneal dialysis. Nephron. 1983;34(3):168–72.
13. Mak SK, Nyunt K, Wong PN, et al. Long-term follow-up of thoracoscopic pleurodesis for hydrothorax complicating peritoneal dialysis. Ann Thorac Surg. 2002;74(1):218–21.
14. Tang S, Chui WH, Tang AW, et al. Video-assisted thoracoscopic talc pleurodesis is effective for maintenance of peritoneal dialysis in acute hydrothorax complicating peritoneal dialysis. Nephrol Dial Transplant. 2003;18(4):804–8.
15. Jagasia MH, Cole FH, Stegman MH, Deaton P, Kennedy L. Video-assisted talc pleurodesis in the management of pleural effusion secondary to continuous ambulatory peritoneal dialysis: a report of three cases. Am J Kidney Dis. 1996;28(5):772–4.

16. Lampainen E, Khanna R, Schaefer R, Twardowski ZJ, Nolph KD. Is air under the diaphragm a significant finding in CAPD patients? ASAIO Trans. 1986;32(1):581–2.
17. Kiefer T, Schenk U, Weber J, Hubel E, Kuhlmann U. Incidence and significance of pneumoperitoneum in continuous ambulatory peritoneal dialysis. Am J Kidney Dis. 1993;22(1):30–5.
18. Hasbargen JA, Hasbargen BJ. Recurrent culture negative peritonitis cured with hemicolectomy. Perit Dial Int. 1990;10(4):303–4.
19. Imran M, Bhat R, Anijeet H. Pneumoperitoneum in peritoneal dialysis patients; one centre's experience. NDT Plus. 2011;4(2):120–3.
20. Carl R, Kjeldsberg JAK. Body fluids: laboratory examination of amniotic, cerebrospinal, seminal, serous [and] synovial fluids. 3rd ed. Chicago: American Society of Clinical Pathologists Press; 1993.
21. Levy RI, Wenk RE. Chyloperitoneum in a peritoneal dialysis patient. Am J Kidney Dis. 2001;38(3):E12.
22. Frampton JE, Plosker GL. Icodextrin: a review of its use in peritoneal dialysis. Drugs. 2003;63(19):2079–105.
23. Meier MJ, Adams BB. Acute generalized exanthematous pustulosis associated with icodextrin. J Am Acad Dermatol. 2010;63(3):536–7.
24. Queffeulou G, Bernard M, Vrtovsnik F, et al. Severe cutaneous hypersensitivity requiring permanent icodextrin withdrawal in a CAPD patient. Clin Nephrol. 1999;51(3):184–6.
25. Cevher SK, Ozkayar N, Dede F. A case report on allergic rash caused by icodextrin. Case Rep Nephrol Dial. 2015;5(1):26–9.
26. Fletcher S, Stables GA, Turney JH. Icodextrin allergy in a peritoneal dialysis patient. Nephrol Dial Transplant. 1998;13(10):2656–8.
27. Biblaki DN, Filiopoulos VC, Vlassopoulos DA. Icodextrin skin rash incidence. Kidney Int. 2015;87(6):1258.
28. Wolfson M, Piraino B, Hamburger RJ, Morton AR, Icodextrin Study Group. A randomized controlled trial to evaluate the efficacy and safety of icodextrin in peritoneal dialysis. Am J Kidney Dis. 2002;40(5):1055–65.
29. Garcia-Lopez E, Lindholm B. Icodextrin metabolites in peritoneal dialysis. Perit Dial Int. 2009;29(4):370–6.
30. Goffin E, Tintillier M, Cosyns JP, Devuyst O. Sterile chemical peritonitis secondary to icodextrin: immunohistopathological description. Perit Dial Int. 2002;22(6):723–6.

Hernias, Hydrothorax, and Other Leaks 15

Rafia Chaudhry

Introduction - Intra-abdominal Pressure

Increased intra-abdominal pressure (IAP) is a risk factor for a number of PD complications, including fluid leaks, cardiopulmonary complications, hernias, and hemorrhoids [1]. IAP varies with PD mechanics and patient-related factors. PD-related factors include dialysate volume, particularly an extreme increase in volume by overfill (see Chap. 10), a potential complication of automated peritoneal dialysis (APD). Patient-related factors include body mass index (BMI), the position of the patient (where the order of increasing IAP is from supine to standing to sitting position), and routine actions such as coughing, lifting weight, and intra-abdominal straining (with physiologic actions such as defecation). Coughing generated the highest IAP in all positions [1].

Hernias

The incidence of hernias in PD patients has been reported at 0.08/patient/year [2], with a widely variable reported prevalence. The highest reported prevalence is 45% in patients with autosomal dominant polycystic kidney disease (ADPKD) [3].

Abdominal wall hernias resulting from initiation of PD are mostly small and asymptomatic initially, with a gradual increase in size and complications. One study reported the location in order of decreasing frequency as umbilical, incisional, inguinal, and peri-catheter hernias [2]. The mean time from the start of PD to the development of hernia was 16.6 ± 25 months, although hernias have been found within the first 3 months of PD initiation. The mean dialysate exchange volume when a hernia appeared was 2100 ± 200 mL, although exchange volume did not

R. Chaudhry (✉)
University of California, San Francisco, San Francisco, CA, USA
e-mail: rafia.chaudhry@ucsf.edu

S. Z. Fadem et al. (eds.), *Complications in Dialysis*,
https://doi.org/10.1007/978-3-031-44557-6_15

seem to have a statistically significant correlation with the risk of development of a hernia [2].

Observational studies evaluating independent risk factors for development of hernias, are small and must be interpreted with caution. ADPKD was the only independent risk factor for hernias (particularly inguinal hernias) identified by one study of 142 PD patients (72 patients on CAPD, 8 APD and 62 utilizing a combination of both) [2]. Body surface area < 1.675 m^2 is identified as an independent risk factor [4]. As mentioned, CAPD as opposed to APD is characterized by increased IAP due to physical activity while full, and during ultrafiltration. Therefore, patients with asymptomatic early or pre-existing small hernias may benefit from APD overnight, or CAPD with lower volume per exchange rather than staying on ambulatory dialysis. Patients using low-volume ambulatory PD may require an increased frequency of exchanges to meet small solute clearance needs. Regardless of these strategies, there must be close observation of hernia progression.

Leaks

Dialysate leakage can occur into anatomically susceptible areas, including into the abdominal wall resulting in abdominal wall or genital edema, retroperitoneal, across the diaphragm into the chest (hydrothorax, discussed in the section below), via a patent processus vaginalis, in the peri-catheter area into the exit site, or through prior surgical incision sites. The reported prevalence of peritoneal leaks is widely variable, with an incidence of 0.13/patient/year [2] and more than 5% in CAPD patients [5].

Peri-catheter leaks are the most frequent leaks [2] and are likely to occur in the immediate post-catheter placement period. This highlights the significance of the proceduralist's technique for PD catheter placement, and the correct placement of the deep cuff into the subaponeurotic area [6]. When initiating PD in an urgent start situation, specific alterations in "routine" training should occur, such as low-volume and more frequent exchanges, delaying ambulation, and avoiding aggressive ultrafiltration. In routine training (2–4 weeks post PD catheter placement), initial low-volume and supine exchanges should be attempted, with a gradual increase in fill volume and awareness of patient positions to minimize the increase in IAP (e.g., avoiding straining at stool). Additionally, in situations where the patient may tolerate reasonable fill volume (1.5–2 L), i.e., in standing positions, but develops a persistent cough, strategies to decrease dialysate volume and return to supine exchanges must be attempted. Similarly, patient education to avoid constipation or straining during defecation, draining peritoneal fluid prior to emptying bowels, and regular use of stool softeners, cathartics, and bulking agents can minimize risk of peri-catheter leaks. Strenuous exercise should be performed with an empty peritoneal cavity [1].

Abdominal wall or peri-catheter leak can present as abdominal wall swelling or skin bogginess, with increased abdominal wall edema in the absence of peripheral edema, subsequently resulting in diminished effluent return and weight gain.

Specifically, peri-catheter leaks will present as wetness or swelling around the catheter exit site; this can later extend further out into the abdominal wall and cause bulging confined to a certain space.

The first step in evaluating for an abdominal wall or peri-catheter leak should include a physical examination with the patient standing in a well-lit examination room to detect any abdominal wall edema, which can have a *peau de orange* appearance, or look for asymmetrical new bulges at the flanks. Other clinical indicators of dialysate leakage into anatomical spaces include volume overload due to diminished effluent volume in the absence of any change in transport status as determined by the modified peritoneal equilibration test (PET) (see Chap. 12). This PET is used to assess ultrafiltration failure. Imaging studies can be diagnostic for leaks and include an ultrasound around the exit site. The nephrologist should specify to the ultrasonographer that images of the abdominal wall are the area of focus rather than the intrabdominal area. The computerized tomography (CT) scan is a more complicated but also more specific diagnostic technique, with iodinated contrast added into the dialysate (100 mL iodinated contrast in 2 L dialysate bag) before it is instilled into the abdominal cavity. After instillation, the patient should ambulate, sit, and stand for at least 30 min total before imaging. These activities allow the leaking pathway to be filled with contrasted dialysate to be defined by the CT images. Non-contrasted magnetic resonance imaging (MRI) with plain dialysate can also be utilized. These imaging studies should be discussed with radiologists, surgeons, and proceduralists placing PD catheters for a multi-specialty interpretation of the clinical problem and correlation with imaging findings. Subsequently, surgical intervention to address the abdominal wall defect resulting in the leak can be planned.

Hydrothorax

Hydrothorax is a rare but recognized complication of PD, with the prevalence of diaphragmatic leaks reported at 1.6% in one large Japanese CAPD cohort [7]. The timing of presentation can vary from 1 to 7 days after initiation of PD to years later. The mechanism of development of these diaphragmatic peritoneal-pleural communication leaks is poorly understood but hypothesized to result from underlying congenital or acquired defects of the diaphragm. In many cases, an obvious defect may not be found. Subsequently, negative pressure in the pleural cavity during inspiration and positive pressure in the abdominal cavity because of dialysate promotes movement of dialysate into the pleural space resulting in hydrothorax. While left-sided and bilateral hydrothorax have been reported, 90% of the cases will have unilateral right-sided pleural effusions. Presenting symptoms can include acute or chronic progressive dyspnea, often disproportionate to overall body volume overload and peripheral edema, decreased ultrafiltration, and chest discomfort. However, the majority may remain asymptomatic despite a large pleural effusion, highlighting the significance of a thorough physical examination at every PD visit. The physical examination will reveal decreased tactile fremitus to palpation, dullness to percussion, and decreased breath sounds over the area of the pleural effusion. Further investigations should include imaging studies such as a chest X-ray, CT, or MRI. The choice of initial imaging modality should consider factors such as cost, complications of using of iodinated dye or gadolinium, and the impact on residual kidney function. Thus, a standard upright and lateral decubitus chest X-ray is the first imaging modality that one should use. The diagnostic thoracentesis should demonstrate an elevated glucose level in the pleural fluid period. The pleural fluid glucose level may be affected by sustained systemic hyperglycemia or absorption from the effusion, so must be interpreted cautiously. Some case studies have established peritoneal-pleural communications by performing scintigraphy of the intraperitoneal cavity using technetium 99mm [8] in the dialysate. This is a relatively safe, non-invasive, and cost-effective technique to establish that the effusion is from the peritoneal cavity fluid. Radiation exposure is low [7]. Following intraperitoneal administration of the radioisotope into dialysate and after exerting the same physical activities described above in the radiographic imaging to detect leaks, subsequent images are taken at 1- or 2-h intervals and again 24 h later. Detection of radioisotope in the pleural cavity is diagnostic [7].

Hydrothorax complicating PD has often forced patients to be transitioned to hemodialysis, particularly those with persistent pleural defects. However, treatment options to address the diaphragmatic leak in order to continue PD have been successful in approximately 50% of patients experiencing hydrothorax. These therapeutic strategies include chemical pleurodesis or video-assisted thoracoscopic surgery with mesh repair or resection of the diaphragmatic defect, with the latter reported to be more successful in resolution of the diaphragmatic leak [7, 9, 10].

Conclusion

IAP and hydrothorax can complicate PD and must recognized, evaluated and treated accordingly. IAP can result in a hernia that if asymptomatic may respond to a change in the dialysis prescription. IAP can also lead to a leak. Many leaks are preventable, but if present are often repairable with surgical intervention. Hydrothorax is uncommon but may present as an unexplained pleural effusion, and may be accompanied by shortness of breath. It is related to a diaphragmatic leak, and may respond to chemical pleurodesis or thorascopic surgery.

References

1. Twardowski ZJ, Khanna R, Nolph KD, Scalamogna A, Metzler MH, Schneider TW, Prowant BF, Ryan LP. Intraabdominal pressures during natural activities in patients treated with continuous ambulatory peritoneal dialysis. Nephron. 1986;44(2):129–35. https://doi.org/10.1159/000184217.
2. Del Peso G, Bajo MA, Costero O, Hevia C, Gil F, Díaz C, Aguilera A, Selgas R. Risk factors for abdominal wall complications in peritoneal dialysis patients. Perit Dial Int. 2003;23(3):249–54.
3. Morris-Stiff G, Coles G, Moore R, Jurewicz A, Lord R. Abdominal wall hernia in autosomal dominant polycystic disease. Br J Surg. 1997;84:615–7.

4. Bleyer AJ, Casey MJ, Russell GB, Kandt M, Burkart J. Peritoneal dialysate fill-volumes and hernia development in a cohort of peritoneal dialysis patients. Adv Perit Dial. 1998;14:102–4.
5. Leblanc M, Ouimet D, Pichette V. Dialysate leaks in peritoneal dialysis. Semin Dial. 2001;14(1):50–4. https://doi.org/10.1046/j.1525-139x.2001.00014.x.
6. Winchester JF, Kriger FL. Fluid leaks: prevention and treatment. Perit Dial Int. 1994;14(Suppl 3):S43–8.
7. Nomoto Y, Suga T, Nakajima K, Sakai H, Osawa G, Ota K, Kawaguchi Y, Sakai T, Sakai S, Shibata M, et al. Acute hydrothorax in continuous ambulatory peritoneal dialysis—a collaborative study of 161 centers. Am J Nephrol. 1989;9(5):363–7. https://doi.org/10.1159/000167997.
8. Carballeira GI, Sánchez RR, Azancot AM, Espinosa BJ, Moltó VM, Domènech CJ. Scintigraphy of the intraperitoneal cavity using technetium 99m as a diagnostic technique for diaphragmatic leaks in peritoneal dialysis: regarding two cases. Nefrologia. 2009;29(3):263–5. Spanish. https://doi.org/10.3265/Nefrologia.2009.29.3.5285.en.full.
9. Lang CL, Kao TW, Lee CM, Tsai CW, Wu MS. Video-assisted thoracoscopic surgery in continuous ambulatory peritoneal dialysis-related hydrothorax. Kidney Int. 2008;74(1):136. https://doi.org/10.1038/sj.ki.5002723.
10. Tsunezuka Y, Hatakeyama S, Iwase T, Watanabe G. Video-assisted thoracoscopic treatment for pleuroperitoneal communication in peritoneal dialysis. Eur J Cardiothorac Surg. 2001;20(1):205–7. https://doi.org/10.1016/s1010-7940(01)00751-5.

Peritoneal Dialysis: Psychosocial Adaptations and Burnout

16

Rachel B. Fissell

Introduction

Most PD patients and their families or home partners specifically choose peritoneal dialysis (PD) over hemodialysis (HD). Often there is an expectation of a higher quality of life with PD than with HD. For many patients, this is the case. However, clinical factors or early catheter problems may complicate the original plan and lead to unmet positive expectations. For example, an incident patient anticipating only nocturnal PD may have lower-than-expected residual kidney function, so an unplanned and unwelcome daytime exchange may be necessary. Also, maintaining PD requires daily consistency and lifestyle adaptation that patients and their home dialysis helpers may only fully appreciate once they have finished training and are responsible for their own treatments in their own homes.

Adapting to PD

Patients must learn to live with and care for their PD catheter, which requires mental and physical adjustments. They may experience relatively minor complications such as flow restriction, exit-site leak, or drain pain [1, 2]. Major complications, such as peritonitis, omental wrap, or hernia, may require hospitalization or surgery [3]. Even a motivated patient with a strong support system can find these complications painful and frightening. Adjustments must be made in a patient's home to accommodate PD. In a recent study, "space taken up by PD supplies" was commonly rated as a disadvantage to PD and was associated with the transition to HD

R. B. Fissell (✉)
Division of Nephrology and Hypertension, Vanderbilt University Medical Center, Nashville, TN, USA
e-mail: rachel.fissell@VUMC.org

S. Z. Fadem et al. (eds.), *Complications in Dialysis*,
https://doi.org/10.1007/978-3-031-44557-6_16

[4]. Most regimens require dialysis at least 5 days a week. Patients and their partners are responsible for recording daily vital signs and body weight and for using consistent sterile techniques to prevent peritonitis. Daily attention, concentration, and focus are necessary. In a recent qualitative study, patients and their care partners described PD as an unrelenting responsibility [5].

Fundamental activities of daily living, such as sleeping and eating, are affected by PD. Many PD patients in high-income countries are maintained on automated PD (APD) instead of continuous ambulatory PD (CAPD). Most APD patients dialyze at night. Sleeping while using the cycler is an acquired skill. Machine alarms may impair sleep quality. Some APD patients have described difficulty sleeping simply because of anticipation that a cycler may alarm [6]. CAPD patients have also reported difficulties with sleep. In a recent study, over half of both APD and CAPD patients reported moderate to severe sleep problems [7]. Another qualitative study focused on sleep concluded that sleep disturbances in both HD and PD patients were pervasive and had negative effects on all aspects of patients' lives, including the ability to do daily tasks, maintain relationships, and emotional and physical well-being [8]. Eating is another fundamental human task that may be affected by PD. Successful PD maintenance usually requires adjustments in eating schedules and in living with new symptoms related to eating caused by indwelling dialysate. It may cause fullness and reflux that interfere with appetite and feeling full and satisfied. Glucose absorption from dialysate may lead to labile blood glucose levels and necessitate changes in insulin doses [9, 10]. These factors could affect patient hunger, satiety, and nutrition. Several surveys of PD patients document the frequent presence of gastrointestinal (GI) symptoms. Patients specifically related the onset of symptoms to starting dialysis [11]. Patient-reported GI symptoms have also been correlated with lower quality of life [12]. A careful qualitative study found that GI symptoms and diet and fluid restrictions have psychosocial consequences resulting in multiple losses of autonomy for PD patients [13]. This study found that PD patients found strategies to regain control and advises clinicians to partner with patients to support their autonomy in the setting of dietary adjustments and restrictions.

Adjustments to basic tasks such as eating and sleeping may become a burden for patients and their care partners, especially when first starting PD. Uncertainty about the future, fear of peritonitis, and procedures needed to treat complications may also cause stress and decrease quality of life. It is not surprising that the emotional challenges of PD can lead to depression and burnout in many PD patients, their families, and care partners. A recent extensive qualitative study focused on burnout and identified several themes contributing to a higher risk for transfer to HD. Patients from Australia, Hong Kong, and the United States described feeling overwhelmed by the daily burden, a perception that their life was coming to a halt, tolerating the PD regimen for survival, and a sense of isolation, and having to bear the burden and uncertainty of what to expect from PD alone [5]. In another multinational sample from Australia, New Zealand, Canada, Japan, the United Kingdom, and the United States, over half the PD patients reported depressive symptoms, and 11–22% reported symptoms that scored >15 on the Center for Epidemiologic Studies Depression Scale (CESD), indicating risk for clinical depression [14].

Solutions to these emotional challenges exist. Those who successfully adapt report establishing a new normal and often rely on family and faith to build resilience [5]. Part of how many patients adapt to PD is by building a network of partners and helpers. PD nurses are a crucial part of this support network. Burnout among PD home partners is prevalent. Awareness and communication with the team at the home unit can identify those partners who may benefit from respite. The psychological well-being of both patients and their partners may be improved with models of care that are different from those currently in use for most patients. An NKF-KDOQI conference recommended the establishment of predialysis education programs for partners and patients together to better support their teamwork in completing PD procedures and handling challenges after PD is begun [15]. Recent qualitative data highlights clinical milestones such as initiating dialysis when psychological distress may be most intense, and patients and their families may benefit from an intervention such as counseling [16]. Of note, assisted PD provides not only physical but also emotional support and may be cost-effective, particularly in the elderly [17]. A feasibility program in the United States showed that assisted PD enabled incident patients to remain on PD after a complication [18]. In Shanghai, a recent multi-center prospective cohort study of a Family-Community-Hospital comprehensive management plan demonstrated improved psychological health, cost-savings, and similar outcomes to the usual model of care [19].

Conclusion

PD is under-utilized in several countries. Many patients could benefit from the autonomy and more flexible schedule that PD provides. Improved support for potential psychological challenges and burnout could increase the proportion of patients and families who commit to home dialysis and help patients and care partners who have chosen PD to remain on PD. A programmatic commitment to this process should be a very high priority.

References

1. Oliver M, Perl J, McQuillan R, et al. Quantifying the risk of insertion-related peritoneal dialysis catheter complications following laparoscopic placement: results from the North American PD Catheter Registry. Perit Dial Int. 2020;40(2):185–92.
2. Blake P. Drain pain, overfill, and how they are connected. Perit Dial Int. 2014;34:342–4.
3. Esagian SM, Sideris GA, Bishawi M, et al. Surgical versus percutaneous catheter placement for peritoneal dialysis: an updated systematic review and meta-analysis. J Nephrol. 2021;34(5):1681–96.
4. Sukul N, Zhao J, Fuller D, et al. Patient-reported advantages and disadvantages of peritoneal dialysis: results from the DOPPS. BMC Nephrol. 2019;20(1):116.

5. Oveyssi J, Manera KE, Baumgart A, et al. Patient and caregiver perspectives on burnout in peritoneal dialysis. Perit Dial Int. 2021;41(5):484–93.
6. Domenici A, Giuliani A. Automated peritoneal dialysis: patient perspectives and outcomes. Int J Nephrol Renovasc Dis. 2021;14:385–92.
7. Guney I, Solak Y, Atalay H, et al. Comparison of effects of automated peritoneal dialysis and continuous ambulatory peritoneal dialysis on health-related quality of life, sleep quality, and depression. Hemodial Int. 2010;14:515–22.
8. DeSilva I, Evangelidis N, Hanson CS, et al. Patient and caregiver perspectives on sleep in dialysis. J Sleep Res. 2021;30(4):e13221.
9. Oei E, Samad N, Visser A, et al. Use of continuous glucose monitoring in patients with diabetes on peritoneal dialysis: poor correlation with HbA1c and high incidence of hypoglycaemia. Diabet Med. 2016;33(9):e17–20.
10. Skubala A, Zywiec J, Zelobowska K, et al. Continuous glucose monitoring system in 72-hour glucose profile assessment in patients with end-stage renal disease on maintenance continuous ambulatory peritoneal. Med Sci Monit. 2010;16(2):CR75–83.
11. Salamon K, Woods J, Pau E, Huggins C. Peritoneal dialysis patients have higher prevalence of gastrointestinal symptoms than hemodialysis patients. J Ren Nutr. 2013;23(2):114–8.
12. Yi C, Wang X, Ye H, et al. Patient-reported gastrointestinal symptoms in patients with peritoneal dialysis: the prevalence, influence factors and association with quality of life. BMC Nephrol. 2022;23(1):99.
13. Duncanson E, Chur-Hansen A, Jesudason S. Psychosocial consequences of gastrointestinal symptoms and dietary changes in people receiving automated peritoneal dialysis. J Ren Care. 2019;45(1):41–50.
14. Brown EA, Zhao J, McCullough K, et al. Burden of kidney disease, health-related quality of life, and employment among patients receiving peritoneal dialysis and in-center hemodialysis: findings from the DOPPS program. Am J Kidney Dis. 2021;78(4):489–500.
15. Chan CT, Wallace E, Golper TA, et al. Exploring barriers and potential solutions in home dialysis: an NKF-KDOQI conference outcomes report. Am J Kidney Dis. 2019;73(3):363–71.
16. Duncanson E, Chur-Hansen A, Jesudason S. Patient perspectives of coping with automated peritoneal dialysis. Perit Dial Int. 2022;42:344–52.
17. Dimkovic N, Aggarwal V, Khan S, et al. Assisted peritoneal dialysis: what is it and who does it involve ? Adv Perit Dial. 2009;25:165–70.
18. Hussein WF, Bennett PN, Anwaar A, et al. Implementation of a staff-assisted peritoneal dialysis program in the United States. Clin J Am Soc Nephrol. 2022;17:703–5.
19. Ma X, Tao M, Hu Y, et al. Clinical outcomes, quality of life, and costs evaluation of peritoneal dialysis management models in Shanghai Songjiang District: a multicenter and prospective cohort study. Ren Fail. 2021;43(1):754–65.

Complications of Home Hemodialysis 17

Stephen Z. Fadem and Sylvia Donato-Moore

Introduction

Although not as frequently selected as a treatment option, home hemodialysis provides distinct advantages to patients but also presents a different set of challenges. Its complications intersect those of dialysis in-center. This chapter will discuss complications that are more common in the home setting.

Some patients are able to successfully train to perform dialysis at home (HHD) with a partner. They achieve a level of independence in doing so but lose the advantage of having a team of highly trained nurses and technicians constantly monitoring their care. HHD is not a novel therapy and has been available for as long as in-center hemodialysis (ICHD) has. Its use was widespread when the legislation was enacted to fund benefits for dialysis patients but dropped for several years. It has been making a resurgence because newer dialysis machines are more "user-friendly." The increased acceptance of remote patient monitoring and telehealth promises to increase its acceptability.

There are two machines that are currently used for home patients—the Fresenius 2008K @home (See Fig. 17.1) and the NxStage (see Fig. 17.2). The Fresenius machines that are in use for ICHD have been modified to make them simpler to use but still have the robustness and versatility of the in-center models. They require a home water purification system and use the same hemodialyzers used in dialysis centers. They have a long training period and are directly supported by the home dialysis team.

S. Z. Fadem (✉)
Section of Nephrology, Department of Medicine, Baylor College of Medicine, Houston, TX, USA
e-mail: fadem@bcm.edu

S. Donato-Moore
DaVita Med Center at Home, Houston, TX, USA

S. Z. Fadem et al. (eds.), *Complications in Dialysis*,
https://doi.org/10.1007/978-3-031-44557-6_17

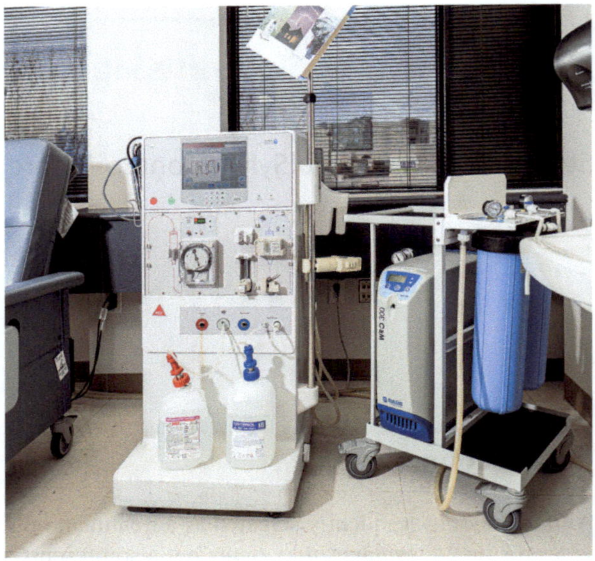

Fig. 17.1 The Fresenius 2008K@home has been modified to make it simpler to use in the care of home dialysis patients. (Photograph by Stephen Z. Fadem)

The NxStage is also a Fresenius product. It uses a cartridge-based dialyzer (see Fig. 17.3) and has a self-contained water purification system. It has been specifically designed for home therapy but is small enough to be used when traveling. It can be used during the day or for nocturnal dialysis. Nocturnal patients are required to have a partner. Its complications are similar to those with conventional dialysis. The machine is fully supported by an internal NxStage team.

Newer models are on the horizon. The Tablo Hemodialysis System is a compact machine that uses cartridge dialyzers and a self-contained water purification system. It has a touch-screen and 3-D animation, walking patients through the setup process. It was cleared by the FDA in 2020 and engages cloud communication and remote patient monitoring. It offers flexibility and claims to be easy to learn with a short training time [1].(Source: https://www.outsetmedical.com/tablo).

Although it is widely known as a local drug store, CVS has partnered with the inventor, Dean Kamen, developer of the Segway and the Baxter HomeChoice Peritoneal Dialysis system, to create a unique home dialysis machine—the HemoCare home dialysis device. The machine is currently being tested. (Source: https://www.cvskidneycare.com/).

Home hemodialysis offers several distinct advantages to the patient. However, in patients who are successfully performing HHD, transitioning back to hemodialysis has been associated with higher mortality, particularly in the first 30 days (Hazard Ratio—HR 3.93, 95% CI 2.09–7.40; $P < 0.001$). This risk persisted. The investigators note that at the onset, the HHD patients had the necessary clinical and socioeconomic qualities to qualify them for success [2]. Thus, failure would denote deterioration in health status that could be secondary to the associated development

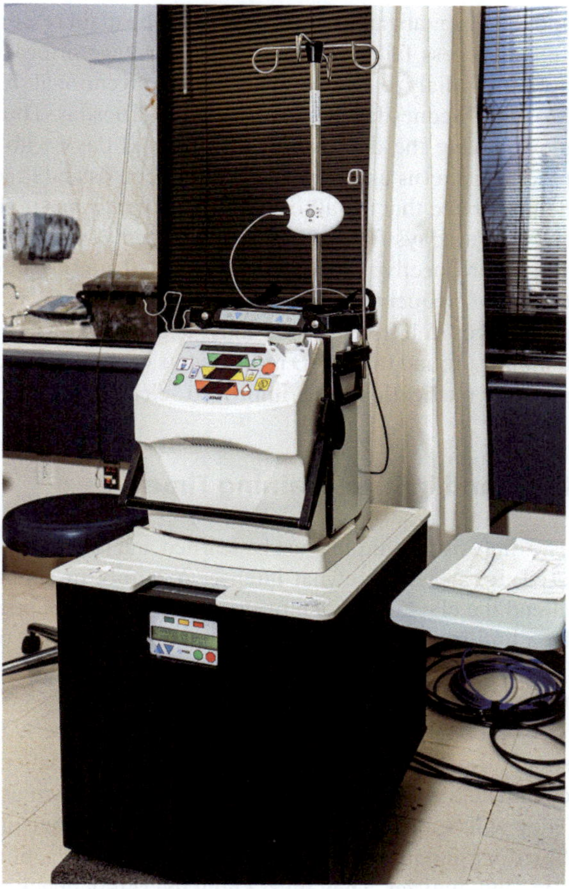

Fig. 17.2 The NxStage sits atop a cart that contains its water purification system. (Photograph by Stephen Z. Fadem)

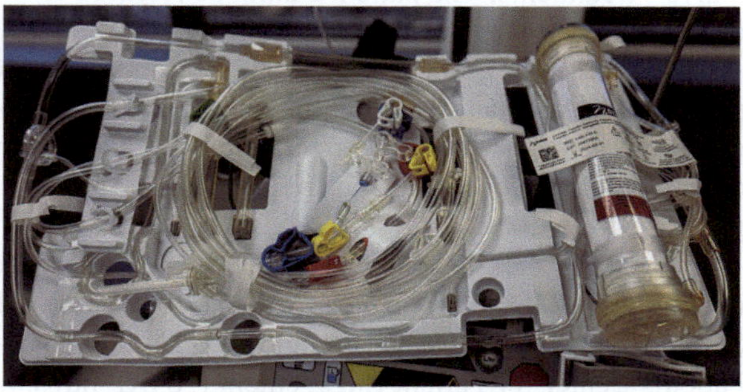

Fig. 17.3 The NxStage 172 C Cartridge dialyzer. (Photograph by Stephen Z. Fadem)

of comorbidities and medical instability. Caregiver burnout and patient wishes are also reasons why patients return to the in-center hemodialysis [3].

For those who overcome the barriers, travel time to dialysis decreases while increased time actually receiving therapy increases. Blood pressure is improved, and the hospitalization rate decreases. The main reason for hospitalization is arteriovenous access failure [4]. Another advantage afforded those selecting HHD is the option to dialyze every other day. Conventional ICHD offers two alternatives, Monday-Wednesday-Friday (MWF) or Tuesday-Thursday-Saturday (TTS) schedules, leaving the disadvantage of going 2 days without treatment. An analysis of practice patterns using the Dialysis Outcomes and Practice Patterns Study (DOPPS) demonstrated that the all-cause mortality rate was higher on Mondays for the MWF and on Tuesdays for the TTS group, especially for cardiovascular events [5, 6].

In a prospective randomized controlled study, Culleton et al., who compared the effects of frequent nocturnal hemodialysis (NHD) with conventional hemodialysis on changes in left ventricular mass and health-related quality of life (HRQoL) over 6 months, found that NHD reduced left ventricular mass, reduced the need for blood pressure medications, and improved selected measures of HRQoL [7].

Long and Intense Training Time

The dialysis technique must be learned and rehearsed. Depending upon the machine used, it can be somewhat intense. A family or support person is also required to attend the classes and demonstrate competence in operating the machine. This may be a limiting factor for patients in cognitive decline or who lack a suitable partner. Thus HHD tends to self-select those patients who are healthier, have good cerebral function, and have a stable home situation.

Complications arise when people are not properly trained and do not fully understand all of the procedures. Not only must the patient and support person learn to cannulate the arteriovenous (AV) access, but they must also learn sterile techniques. They will be required to have a working knowledge of how their dialysis equipment functions and must demonstrate know-how at attaching the blood tubing, water system, and dialyzer. They must know the safety check procedure and how to monitor dialysis treatments. The patient cannot be released for independent dialysis until he or she can demonstrate full proficiency.

The success of a home as measured by incident-free retention is a function of preparation. Adequate training time must be provided to allow the patient and caregiver to practice skills under supervision and address any vascular access issues or other concerns. Consistent and frequent follow-ups by the home dialysis care team greatly aid retention.

The patient should be able to talk with other patients and caregivers who are also undergoing HHD. Support networks can be found online and include the Renal Support Network (RSN http://rsnhome.org), the American Association of Kidney Patients Center for Patient Engagement (AAKP https://aakp.org/center-for-patient-engagement-and-advocacy/support-groups/), The National Kidney Foundation (NKF https://www.kidney.org/treatment-support). Large dialysis organizations such as DaVita (http://mydavita.com) and Fresenius (**https://www.freseniusmedicalcare.com/en/patient-support**) also have support resources.

The Optimal Need for a Partner

A partner can be an immediate family member or a friend. It is a long-term and continuous time commitment. The difficulty arises when the partner is unavailable to provide support, and the patient will, in those circumstances, need to arrange for the dialysis treatment to occur in a backup facility.

In some instances, the caregiver makes an error or does not follow the procedure as originally taught. In those circumstances, retraining sessions might be necessary.

A more serious problem is caregiver burnout. In a focused narrative, concerns were raised by patients and caregivers over the risk of complications or incorrectly performing the procedure. Psychosocial issues included quality of life, perceived financial burdens, social isolation, sleep disturbances, fatigue, and anxiety [8].

A few patients, with the permission of their physician and proper preparation and education, perform their therapy alone. It may be a personal preference, or the patient may not have a suitable partner available. Patients committing to solo dialysis (SOLO) must be able to self-cannulate their AV access.

Lack of Home Supervision and Caregiver Burnout

When in the dialysis facility, highly trained licensed personnel are involved in the put-on, management, and take-off of the patient. They set up the machine, provide its maintenance, and assume full control. With home care, the patient must provide all of the steps from beginning to end without any supervision. In a self-reported questionnaire, 91% of patients elected against HHD because they were already satisfied with their care and desired the supervisory environment of an ICHD program. 54% reported they did not want medicalization of their home [9]. Caregivers for either HHD or home PD tended to be women (84%), married with a mean age of 46 ± 2. 38% were wives, and 27% were other relatives. Using the SF-36 quality of life survey, the dimensions of Environment and Disappointment were highest. Wives perceived a higher burden when compared with other caregivers (sons, daughters, or mothers) (2.25 ± 0.09 vs. 1.96 ± 0.06; $P < 0.0.01$). Caregivers also have more psychopathological disorders than physical ailments and visit the doctor more frequently. HHD places significant strain on a family and can be associated with marital discord. The levels of depression between spouse and patient are related. Socioeconomic conditions play a big role [10].

Frequent Hemodialysis: Pros and Cons

One distinct advantage of home dialysis is the opportunity to increase the treatment frequency. A large clinical trial, the Frequent Hemodialysis Network (FHN) trial, randomized hemodialysis patients to six times per week—the frequent hemodialysis group (FHG) vs. three times per week—the conventional hemodialysis group (CHG) for 12 months. Kt/V was increased in the FHG (3.54 ± 0.56 vs. 2.49 ± 0.27).

The hazard ratio (HR) for death or increased left ventricular mass was reduced to 0.61 (95% CI 0.46–0.82). Blood pressure and phosphorus control also improved. The drawback of frequent hemodialysis was the increased number of vascular access interventional procedures. (HR 1.71; 95%CI 1.08–2.73) [11]. In a further study, 87 patients were randomized to thrice weekly or six hemodialysis sessions per week. This study did not find a significant effect of nocturnal hemodialysis on left ventricular mass or death. In this frequent hemodialysis group, there was a trend toward increased vascular access events [12].

Air Emboli

In a systemic review, there were six cases out of 183,603 patients. While this may appear to be a small number, it reflects a catastrophe that often results in a stroke [13]. An air embolism can occur if alarm detectors have been bypassed. In a disconnection mishap, air can enter the venous line and travel into the brain leading to acute hypoxia. These events are catastrophic and can be fatal [14]. Patients are extensively trained to follow protocols, ensure lines are secured, and to know the procedures to follow if an air embolus is suspected.

Arteriovenous Access Catastrophes

Blood loss from a bleeding AV access is the most common complication of HHD and potentially the most catastrophic. If a fistula needle is dislodged or a catheter connector becomes disconnected, at 400 ccs per minute blood flow, it is a matter of minutes before substantial blood is lost, and the patient loses over 40% of blood volume and develops hemorrhagic shock. If the access is improperly taped or the Luer lock tubing connector is not secure, severe blood loss can occur. Bleeding has also been associated with the use of short fistula needle lengths less than 2.5 cm.

Contributing factors include ignoring alarms, not following the prescribed protocol, improperly connecting the arterial or venous tubing to the dialyzer head, improper clamp placement, and incorrectly positioning or failing to use the wetness detector. Connector device malfunction can also cause line disconnection problems [15].

During the dialysis treatment, the patient can develop a hypotensive episode leading to acute confusion. Thrashing can cause the poorly taped fistula to become dislodged. In the dialysis center, the patient is required to keep the dialysis access uncovered so that nurses and technicians can inspect it at regular intervals and ensure that it remains secure. Home dialysis patients are at a disadvantage in that they may not be supervised.

Abnormal bleeding during the dialysis can be determined by either an enuresis alarm pad or a Redsense blood loss sensor. The enuresis pad has the advantage that it is easy to use and allows the AV access to be fully visible. It is used for regular home treatments.

When the patient is less optimally supervised or must dialyze at night, the risk of inadvertent dislodgement leading to excessive blood loss and even shock or death is higher. Thus, the procedure is to use the Redsense Blood loss sensor https://redsensemedical.com/products/alarm-unit/. It completely covers the AV access and does not offer the same flexibility with regard to adjusting needles. (See Fig. 17.4).

NxStage has a cartridge (172-C) with a secure clip on the venous line that can be pushed up against the rotating Luer lock connector to avoid line disconnection. This can be used for daily dialysis, specifically for SOLO and NHD.

A clamp has been developed and can be used in nocturnal care. It can automatically deploy if a blood leak is detected. This device is burdensome but does offer additional safety [16].

Infections

The buttonhole technique is an alternate method of cannulating an AV fistula. With the conventional rope ladder cannulation techniques, a sharp needle is inserted into a new site on the fistula. With the buttonhole technique, a dull needle can be used through a tunneled track, which allows a conduit for blood transport, but seals when the needle is removed. The tunnel is created by granulation tissue formation and is similar to having a pierced ear. In the rope ladder technique, the needle cannulation is performed at a different site for each treatment. The new cannulation site is spaced, like the rungs of a ladder. The medical literature demonstrates an increased incidence of infection, with hazard ratios greater than three when the buttonhole

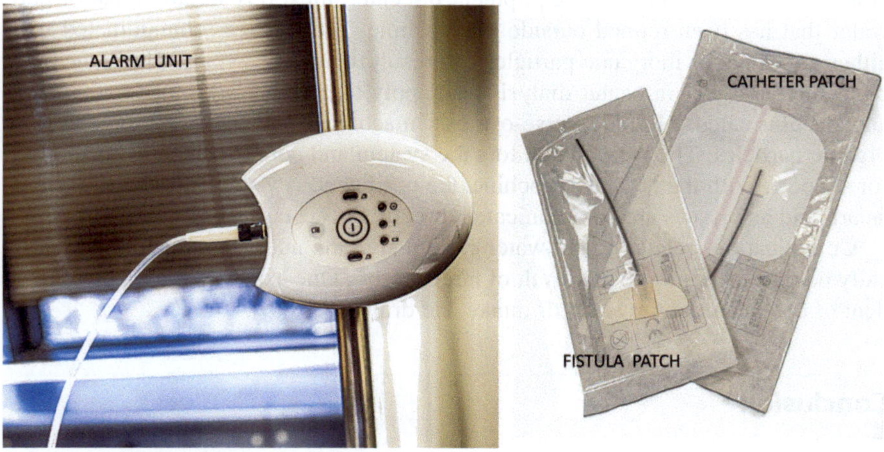

Fig. 17.4 The Redsense is an alarm system that monitors the AV access or the catheter bloodline during hemodialysis. It consists of sensor patches containing an optical fiber and an absorbent sponge. The patches are placed in contact with the bloodline or the AV access, and if a disconnect or dislodgement occurs, the wet patch transmits a signal to the alarm that alerts the patient or caregiver

cannulation technique is compared with the conventional cannulation style—the rope ladder method. Evidence does not support that it prolongs the life of the access or reduces pain. When several people cannulate the fistula, false buttonhole tracks can develop, further increasing the chance of an infection [17]. Although it has fallen out of favor, it remains popular in the HHD setting where the patient has total control of the site, in contrast to having a technician or multiple technicians cannulate their access. The use of antibiotic creams may reduce the incidence of infection.

Machine Failure

In the dialysis center, an alarming machine or one that fails predialysis testing can simply be pulled offline and replaced with another. Biomedical technicians are readily available and highly trained to quickly recognize when the dialysis machine malfunctions. Part of the education process is to instruct the patient on how to quickly spot when a machine is not functioning properly. By the time the training program is complete, the patient must be aware of all alarms on the machine and what maintenance is required to ensure they are always operating properly and to never ignore them. Also, the patient must be able to call appropriate support personnel, either at NxStage or the dialysis facility, if the machine is not operating as it should.

Water Quality

Home dialysis machines, like equipment in-center, must rely on an intake of pure water that has been refined outside the machine. Water that is contaminated with either microbial or inorganic particles can result in adverse events. The same principles that apply to in-center dialysis also apply to home. Water must be softened and dechlorinated. Home reverse-osmosis machines then remove inorganic and organic particles. The patient monitors the system and contacts the dialysis facility for support. With the NxStage machine, the purification system is self-contained in a cart, and any issues are communicated directly to NxStage.

Complications related to the water system are rare, and when they have historically occurred, they were the result of human error. One example is a reported incident of an inadvertent reversal of intake and drain lines [15].

Conclusion

HHD is again emerging as a promising alternative to ICHD as a result of innovative new dialysis machines that are easier to set up and offer more safety features, including remote monitoring. While many of the complications of HHD parallel those of ICHD, some are unique. HHD patients must be well-trained and follow procedures and techniques meticulously. A caregiver is also required, and burnout may occur. A catastrophic bleeding episode can occur if the cannulation needles become dislodged or the tubing becomes disconnected. Adherence to protocols is thus essential to ensure that connectors are secured. Sensing devices can reduce this risk. The buttonhole technique is a popular means of cannulation, but it has a high infection rate when compared with the conventional rope and ladder technique. Air entry into the dialysis tubing can be prevented by fastidiously following procedures. Machine failure and water quality are infrequent but potential sources of complications. Again, careful adherence to techniques is necessary for their prevention.

References

1. Zaman T, Moore K, Jellerson J, Chahal Y, Schumacher J, Dalessandri-Silva C, et al. Extension of Tablo TrEatmeNt Duration (XTEND) study: successful 24 h prolonged therapy with Tablo in critical patients. BMC Nephrol. 2022;23(1):338. https://doi.org/10.1186/s12882-022-02968-4.
2. Semple DJ, Sypek M, Ullah S, Davies C, McDonald S. Mortality after home hemodialysis treatment failure and return to in-center hemodialysis. Am J Kidney Dis. 2022;79(1):15–23.e1.
3. Shah N, Reintjes F, Courtney M, Klarenbach SW, Ye F, Schick-Makaroff K, et al. Quality assurance audit of technique failure and 90-day mortality after program discharge in a Canadian Home Hemodialysis Program. Clin J Am Soc Nephrol. 2017;12(8):1259–64. https://doi.org/10.2215/cjn.00140117.
4. Connaughton DM, Jamal A, McWilliams J, O'Kelly P, Ormond J, Butler A, et al. Home haemodialysis in Ireland. Ir J Med Sci. 2013;182(1):91–6. https://doi.org/10.1007/s11845-012-0835-4.
5. Vanholder R, Eloot S, Neirynck N, Van Biesen W. Home haemodialysis and uraemic toxin removal: does a happy marriage exist? Nat Rev Nephrol. 2012;8(10):579–88. https://doi.org/10.1038/nrneph.2012.189.
6. Fayed A, Tarek A, Refaat MI, Abouzeid S, Salim SA, Zsom L, et al. Retrospective analysis of nontraumatic subdural hematoma incidence and outcomes in Egyptian patients with end-stage renal disease on hemodialysis. Ren Fail. 2021;43(1):1322–8. https://doi.org/10.1080/0886022x.2021.1979038.
7. Culleton BF, Walsh M, Klarenbach SW, Mortis G, Scott-Douglas N, Quinn RR, et al. Effect of frequent nocturnal hemodialysis vs conventional hemodialysis on left ventricular mass and quality of life: a randomized controlled trial. JAMA. 2007;298(11):1291–9. https://doi.org/10.1001/jama.298.11.1291.
8. Jacquet S, Trinh E. The potential burden of home dialysis on patients and caregivers: a narrative review. Can J Kidney Health Dis. 2019;6:2054358119893335. https://doi.org/10.1177/2054358119893335.
9. Diebel L, Jafari M, Shah S, Day C, McNaught C, Prasad B. Barriers to home hemodialysis across Saskatchewan, Canada: a cross-sectional survey of in-center dialysis patients. Can J Kidney Health Dis. 2020;7:2054358120948293. https://doi.org/10.1177/2054358120948293.
10. Belasco AG, Sesso R. Burden and quality of life of caregivers for hemodialysis patients. Am J Kidney Dis. 2002;39(4):805–12. https://doi.org/10.1053/ajkd.2002.32001.
11. In-center hemodialysis six times per week versus three times per week. N Engl J Med. 2010;363(24):2287–2300. https://doi.org/10.1056/NEJMoa1001593.
12. Rocco MV, Lockridge RS Jr, Beck GJ, Eggers PW, Gassman JJ, Greene T, et al. The effects of frequent nocturnal home hemodialysis: the frequent hemodialysis network nocturnal trial. Kidney Int. 2011;80(10):1080–91. https://doi.org/10.1038/ki.2011.213.
13. Gupta A, Zimmerman D. Complications and challenges of home hemodialysis: a historical review. Semin Dial. 2021;34(4):269–74. https://doi.org/10.1111/sdi.12960.

14. Tennankore KK, d'Gama C, Faratro R, Fung S, Wong E, Chan CT. Adverse technical events in home hemodialysis. Am J Kidney Dis. 2015;65(1):116–21. https://doi.org/10.1053/j.ajkd.2014.08.013.
15. Pauly RP, Eastwood DO, Marshall MR. Patient safety in home hemodialysis: quality assurance and serious adverse events in the home setting. Hemodial Int. 2015;19(Suppl 1):S59–70. https://doi.org/10.1111/hdi.12248.
16. Kennedy C, McGrath-Chong M, Arustei D, d'Gama C, Faratro R, Fung S, et al. A prototype line clamp for venous access bleeding in hemodialysis: a prospective cohort study. Hemodial Int. 2019;23(2):151–7. https://doi.org/10.1111/hdi.12737.
17. MacRae JM. Should buttonhole cannulation of arteriovenous fistulas be used? CON. Kidney360. 2020;1(5):322–5. https://doi.org/10.34067/kid.0000602019.

Medication Errors in Dialysis Patients 18

Karen Ugwu and George R. Aronoff

Introduction

The inflated medication burden and complexity of medication regimens for individuals with end-stage kidney disease (ESKD) who are receiving dialysis treatment are unlike any other chronic conditions. In addition to the cumbersome care plans and needing to dialyze multiple times a week, dialysis patients are also often inflicted by several other comorbid conditions. On average, ESKD patients have six comorbid conditions and are prescribed approximately 10–12 different medications, which contribute to a high pill burden with the need for frequent dose adjustments and monitoring [1, 2]. Many different medications are eliminated through the kidney, which further exacerbates the risk of medication-related complications in dialysis patients [3]. As kidney disease progresses, secondary complications like anemia, cardiovascular disease, hyperparathyroidism, and hyperphosphatemia may develop, further convoluting treatment plans. Advanced age in kidney disease is another level of complexity to manage due to worsening cognitive impairment, reduced muscle mass, and malnutrition affecting older adults. These factors can further enhance the effects of alterations in medication pharmacokinetics and pharmacodynamics.

Because the kidneys play such a key role in the disposition of drugs, novel strategies to facilitate ESKD-specific care should be promoted in this patient population. Medication errors in dialysis patients have the potential to exacerbate illness severity, increase unnecessary clinic visits and hospital admissions, and accelerate kidney disease progression. In order to decrease the frequency of adverse drug events and improve the quality of care in this high-risk population, system-wide strategies

K. Ugwu (✉)
Value-Based Care, Panoramic Health, Tempe, AZ, USA

G. R. Aronoff
DaVita Kidney Care, Denver, CO, USA

S. Z. Fadem et al. (eds.), *Complications in Dialysis*,
https://doi.org/10.1007/978-3-031-44557-6_18

must be developed and implemented, including leveraging computerized clinical decision support and renal pharmacist expertise across the broad landscape of the healthcare system. Overall, individuals with ESKD disease rely on close and intentional management to help prevent adverse drug reactions and emergency room visits while also prolonging and improving their quality of life.

Pill Burden, Polypharmacy, and Prescribing Cascades

The daily pill burden in the dialysis population is one of the highest reported in any chronic disease state, and a high pill burden is also associated with lower health-related quality of life (HRQOL) [4]. Besides contributing to a lower quality of life, taking multiple medications can increase the risk for medication-related problems, circumstances where drug therapy has the potential to interfere with desired patient outcomes. Some examples of common medication errors that may be identified in this population include medications that are inappropriately dosed for individuals on dialysis, medications that are contraindicated in ESKD, medications without an indication, indications without corresponding medications, and duplications in therapy.

Besides having to take multiple tablets and capsules each day, dialysis patients are also often plagued with large, difficult-to-swallow pills, such as phosphate binders. Phosphate binders, which make up approximately half of an ESKD patient's daily pill burden, are used to help regulate serum phosphorus levels, with multiple tablets needing to be taken with meals multiple times a day. Research shows that factors associated with medication-related problems in dialysis patients include having more than three comorbid conditions, four medication changes over the past year, five or more medications in the drug regimen, 12 or more medication doses per day, not adhering to the medication regimen, taking medications that require monitoring, and the presence of diabetes [4]. It is important to be aware that a high pill burden can decrease an individual's adherence to therapy, leading to additional medications being prescribed in order to achieve healthcare goals in an ESKD patient. When prescribers thoroughly understand the medication complexities that ESKD patients are faced with, they can more easily adopt and execute deprescribing and medication optimization practices while becoming more vigilant partners in the patient's course of care.

Polypharmacy can be defined as the concurrent use of more than one drug to treat a single condition. With an average of 4.7 prescribers and 19 pills per day [5], it is no surprise that there is a high prevalence of polypharmacy among patients with ESKD. Minimizing polypharmacy can be targeted at the transition of care points (e.g., post-hospitalization) to help improve clinical outcomes. Additionally, medication adherence, cost-effectiveness, patient quality of life, and clinical goals must be taken into account prior to prescribing medications to dialysis patients. In prescribing cascades, adverse drug events are misinterpreted as new medical conditions, and patients are prescribed additional medications to treat those symptoms. A classic prescribing cascade example is when patients develop a cough after starting on an angiotensin-converting enzyme (ACE) inhibitor for hypertension and are then prescribed a cough suppressant to help treat the cough. Clinicians with the knowledge of hallmark medication side effects are best suited to pinpoint adverse drug event etiologies and make adjustments accordingly. In that scenario, cough is one of the potential side effects of ACE inhibitors, so there is a likelihood that the angiotensin-converting enzyme inhibitor led to the cough. Experienced clinicians would know to consider whether the patient's ACE inhibitor should be discontinued and switched to an alternative medication, such as an angiotensin II receptor blocker (ARB), in order to avoid the side effect while still treating the chronic condition.

The Economic Impact of Medication Errors

A vast majority of patients with ESKD receive their health insurance through Medicare, which provides coverage for individuals of all ages with kidney failure. In 2015, the total fee-for-service spending for ESKD beneficiaries was $33.9 billion [6]. Also, the financial burden of care for individuals with ESKD accounts for more than 7% of Medicare spending despite only making up around 1% of the Medicare population. Inpatient care for this patient population has drastic financial implications with one-third of the ESKD Medicare budget being spent on hospital admissions [6]. Additionally, among the 77% of ESKD patients enrolled in Medicare part D, the total estimated spend for prescription medications was $2.7 billion in 2014 [7].

Impacts due, specifically, to medication errors in severe kidney disease are substantial to the American healthcare system. Chronic kidney disease is frequently unrecognized, which compounds the risk of harm as the kidneys often play a key role in the disposition of drugs. In fact, historical studies have shown that 15–67% of prescriptions for patients with impaired kidney function contain errors such as contraindications, inadequate lab monitoring, inappropriate medications, improper doses, and inappropriate intervals [8, 9]. Older age further complicates care as kidneys become increasingly more susceptible to decline. Factors contributing to the high cost of healthcare in older adults who require dialysis therapy include cognitive impairment and an increased risk for falls which can make medication use more dangerous. A University of North Carolina Hospitals study on 30-day readmission predictors among hemodialysis patients showed that patients taking 10 or more medications had a 1.7 times higher chance of being readmitted to the hospital [6]. Ongoing medication management, as well as deprescribing efforts, is of immense benefit for ESKD patients and the healthcare system in helping to reduce emergency department visits.

ESKD patients are admitted to the hospital two times per year on average, and, upon discharge, over 33% of them are readmitted within a month's time span. This readmission rate is more than 50% that of Medicare beneficiaries that do not have kidney disease [6]. Factors that have been shown to increase the risk for hospital admissions due to adverse drug events include female gender, being 65 years old or more, and having hemodialysis as a modality. Of note, the impact of warfarin use on increased readmission risk exceeded the risk of having a catheter as vascular access and taking 10 or more medications in the Chan et al. study [10]. There is certainly a wealth of opportunity for improvement in this patient population, both from clinical and financial standpoints. After a patient is discharged, a multi-pronged approach involving patients, nephrologists, nurses, social workers, dietitans, and pharmacists is beneficial to all stakeholders, including payors, for improved health outcomes and reduced spend.

Medication Complications in ESKD

Some of the types of medication mishaps leading to complications that occur in the dialysis population include patients receiving incorrect medications or doses, taking medications at the wrong time, not receiving necessary medications, and omitting the reconciliation of medications after a transition of care event. There are several places where medication errors occur for patients with ESKD, including, but not limited to, skilled nursing facilities, dialysis centers, during hospital stays, and even at home. In a small retrospective, single-center 2018 study, the University of California, San Diego Health (UCSDH) added a pharmacist to the interdisciplinary care team and found that medication discrepancies and medication-related problems for in-center hemodialysis patients were reduced by approximately 50% between pharmacist encounters (Fig. 18.1).

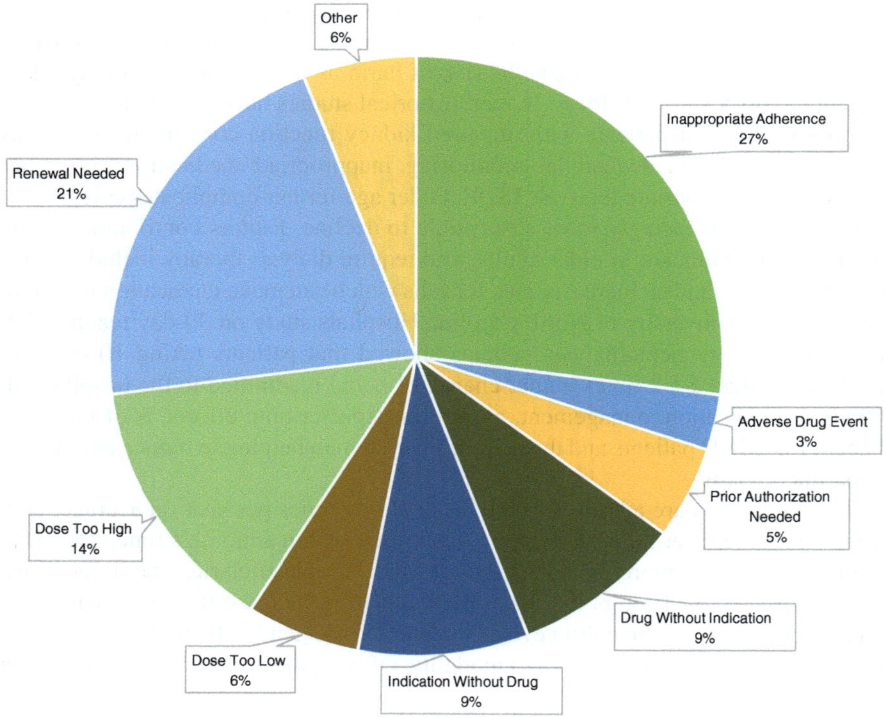

Fig. 18.1 Types of medication-related problems (Source: Dyer et al. [11])

Although there are many avenues for medication errors to occur, prescribing is a prime juncture for kidney patients. Prescribing errors are often multifactorial and failure to recognize and amend inaccuracies at the prescribing point can lead to a cascade of unwanted consequences. Heavy workload pressures, fatigue, and lack of training or experience are some limitations that prescribers face which lead to unintended patient harm. Computerized Physician Order Entry (CPOEs) systems are tools that allow prescribers to enter in prescriptions for drugs through a computer application instead of handwritten on paper. By eliminating legibility concerns and incorporating automated patient safety features, CPOEs have helped to transcend prescribing while improving workflows.

Though the concept of computerized physician order entry is an incredible advancement in the world of healthcare, it is not without its limitations. Novel types of errors have transpired with the emergence of decision support tools within CPOEs. One common example of a CPOE nuisance that is often voiced by prescribers is alert fatigue due to the numerous general cautions that are programmed within the system to automatically appear when certain drugs are selected. The prescriber must then acknowledge that they have read the alert and agree that they understand the potential risk before being able to move forward and create the prescription. Over time, prescribers may get so used to seeing system-generated warnings that it becomes excessive or numbing to a point that they find themselves skipping through the alerts without taking time to analyze and apply them; this can lead to unintentional oversight on a patient that is still prescribed a medication even though the system flagged a caution that was relevant for the patient (e.g., active drug–drug interaction, patient allergy, etc.). One qualitative study that looked to explore the causes and contributing factors associated with prescribing errors reported by multidisciplinary prescribers working within a CPOE system discovered that inadequate access to a medication history of patients across healthcare sectors leads to prescribing errors [12]. The design of CPOEs or user interfaces can also be a hindrance to patient safety when users accidentally select incorrect dropdown options from electronic lists. Other problems with usability, including burdensome documentation methods, inconvenient workflow arrangements, and lack of interoperability with patient record systems, may enhance provider frustration and burnout, with potential implications for patient safety [13].

There are several avenues for prescribing errors to occur, such as at the time of prescribing, during the transcribing or dispensing process, when the medication is being administered, and when the list of medications that the patient is taking is being reconciled. Medication errors are most common at the ordering or prescribing stage, and prescription errors make up 70% of medication errors that could potentially result in adverse effects [14]. When clinicians write prescriptions for patients, it is important for them to identify drug interactions and/or allergies that the patient might have. By pinpointing and preventing the issue from happening, prescribers can avoid unnecessary medication-related problems further downstream for a patient. Many CPOE systems incorporate tools that are useful in assisting prescribers by proactively identifying and flagging any drug–drug or drug–allergy interactions automatically from the patient profile. Not only does this feature save time, but it also allows for an added measure of security. Heavy workload, time pressures, and fatigue, are common contributors to errors that occur during the prescribing process.

After a prescription is sent to the pharmacy, and during the transcribing process, another potential mistake may present itself when the prescription order is misread or misinterpreted. Omitting transcriptions, typing errors, and the use of abbreviations can be detrimental actions in the process of preparing a medication for dispensing. While dispensing, there may be unintended errors that also result in consequences for the patient, such as look-alike or sound-alike (LASA) medications. LASA errors lead to the selection of the incorrect medication from a shelf or from an electronic record [15]. Employing risk reduction strategies and best-demonstrated practices such as barcode scanning technology and tall man lettering can improve dispensing outcomes. Institutions can also look to pre-build order sets with medication indications to guide prescriber selection among problematic LASA names like hydrOXYzine (for pruritus) versus hydrALAZINE (for hypertension) [16]. This will help clinicians avoid confusion between similar sounding and looking medications since many LASAs have different indications.

When patients or their caregivers fail to comply with the prescription as it was written, adverse drug reactions can occur. Examples of these instances include taking the wrong dose, using the inappropriate route of administration, and incorrectly timing when the medication should be taken. Confusion between brand and generic drug names can also pose difficulties during medication reconciliation and treatment. Patients with poor eyesight may have trouble reading the label on their prescription medication bottle in order to select the correct medication or follow the prescribed directions, while patients with functional decline may have difficulty opening or even administering certain medications. Functional decline is a common contributor to fall risk in ESKD, and mortality risk increases by nearly 50% for those who experience falls [17]. Proactive prevention, identification, and resolution are essential to making sure that avertible adverse events are minimized.

Patient Case Scenarios

Medication-related problems might not always be easy to spot, but there are key signs, symptoms, and manifestations that should always be identified and addressed to help prevent an unnecessary adverse drug event. Medication errors can happen when a medication is prescribed, prepared, or dispensed improperly, as well as when drug information is entered into a computer system inaccurately, or when a patient takes a medication incorrectly. Errors can happen with prescription drugs, over-the-counter medications, vitamins, and even supplements (Table 18.1).

It is important that lab values be assessed when evaluating and prior to prescribing medication therapy. In a pooled analysis of medication-related problems in hemodialysis patients, the top two categories identified were inadequate laboratory monitoring of medications (23.5%) and inappropriate drug dosing (20.4%) [1]. In many cases, when reviewing a patient's labs, it is prudent to analyze a trend of laboratory results as opposed to a single lab value. Similar to how a blood pressure log can better guide therapeutic changes for antihypertensive drug therapy than one single blood pressure reading, trending lab values help paint the patient picture

Table 18.1 Patient case examples

Scenario	Problem	Commentary
A 55-year-old hemodialysis patient was prescribed cephalexin 500 mg by mouth daily (take after dialysis on Tuesday/Thursday/ Saturday) for 2 weeks	The prescription was misinterpreted and filled as: take 6 tablets on Tuesday/Thursday/ Saturday for 2 weeks. The patient noticed the discrepancy and called the prescriber to confirm that the medication is supposed to be taken every day for 2 weeks, and, on dialysis days (Tuesdays, Thursday, and Saturdays), it should be taken after the dialysis session	It is prudent to take cephalexin after a dialysis session because this medication is dialyzable. Taking this antibiotic after dialysis will prevent it from being dialyzed and removed whereas taking it before a dialysis session would lead to unnecessary waste and the potential for treatment failure. If this error was missed, it may have led to the patient not receiving an adequate course of treatment to treat the infection as well as undesirable side effects from taking high doses at a time
A 63-year-old dialysis patient was prescribed rosuvastatin 20 mg daily to help with hyperlipidemia	The patient complained of muscle tenderness, cramps, and weakness after starting the statin. Rosuvastatin serum concentrations are increased by approximately 50% in hemodialysis patients compared to patients with normal renal function.	In dialysis-dependent adults, KDIGO guidelines (Kidney Disease: Improving Global Outcomes) recommend avoiding the initiation of statins due to the lack of additional benefit in this population. Patients receiving statins should be monitored for symptoms of myopathy or rhabdomyolysis. If these conditions are suspected, the statin should be discontinued.
A 71-year-old peritoneal dialysis patient was taking glimepiride 2 mg daily for diabetes management	During a comprehensive medication review, the patient noted having a couple recent episodes of shakiness and light-headedness. Upon analysis, it was discovered that the patient's most recent A1c result was 6.1%. Long duration sulfonylureas, like glimepiride, increase the risk of severe prolonged hypoglycemia in older adults.	For patients with ESKD, the National Kidney Foundation (NKF) recommends not to treat A1c lab values that are less than 7% due to the increased risk of hypoglycemic episodes [18]. The risk of hypoglycemia may outweigh the benefits of stringent control in patients with severe kidney impairment. A1c goals in individuals with kidney impairment can be more flexible, especially after patient-specific factors, like age, are accounted for. Patients should be educated on how to prevent and navigate a hypoglycemic episode.

(continued)

Table 18.1 (continued)

Scenario	Problem	Commentary
A 42-year-old, new to dialysis, patient was recently prescribed calcium acetate 667 mg (two capsules with each meal) to help with hyperphosphatemia	The patient's phosphorus levels continued to rise over time despite the patient taking calcium acetate regularly. During a medication reconciliation, it was discovered that the patient was taking this medication upon waking up, midday, and before bed, without regard to meals. Additionally, the patient's first meal of the day occurred many hours after waking and their last meal of the day was typically well before bedtime.	Phosphate binders work best when taken within 10–15 min before or immediately after eating meals and snacks; their mechanism of action is to bind phosphorus in the intestine and help eliminate it from the body. Patients should be counseled to only take binders with meals versus on an empty stomach in order for the medication to be most effective.
Apixaban 5 mg twice daily was prescribed to an 81-year-old dialysis patient for stroke prophylaxis. The patient was also taking over-the-counter extra strength aspirin daily to help with muscle aches.	The patient's caregiver reported that the patient was experiencing gum bleeding when brushing or flossing. The patient also experienced instances of easier bruising than normal.	Dialysis patients are at a greater risk of serious bleeding due to several factors, including uremic platelet dysfunction, anemia, and heparin use. When initiating concurrent anticoagulant and antiplatelet therapy in ESKD patients, especially in older adults, the risk versus benefit ratio must always be considered in order to minimize thrombotic risk while also reducing bleeding events. Gum bleeding and easy bruising may be indicators of abnormal and excessive bleeding and should be addressed immediately. Apixaban dosing should be limited to no more than 2.5 mg twice a day in individuals who meet any two of the following characteristics: age 80 years and older; body weight 60 kg or less; or serum creatinine 1.5 mg/dL or greater [19]. Additionally, long-term aspirin at doses greater than 160 mg a day has been shown to increase the risk of bleeding without providing increased efficacy.

(continued)

Table 18.1 (continued)

Scenario	Problem	Commentary
A 59-year-old ESKD patient complained of extremely painful diabetic neuropathy and was prescribed extended-release oxycodone. The patient was also taking alprazolam to help with generalized anxiety.	The patient reported having problems with balance and hand coordination along with bouts of extreme light-headedness.	Concurrent use of opiate agonists with benzodiazepines may cause respiratory depression, hypotension, profound sedation, and even death. If alternative treatment options are inadequate, and concurrent use is necessary, the lowest effective doses and shortest treatment duration should be used to achieve the desired clinical effect. Patients should be educated about the risks and symptoms of respiratory depression and sedation. Rescue medications, like naloxone, should be provided, especially for high-risk patients and their caregivers, in the event of an opioid overdose. When discontinuing oxycodone therapy in patients who are opioid-dependent, the dose should be tapered gradually by 10–25% every 2–4 weeks. Individuals who have been taking opioids for shorter periods of time may tolerate a more rapid taper [20, 21].

more accurately than one moment in time. In ESKD patients, phosphate binders are frequently used to help reduce elevated serum phosphorus levels. Because phosphorus levels can fluctuate based on phosphate intake (e.g., phosphate-containing laxatives or enemas) it is wise to obtain more than one trend of phosphate levels before prematurely adjusting the dose of the medication.

Clinicians should be cognizant of dose adjustments and medication changes needed for individuals who have recently started dialysis therapy because there may still be residual renal function (RRF). The ability of native kidneys to eliminate water and uremic toxins describes the residual renal function, and it is typically measured and estimated by calculating the average creatinine level and urea clearance within a 24-h period. Besides restricting fluid intake, diuretics play a key role in volume control. Furosemide is a common diuretic medication that patients with chronic kidney disease take to help eliminate extra fluids in their bodies. Once a CKD patient transitions to ESKD, a low or moderate dose of furosemide may no longer be effective at producing the diuretic effect necessary. By up-titrating the dose of furosemide to a more optimal level, patients with severe kidney impairment can have a more pronounced effect to best achieve diuresis. In fact, a long-term study on continuous ambulatory peritoneal dialysis (CAPD) patients showed that a furosemide dose of 250 mg per day had zero impact on the rate of residual renal function decline but led to a clinically significant preservation of urine volume after one year without any observed side effects [22]. Because preservation of residual renal function is associated with improved survival and decreased mortality in both hemodialysis and peritoneal dialysis patients, it is important to adopt methods that support the prolongation of all lasting levels of kidney functionality.

Drug pharmacokinetics may be altered in those with kidney impairment who require dialysis, so lower dose or less frequent dosing may be required in certain instances, whereas some drugs will be contraindicated and should be discontinued altogether. A United States study found that one-third of hemodialysis patients are prescribed a medication at a dose that does not align with recommended dosing parameters; adverse effects occur in one fifth of those instances [23]. When dose adjustments are not made in dialysis patients for medications that undergo significant renal clearance, their considerable drop in GFR equates to an increase in drug accumulation and half-life with repeated dosing. These changes are also applicable to drug metabolites that are cleared by the kidney, which may be active or toxic [24]. In theory, the drug's clearance and therapeutic index help determine if a dose adjustment is needed.

Dose adjustments in ESKD can be made by reducing the dose, increasing the interval between doses, or a combination of the two techniques. The proper approach to take depends upon how important it is to have stable serum drug concentrations of the medications in question, such as is the case with maintaining the antimicrobial effect of penicillin; other considerations to assess include patient convenience and being aware of the adverse effects of peak drug concentrations after intermittent dosing [24]. Medications with narrow therapeutic indexes, such as digoxin, may require considerable dose reductions, and hemodialysis can introduce yet another challenge since it is recurrent and has the potential to yield swift drug clearance. This is more relevant for medications taken once a day, especially antibiotics; it is ideal to administer them after hemodialysis sessions. Dose timing can usually remain unchanged for drugs dosed more frequently since adding to the complexity of dosing regimens may further reduce a patient's adherence to medication therapy. In peritoneal dialysis (PD), the timing of administration is a non-factor as the clearance of small molecules is slower and more evenly dispersed than in hemodialysis [24, 25].

In practice, anticoagulants, gabapentinoids, opioids, and anti-infective agents are common culprits in prescribing errors, as these agents typically need to be used with caution in those with severe kidney impairment. A striking observation in the Chan et al. study was that anticoagulants contributed toward a significant percentage (~19%) of adverse drug events resulting in emergency department visits among dialysis patients [26]. Atrial fibrillation is the most common indication for anticoagulant use, and with the high burden of cardiovascular disease in dialysis patients, warfarin has been the mainstay of anticoagulation therapy, working to reduce the risk of blood clotting for stroke prevention and treatment of venous thromboembolism. Bleeding is the main adverse effect associated with anticoagulant use, and those with renal impairment are even more susceptible to the risk due to factors like inflammation, uremia, and insufficient platelet functioning. The American Heart

Association identified older adults and patients with chronic kidney disease as high-risk groups for medication errors and agreed with the Institute for Safe Medication Practices (ISMP) in their classification of antithrombotic drugs as high-alert pharmacologic treatments that have the highest risk of causing injury when used inappropriately [27, 28].

Another limitation of warfarin therapy is its heavy reliance on frequent INR lab monitoring in order to help guide dosing adjustments. Vitamin K intake fluctuations can cause the instability of INR levels leading to the need for a warfarin dosage change. For ESKD patients, INR levels are not commonly monitored at their dialysis clinic, adding to the inconvenience of having to coordinate multiple different clinicians and outpatient visits. Unlike warfarin, novel oral anticoagulants (NOACs), which are newer agents also used to prevent blood clotting, do not require any additional monitoring. Apixaban (Eliquis™) is a NOAC that is currently approved for use in dialysis patients, despite very limited studies conducted in this patient population. Since there are no reliable monitoring tests that can allow for dose adjustments in individuals with ESKD, and dialysis patients are already prone to bleeding, there is an elevated risk for inappropriate dosing in dialysis patients, which could lead to bleeding episodes and in turn, hospital admissions.

A difficult area of treatment for ESKD patients is percutaneous coronary intervention (PCI) because several antithrombotic medications are not recommended for use in dialysis patients. The Journal of the American Medical Association (JAMA) published a study about 22,778 dialysis patients who received a percutaneous coronary intervention (PCI) in the United States during a four-year period; it was found that more than 22% of the patients received a contraindicated antithrombotic medication, an error that was associated with an increased risk of in-hospital major bleeding [29]. Both eptifibatide, a platelet glycoprotein IIb/IIIa inhibitor, and enoxaparin, a low-molecular-weight heparin, are anticoagulants that are cleared by the kidney and increase the risk of bleeding complications in dialysis patients [30–32].

Often, patients on dialysis suffer from the sub-optimal treatment of their comorbid pain. In fact, pain is the most commonly reported symptom of patients with ESKD [33]. Acetaminophen, which is predominantly metabolized by the liver, is the preferred simple analgesic since it is relatively safe and can be taken without dose modification [33–35]. Non-steroidal anti-inflammatory drugs (NSAIDs) should be avoided or reserved for very short-term treatment if better alternatives are not available. Cyclo-oxygenase-2 (COX-2) inhibitors, specifically, have been shown to elevate the risk of myocardial infarction seen in the general population, so should be avoided in dialysis patients who are already at a substantially higher baseline cardiovascular risk [36, 37]. If indicated, topical NSAIDs are a safe option since systemic absorption is minimal [25].

The etiology of the pain is multifactorial and related to comorbidities, complications of renal failure (e.g., bone disease, calciphylaxis, peripheral neuropathy), and the dialysis procedure (e.g., needle insertion, osmolar shift cramps, dialysate infusion pain, etc.) [38]. Understanding the etiology of the dialysis patient's pain is the first step to determining the right treatment option. Neuropathic pain is a common comorbidity of ESKD [39], and for dialysis patients with neuropathies, gabapentinoids are the pharmacotherapeutic option of choice. Both gabapentin and pregabalin are gabapentinoids that are effective against nerve pain and can also double in helping to treat uremic pruritus. However, they are extensively cleared by the kidney and reducing the dose in dialysis patients is necessary to avoid the adverse effects of dizziness and sedation. To avoid drug wasting, doses should be taken after hemodialysis sessions [35].

If used with extreme caution, and for shorter term therapy, certain opioid medications can be a good option for moderate to severe pain. Morphine and codeine are not recommended opioid choices in severe kidney impairment due to their active metabolites which are renally excreted and increase the risk for toxicity. Hydromorphone-3-glucuronide, the active metabolite of hydromorphone, can accumulate, but is much less likely to cause adverse effects than the others, making it the more preferred oral opioid option [40]. Regardless of the opioid agent prescribed, it is always prudent to initiate at the lowest effective dose and closely monitor when increasing the doses. Key strategies to remember when initiating or continuing opioid therapy in the dialysis population are to individualize dosing for each patient, consider the severity of pain, assess the patient response over time, understand their prior analgesic treatment experience, and become familiarized with risk factors for addiction, abuse, and misuse. The ideal technique is to use the lowest effective dose for the shortest duration consistent with individual treatment goals (Table 18.2).

One notable limitation for individuals with ESKD taking opioids to alleviate pain is the opioid-induced constipation that is associated with these agents. More than 50% of patients on dialysis report having constipation [33]. Docusate, lactulose, senna, and bisacodyl are appropriate treatments for constipation, and preparations containing polyethylene glycol can be used safely as laxatives or bowel preparation. Conversely, saline laxatives that consist of magnesium or phosphate salts are contraindicated in patients on dialysis due to the risk of severe electrolyte disturbances; sodium phosphate-containing bowel preparations (e.g., Fleet) can cause severe hyperphosphatemia and calcium phosphate deposition [41].

Many antibiotics, like quinolones, sulfamethoxazole with trimethoprim, glycopeptides, and aminoglycosides, require dose reductions in ESKD patients on dialysis. Trimethoprim should be avoided in this patient population due to the risk for hyperkalemia and bone marrow suppression. Nitrofurantoin is primarily excreted by the kidneys and thus relies on urinary concentration to achieve its effect. Although rare, it has also been associated with neurotoxicity and life-threatening pulmonary toxicity. Despite recent support for extending its use in chronic kidney disease, it should be avoided in dialysis patients on dialysis [42, 43]. Penicillin and cephalosporin vary in the need for dose adjustment in ESKD and have wider therapeutic indexes, but, typically, once-daily doses should be prescribed for after hemodialysis sessions, as they can be washed out during treatment. The antiviral medications, acyclovir, famciclovir, and valacyclovir, are extensively renally excreted and accumulate rapidly in patients on dialysis leading to the risk for severe neurological toxicity [44]. These antivirals should only be prescribed after discussion with the patient's nephrologist, with appropriate dose reduction, and close clinical monitoring and follow-up.

Table 18.2 Analgesic treatment options in dialysis patients [24]

Drug	Clearance	Suggested starting dose	Comments
Hydromorphone	Its major renally excreted metabolite hydromorphone-3-glucuronide is inactive	0.5–1 mg orally four times a day	Preferred oral opioid in dialysis patients
Oxycodone	Both oxycodone and its active metabolite oxymorphone are renally excreted	2.5–5 mg orally three times a day	Use controlled-release preparations with caution
Tramadol	Active renally excreted metabolite O-desmethyltramadol	50 mg orally twice a day	Maximum 100 mg twice a day Avoid controlled-release preparations
Buprenorphine	Hepatic metabolism with no accumulation of metabolites	5 mcg/h (transdermal)	Not dialyzed
Fentanyl	Hepatic metabolism with no active metabolites	12 mcg/h (transdermal)	Not dialyzed Use with caution in opioid-naïve patients
Gabapentin	Renal excretion	100 mg orally at night on dialysis days	Large-dose reductions required Can treat uremic pruritus and restless legs syndrome
Pregabalin	Renal excretion	25 mg orally at night on dialysis days	Large-dose reductions required Can treat uremic pruritus and restless legs syndrome
Morphine	Metabolized to renally excreted glucuronide metabolites (M-6-G and M-3-G) M-6-G is active and accumulates within the central nervous system, M-3-G lacks analgesic activity but may cause hyperalgesia and allodynia	2.5 mg orally three times a day	Avoid if possible Could be used for emergency analgesia if hydromorphone or fentanyl not immediately available
Codeine	Renally excreted active metabolites	–	Avoid
Acetaminophen	Hepatic clearance	1 g orally 3–4 times a day	Preferred simple analgesic

Source: Smyth et al. (2016) [24]

ESKD patients who are diabetic have reduced insulin clearance, so may be more susceptible to hypoglycemia with both insulin and sulfonylureas (e.g., glyburide). These individuals may also be at increased risk of hypoglycemia unawareness due to concurrent comorbidities and other medications. Glipizide is the preferred sulfonylurea due to its short half-life and no active metabolites. Regardless of the sulfonylurea that is selected, it should be initiated at a low dose and titrated up gradually as necessary. The dipeptidyl peptidase-4 (DPP-4) inhibitors vary in their suitability for use in dialysis patients, so prescribers should exercise sound clinical judgment. In the general population, metformin is typically considered the first-line therapeutic agent in diabetes, but in ESKD, metformin is contraindicated due to the risk of lactic acidosis. Thiazolidinediones (TZDs) are not renally excreted, but are associated with fluid retention, so are not recommended in dialysis. Sodium-glucose co-transporter (SGLT2) inhibitors should not be initiated in dialysis patients since they depend on the glomerular filtration of glucose to produce their effect.

Treatment for people on dialysis cannot be blanketed as no two patients are exactly the same. Clinical judgment should always be employed in balancing out the necessary treatment intensity against the risk of toxicity in an individual patient. As a general rule of thumb, "start low, and go slow"; always begin with the lowest effective dose and monitor patients closely for adverse effects, increasing the dose only after a timely interval.

Strategies for Increasing Medication Safety

The advancement of decision support tools and technologies will continue to serve as a safeguard for patients and providers in helping to minimize the risks associated with human error. By incorporating automated alerting into electronic medical records, medication issues can continuously be flagged proactively. Prescriber decision support tools and the use of e-prescribing are additional layers of protection that will ensure optimal patient outcomes. An observational study that assessed the impact of e-prescribing on adverse drug events in Medicare Part D beneficiaries revealed that in patients with 75% or more of their medications e-prescribed, the rate of adverse drug events was significantly lower than beneficiaries with lower e-prescribing levels [45].

Collaborative practice agreements (CPAs) or protocols between physicians and pharmacists are additional tools that can be leveraged and embedded into operational workflows to help pharmacists perform at the top of their licenses while giving time back to physicians to deliver more in-depth and thorough patient assessments. Collaborative practice agreements define certain patient care functions that a pharmacist can autonomously provide under specified situations and conditions. For example, a CPA could enable a pharmacist to prescribe an antiviral product to a patient who tests positive on a rapid diagnostic flu test. A 2010 study

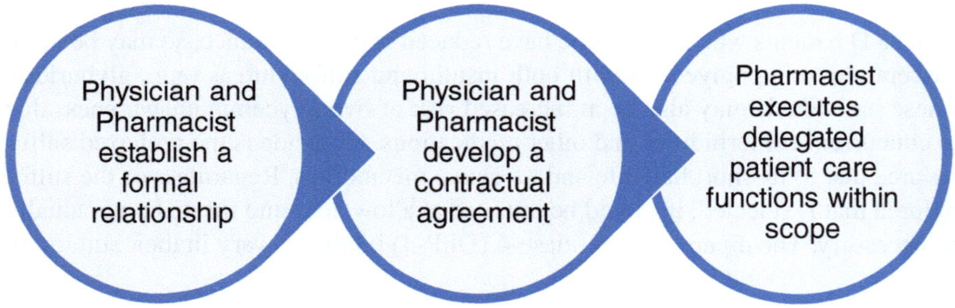
Physician and Pharmacist establish a formal relationship
Physician and Pharmacist develop a contractual agreement
Pharmacist executes delegated patient care functions within scope

Fig. 18.2 Collaborative practice agreement process flow

discovered that patient health improves significantly when pharmacists collaborate with providers to help in managing patient care [46]. Collaborative practice agreements define specific patient care functions that a pharmacist can autonomously provide under agreed upon conditions (Fig. 18.2).

Typically, CPAs are used in the context of authorizing pharmacists to initiate, modify, or discontinue medication therapy within their scope of practice. Pharmacist patient care services provided through collaborative practice agreements have been shown to improve patient outcomes for diabetes, hypertension, anticoagulation, and other chronic diseases [46–48]. As health care delivery systems adopt models of team-based care, pharmacists can be further embedded into the standard model of care for patients with kidney disease. In essence, collaborative practice agreements expand available services to patients and increase the efficiency and coordination of care, thus allowing members of the care team to complement the skills and knowledge of each other and best facilitate patient care.

A quality medication reconciliation leads to an accurate medication list which is the driving force toward an impactful medication review. Medication reconciliation is a critical component of providing quality and effective patient care and can be defined as obtaining a current and precise list of all medications reflecting what a patient is taking and how they are taking it. Components of an ideal medication reconciliation include gathering an accurate medication history, capturing any new updates to the medication list and regimen, and making sure to document any changes in the patient's medical record. For dialysis patients, medication reconciliation is of particular importance due to the high complexity of the disease state.

Medication reconciliation is often confused with medication review. Medication reconciliation can typically be performed by any member of the care team, whereas medication reviews should be reserved for a clinical pharmacist who has more in-depth pharmacotherapy knowledge and experience. During a medication review, a pharmacist should evaluate the medication list for appropriateness, effectiveness, and safety as it relates to the patient's current health status and document and provide any recommendations to the prescribers for consideration. Medication reviews are also a catalyst for ongoing, patient-centered medication therapy management as they help guide the development of treatment plans centered on each patient's medication-related goals. A team approach that includes pharmacists as part of the dialysis team with the dialysis facility as the primary medication home is necessary in ensuring a high standard of care for ESKD on dialysis [5].

Economic analysis suggests that for every dollar spent on pharmaceutical care, the healthcare system saves approximately $4, supporting the idea that all ESKD patients should have a pharmacist as part of their care team [49]. In a randomized controlled trial, patients on dialysis who received medication reconciliation and management of medication-related problems by a clinical pharmacist used 14% less medications and had about half as many hospitalizations than the control group at the end of a 2-year intervention period [50].

Clinicians caring for individuals with severe kidney impairment should establish a culture of safety while instituting patient engagement opportunities. By encouraging patients to know their medications, take them as prescribed, report any side effects, and ask questions, the care team allows the patient to take ownership of their outcomes. When it comes to medication management, best demonstrated practices involve patients keeping a list of the names of all their medications, the doses they take, and the times of day that they take them. It is also important for individuals to not forget to include inhalers, eye drops, over-the-counter medicines, vitamins, and supplements that they take. The patient medication list should be kept on hand, properly updated, and taken to every medically related appointment.

Lastly, standardized policies and procedures for clinical workflows should be incorporated for care teams to provide a baseline standard of care for all ESKD patients. Equipping team members with avenues for error reporting and performing a root cause analysis for all unfavorable events allows for continued growth in the quality of care provided.

Conclusion

Patients with severe kidney impairment have significant clinical challenges and opportunities in medication-related management that place them at increased risk of mortality compared to patients with normal kidney functioning. ESKD introduces an increase in overall medication and financial burden, with complex care plans, numerous healthcare providers, and a reduced quality of life. Combined, these elements lead to unintended medication-related problems that jeopardize therapeutic goals. Continued emphasis on assessing the appropriateness of drug dosing and addressing high pill burden in these individuals is necessary to avoid exposure to potentially harmful medications while also helping to drive down costs to the overall healthcare system. Of note, renal disease is accompanied by alterations in pharmacodynamic and pharmacokinetic parameters, placing dialysis patients at further increased risk for undesirable side effects and accounting for a significant increase in length and frequency of hospitalization.

Medication reconciliation is an effective process to reduce errors and harm associated with inappropriate drug administration practices. The Joint Commission on Accreditation of Health Care Organizations (JCAHO) has shown that medication reconciliation may prevent up to 70% of all potential errors and 15% of all adverse drug events [51]. When medications are accurately reconciled, clinical pharmacists can identify medication-related problems through a structured review of a patient's medication list and communicate with prescribers to switch to therapeutic alternatives or deprescribe medications as necessary to best optimize medication regimens.

Drug treatment is the most common medical intervention for dialysis patients, and medication use is highly complex and multidisciplinary. Strong emphasis should be placed on reducing medication-related problems by establishing a cadence of always ensuring the right patient is receiving the right drug, at the right dose, at the right route, at the right time, and for the right indication. Since patients are cared for by multiple providers, collaboration is needed within this circle of care to prevent errors and provide the best possible care.

References

1. Manley HJ, Cannella CA, Bailie GR, St Peter WL. Medication-related problems in ambulatory hemodialysis patients: a pooled analysis. Am J Kidney Dis. 2005;46:669–80.
2. St Peter WL. Improving medication safety in chronic kidney disease patients on dialysis through medication reconciliation. Adv Chronic Kidney Dis. 2010;17(5):413–9. https://doi.org/10.1053/j.ackd.2010.06.001.
3. Ray K. Medication errors in dialysis patients undergoing PCI. Nat Rev Cardiol. 2010;7:118. https://doi.org/10.1038/nrcardio.2010.7.
4. Chiu YW, Teitelbaum I, Misra M, De Leon EM, Adzize T, Mehrotra R. Pill burden, adherence, hyperphosphatemia, and quality of life in maintenance dialysis patients. Clin J Am Soc Nephrol. 2009;4:1089–96.
5. St Peter WL. Management of polypharmacy in dialysis patients. Semin Dial. 2015;28(4):427–32. https://doi.org/10.1111/sdi.12377.
6. Doshi S, Wish JB. Can emergency department visits for adverse drug reactions in dialysis patients be reduced? Am J Nephrol. 2018;47:435–7. https://doi.org/10.1159/000490064.
7. Pai AB, Boyd A, Depczynski J, Chavez IM, Khan N, Manley H. Reduced drug use and hospitalization rates in patients undergoing hemodialysis who received pharmaceutical care: a 2-year, randomized, controlled study. Pharmacotherapy. 2009;29(12):1433–40. https://doi.org/10.1592/phco.29.12.1433.
8. Wong NA, Jones HW. An analysis of discharge drug prescribing amongst elderly patients with renal impairment. Postgrad Med J. 1998;74(873):420–2. https://doi.org/10.1136/pgmj.74.873.420.
9. Chang F, O'Hare AM, Miao Y, Steinman MA. Use of renally inappropriate medications in older veterans: a national study. J Am Geriatr Soc. 2015;63(11):2290–7. https://doi.org/10.1111/jgs.13790.
10. Flythe JE, et al. Predictors of 30-day hospital readmission among maintenance hemodialysis patients: a hospital's perspective. Clin J Am Soc Nephrol. 2016;11(6):1005–14. https://doi.org/10.2215/CJN.11611115.
11. Dyer SA, Nguyen V, Rafie S, Awdishu L. Impact of medication reconciliation by a dialysis pharmacist. Kidney360. 2022;3:922–5. https://doi.org/10.34067/KID.0007182021.
12. Alshahrani F, Marriott JF, Cox AR. A qualitative study of prescribing errors among multi-professional prescribers within an e-prescribing system. Int J Clin Pharm. 2021;43:884–92. https://doi.org/10.1007/s11096-020-01192-0.
13. Downing NL, Bates DW, Longhurst CA. Physician burnout in the electronic health record era: are we ignoring the real cause? Ann Intern Med. 2018;169(1):50–1.
14. Velo GP, Minuz P. Medication errors: prescribing faults and prescription errors. Br J Clin Pharmacol. 2009;67(6):624–8. https://doi.org/10.1111/j.1365-2125.2009.03425.x.
15. Emmerton LM, Rizk MFS. Look-alike and sound-alike medicines: risks and "solutions". Int J Clin Pharm. 2012;34(1):4–8.
16. Institute for Safe Medication Practices (ISMP). Adopt strategies to manage look-alike and/or sound-alike medication name mix-ups. ISMP medication safety alert! Acute Care. 2022;27(11):1–4.
17. Li M, Tomlinson G, Naglie G, et al. Geriatric comorbidities, such as falls, confer an independent mortality risk to elderly dialysis patients. Nephrol Dial Transplant. 2008;23(4):1396–400.
18. National Kidney Foundation. KDOQI clinical practice guideline for diabetes and CKD: 2012 update. Am J Kidney Dis. 2012;60(5):850–86.
19. Clinical Pharmacology powered by ClinicalKey. Tampa: Elsevier; 2022. http://www.clinicalkey.com.
20. OxyContin (oxycodone HCl extended-release) package insert. Stamford: Purdue Pharma L.P.; 2021.
21. Roxicodone (oxycodone) tablet package insert. Webster Groves: Mallinckrodt Pharmaceuticals; 2021.

22. Medcalf JF, Harris KP, Walls J. Role of diuretics in the preservation of residual renal function in patients on continuous ambulatory peritoneal dialysis. Kidney Int. 2001;59(3):1128–33. https://doi.org/10.1046/j.1523-1755.2001.0590031128.x.
23. Manley HJ, Drayer DK, Muther RS. Medication-related problem type and appearance rate in ambulatory hemodialysis patients. BMC Nephrol. 2003;4:10. https://doi.org/10.1186/1471-2369-4-10.
24. Smyth B, Jones C, Saunders J. Prescribing for patients on dialysis. Aust Prescr. 2016;39(1):21–4. https://doi.org/10.18773/austprescr.2016.008.
25. Floege J, Johnson RJ, Feehally J. Comprehensive clinical nephrology. 4th ed. St Louis: Elsevier; 2010.
26. Chan L, Saha A, Poojary P, Chauhan K, Naik N, Coca S, et al. National trends in emergency room visits of dialysis patients for adverse drug reactions. Am J Nephrol. 2018;47:441–9.
27. Michaels AD, Spinler SA, Leeper B, et al. Medication errors in acute cardiovascular and stroke patients: a scientific statement from the American Heart Association. Circulation. 2010;121(14):1664–82.
28. Federico F. Preventing harm from high-alert medications. Jt Comm J Qual Patient Saf. 2007;33(9):537–42.
29. Tsai TT, Maddox TM, Roe MT, et al. Contraindicated medication use in dialysis patients undergoing percutaneous coronary intervention. JAMA. 2009;302(22):2458–64.
30. Busby LT, Weyman A, Rodgers GM. Excessive anticoagulation in patients with mild renal insufficiency receiving long-term therapeutic enoxaparin. Am J Hematol. 2001;67(1):54–6.
31. Gerlach AT, Pickworth KK, Seth SK, Tanna SB, Barnes JF. Enoxaparin and bleeding complications: a review in patients with and without renal insufficiency. Pharmacotherapy. 2000;20(7):771–5.
32. Thorevska N, Amoateng-Adjepong Y, Sabahi R, et al. Anticoagulation in hospitalized patients with renal insufficiency: a comparison of bleeding rates with unfractionated heparin vs enoxaparin. Chest. 2004;125(3):856–63.
33. Murtagh FE, Addington-Hall J, Higginson IJ. The prevalence of symptoms in end-stage renal disease: a systematic review. Adv Chronic Kidney Dis. 2007;14:82–99. https://doi.org/10.1053/j.ackd.2006.10.001.
34. Bailie GR, Mason NA, Bragg-Gresham JL, Gillespie BW, Young EW. Analgesic prescription patterns among hemodialysis patients in the DOPPS: potential for underprescription. Kidney Int. 2004;65:2419–25. https://doi.org/10.1111/j.1523-1755.2004.00658.x.
35. Davison SN, Ferro CJ. Management of pain in chronic kidney disease. Prog Palliat Care. 2009;17:186–95. https://doi.org/10.1179/096992609X12455871937189.
36. Andersohn F, Suissa S, Garbe E. Use of first- and second-generation cyclooxygenase-2-selective nonsteroidal antiinflammatory drugs and risk of acute myocardial infarction. Circulation. 2006;113:1950–7. https://doi.org/10.1161/circulationaha.105.602425.
37. Cass A, Chadban S, Gallagher M, Howard K, Jones A, McDonald S, et al. Economic impact of end-stage kidney disease in Australia: projections to 2020. Melbourne: Kidney Health Australia; 2010.
38. Wyne A, Rai R, Cuerden M, Clark WF, Suri RS. Opioid and benzodiazepine use in end-stage renal disease: a systematic review. Clin J Am Soc Nephrol. 2011;6(2):326–33. https://doi.org/10.2215/CJN.04770610.
39. Mambelli E, Barrella M, Facchini MG, Mancini E, Sicuso C, Bainotti S, et al. The prevalence of peripheral neuropathy in hemodialysis patients. Clin Nephrol. 2012;77:468–75. https://doi.org/10.5414/CN107188.
40. Davison SN, Mayo PR. Pain management in chronic kidney disease: the pharmacokinetics and pharmacodynamics of hydromorphone and hydromorphone-3-glucuronide in hemodialysis patients. J Opioid Manag. 2008;4:335–6.
41. Heher EC, Thier SO, Rennke H, Humphreys BD. Adverse renal and metabolic effects associated with oral sodium phosphate bowel preparation. Clin J Am Soc Nephrol. 2008;3:1494–503. https://doi.org/10.2215/CJN.02040408.

42. Geerts AF, Eppenga WL, Heerdink R, Derijks HJ, Wensing MJ, Egberts TC, et al. Ineffectiveness and adverse events of nitrofurantoin in women with urinary tract infection and renal impairment in primary care. Eur J Clin Pharmacol. 2013;69:1701–7. https://doi.org/10.1007/s00228-013-1520-x.
43. Singh N, Gandhi S, McArthur E, Moist L, Jain AK, Liu AR, et al. Kidney function and the use of nitrofurantoin to treat urinary tract infections in older women. CMAJ. 2015;187:648–56. https://doi.org/10.1503/cmaj.150067.
44. Strumia S, De Mitri P, Bionda E. Neurotoxicity of acyclovir and valacyclovir in a hemodialyzed patient. Eur J Neurol. 2004;11:68–9. https://doi.org/10.1046/j.1351-5101.2003.00719.x.
45. Gabriel MH, Powers C, Encinosa W, Bynum JP. E-prescribing and adverse drug events: an observational study of the medicare part D population with diabetes. Med Care. 2017;55:456–62.
46. Chisholm-Burns MA, Kim Lee J, Spivey CA, Slack M, Herrier RN, Hall-Lipsy E, et al. US pharmacists' effect as team members on patient care: systematic review and meta-analyses. Med Care. 2010;48:923–33.
47. Chiquette E, Amato MG, Bussey HI. Comparison of an anticoagulation clinic with usual medical care: anticoagulation control, patient outcomes, and health care costs. Arch Intern Med. 1998;158(15):1641–7.
48. Davidson MB, Karlan VJ, Hair TL. Effect of a pharmacist-managed diabetes care program in a free medical clinic. Am J Med Qual. 2000;15(4):137–42.
49. Manley HJ, Carroll CA. The clinical and economic impact of pharmaceutical care in end-stage renal disease patients. Semin Dial. 2002;15(1):45–9.
50. Ernst FR, Grizzle AJ. Drug-related morbidity and mortality: updating the cost-of-illness model. J Am Pharm Assoc (Wash). 2001;41(2):192–9. https://doi.org/10.1016/s1086-5802(16)31229-3.
51. Levanda M. Implementing a medication reconciliation process in a community hospital. Am J Health Syst Pharm. 2007;64:1372–8.

Falls in the Elderly and in Persons with Chronic Disease

19

Stephen Z. Fadem

Introduction

Falls are common, not just in persons with chronic kidney disease but across the population. As will be shown, they have many reasons to occur, and hence there are multiple opportunities to enact preventive strategies.

The World Health Organization states that falls are the second leading cause of unintentional traumatic death and that 684,000 persons die from a fall each year. Each year there are 37.3 million falls that require medical attention (SOURCE www.who.int accessed April 30, 2022). The death rates are highest in persons over 60 years old. As the world population of aging individuals increases, the incidence of chronic kidney disease (CKD) among the elderly also rises. CKD patients often have comorbidities associated with heart disease and diabetes.

Given the high mortality associated with falls, as well as the consequence of human suffering, and the costs incurred, there has been a considerable effort to prevent injury, particularly in the aged patient with kidney disease. This population is particularly vulnerable to falling and sustaining severe injuries due to the fall. But the question is whether kidney function alone is an independent risk factor that leads to falls. A large study that looked at the propensity of falling in 2256 participants with a median age of 79.5 years found that among the 746 patients who experienced a fall, the association was strong with lower urinary tract symptoms odds ratio (OR) 1.56, 95% CI (Confidence Interval) 1.29–1.89) but not with eGFR [1]. Instead, falls in the dialysis population are related to the patient's age and the adverse events associated with dialysis. One study showed that in the elderly hemodialysis (HD) population, the incidence of falls was 38.2% over a 12-month period.

S. Z. Fadem (✉)
Section of Nephrology, Department of Medicine, Baylor College of Medicine, Houston, TX, USA
e-mail: fadem@bcm.edu

S. Z. Fadem et al. (eds.), *Complications in Dialysis*,
https://doi.org/10.1007/978-3-031-44557-6_19

The systemic complications associated with diabetes, the most common cause of end-stage renal disease (ESRD), put this group of patients at risk for falling.

Visual disorders related to retinopathy, microvascular disease, peripheral neuropathy, heart disease, and medication use are but a few of the risk factors that diabetics undergoing dialysis encounter [2]. Muscle atrophy, fatigue, mineral-bone disease, low exercise tolerance, impaired autonomic control, and cardiac dysfunction all occur in kidney disease. Dialysis patients are particularly vulnerable after dialysis therapy; this is related to orthostatic hypotension that frequently occurs in the immediate post-dialysis period. One study demonstrated that the incidence of orthostatic hypotension immediately post-dialysis was 69.6% [3]. Fatigue post-therapy also predisposes the HD patient to a fall post-treatment.

Although age is the primary factor associated with falls, a review of 14 studies performed in HD units demonstrated that the risk of falling includes a past history of falls, frailty, therapy with antidepressant medications, the number of prescribed oral medications, a failed walking test, malnutrition, comorbidities, diabetes, and the level of education. While frailty and age both increase the risk of a fall, elderly patients with good cognitive function have a lower risk of falling. Predictors of falls included postural hypotension, the levels of 25-hydroxyvitamin D, and serum albumin levels. The danger escalates with age; only 30% of persons over 75 are free of falls. Other risk factors for accidental falls are dementia, pneumonia, diabetes, gastrointestinal disorders, and cardiac arrhythmias.

The comprehensive review of 14 studies further demonstrated that 82% of falls occurred at home and 69% indoors. 16% of falls happen in a bathroom. Falls in women were associated with muscle strength reduction or a decrease in bone mineral density. Concerning hemodialysis, it was found that 73% of falls occur after and 27% before dialysis treatments. Quadricep muscle weakness, osteoporosis, malnutrition, and sarcopenia also present a risk for falling in the HD population.

The risk of death was 2.13-fold higher when associated with falls, and there was a 3.5-fold increase in a nursing home placement [4].

Fall Prediction Models

The risk of a fall can be assessed by the Morse Fall Scale (MFS), a simple six-item tool.

1. History of falling (yes = 25 points)
2. Secondary diagnoses (yes = 15 points)
3. Ambulatory aid (bed rest = 0; crutches, cane, walker = 15; furniture = 30)
4. The presence of an intravenous line or heparin lock (yes = 20)
5. Gait disorder (normal, bed rest, or immobile = 0; weak = 10; impaired = 20)
6. Mental status(forgets limitations = 15) [5]

Although the scoring may vary slightly, an MFS score of 1–24 indicates a low risk of falling, while a score of 25–45 indicates moderate risk and the need to implement standard fall prevention interventions. A score of ≥45 indicates a high risk of falling [5].

The dialysis fall risk index (DFRI) developed and validated a seven-item fall risk assessment specifically for dialysis patients. Two hundred fifty-one maintenance HD patients were evaluated over the domains of (1) age, (2) C-reactive protein, (3) nutrition status, (4) gait and balance, (5) hand grip, (6) intra-dialytic hypotension, and (7) fall occurrence. The patients were divided into quartiles based on scoring. The hazard ratio (HR) for quartile three was 2.65 and for quartile four was 3.84 [6].

Mechanical Vs. Non-mechanical Falls (See Fig. 19.1)

Falls that occur in patients with medical conditions are termed non-mechanical falls. Otherwise, a fall is termed mechanical. Well-known examples of mechanical falls are tripping over an object on the floor or slipping on a wet floor. There is considerable overlap since patients with a high risk of falling are more likely to sustain mechanical falls.

Non-mechanical Falls

It appears that non-mechanical falls can be grouped into three major categories:

1. Patients who are frail, who have cognitive decline, or a neurological deficit
2. Patients who are over-medicated
3. Patients with systemic diseases who have trouble with balance, gait, muscle weakness, and vision

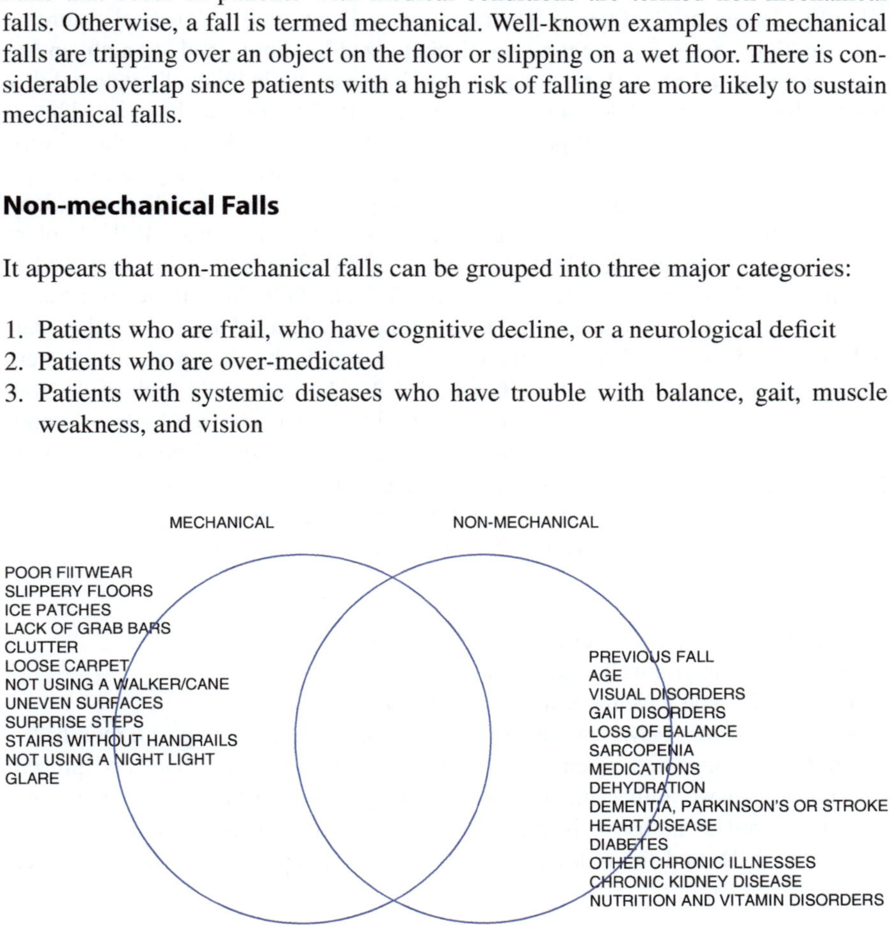

Fig. 19.1 This diagram highlights the two major categories of falls. Patients who have a risk of a non-mechanical fall are more likely to sustain a mechanical fall

Category 1: Frailty, Cognitive Decline, Neurological Deficit

Falls in persons with cognitive decline require urgent attention and create a need for renewed decisions on health care. They confirm a worsening in the individual's independence and increased reliance on caregivers. A major challenge is that once patients fall, they are likely to fall again. The action of a fall in persons with dementia places a burden of added stress on caregivers [7]. Not only families but dialysis personnel can experience stress related to fall incidents.

Frailty

Frailty is a state of vulnerability that results from the loss of physiologic reserve. It is an indicator of functional decline and, although most commonly associated with advancing age, in actuality, is the consequence of the comorbidities that may appear earlier as the result of chronic disease. Its formal definition was developed in 2013 by a Frailty Consensus Conference. Their consensus definition is "A medical syndrome with multiple causes and contributors characterized by diminished strength, endurance, and reduced physiologic function that increases an individual's vulnerability for developing increased dependency and/or death [8]." Frailty can be indexed based on health status deficits. A 40-point index was developed in 2008 and included variables related to independence (assistance in bathing, dressing, eating, ambulating), self-rating of health, weight loss, depression, the presence of chronic disorders (heart attack, CHF, diabetes, arthritis, lung disease), and measurements (BMI, shoulder strength, grip strength, usual and rapid pace) [9]. A modified version was used to evaluate 13,877 participants, among which 2,310 had falls. Indexing demonstrated that increments were associated with falls among middle-aged and older individuals (OR 1.52, 95% CI: 1.45–1.6). This association was high when participants were classed as prefrail (OR 1.75, 95% CI: 1.59–1.93), but especially high in the frail population (3.04, 95% CI: 2.60–3.56) [10]. Frailty is characterized by five components, weight loss, exhaustion, weakness, slowness, and reduced physical activity. Not just the elderly but any individual with a significant weight loss of 5% over a year period should be screened for frailty. Several screening tests are available. The most straightforward assessment is the 5 question "FRAIL" tool:

Fatigue: Are you Fatigued?
Resistance—Can you walk up one flight of stairs?
Aerobic—Can you walk one block?
Illness—Do you have more than five illnesses?
Loss of weight—Have you lost over 5% of your weight in the past 6 months?

Frailty is considered when three or more questions are positive, and prefrail patients will answer either one or two questions positively. Frailty can be managed, and the consensus is that resistance and aerobic exercise, caloric and protein support, vitamin D, and the reduction in polypharmacy have some efficacy in treatment [8].

Cognitive Decline

Dementia is the generic term for the irreversible decline in mental function that is severe enough to interfere with the activities of daily living. It is associated with memory loss, personality changes, and impaired reasoning ability. Mild forgetfulness is not a reason to suspect dementia and is common with normal aging, although severe memory loss is a hallmark of the disease. It has many causes, including Alzheimer's, but it goes beyond just forgetting a name or a place.

Alzheimer's disease is characterized by a slow intellectual decline with executive function impairment in later stages. Vascular dementia can either be of sudden or gradual onset and is related to vascular disease, diabetes, or atherosclerosis. It is characterized by mild memory loss and becomes a fall risk when it starts to impair gait and balance. When dementia is associated with parkinsonism, it is termed Lewy body dementia. This disorder has a poor prognosis. Dementia limited to the frontal lobe may result in memory loss combined with aggression, agitation, and behavioral disorders [11].

On the other hand, the deficits associated with mild cognitive impairment (MCI) may include difficulties with thinking, reasoning, language, and judgment. MCI does not predispose one to falls until it begins to interfere with activities of daily living.

When considering dementia, it is critical to contemplate not just cognitive functioning but activities of daily living, physical health, psychological symptoms, social support, and the utilization of formal and informal health care. Ranking programs have been developed to categorize dementia based on these dimensions. For practical purposes, the composite of these dimensions must be considered when assessing fall risks [12]. This is because planning, assistance, and support depend upon the patient's own abilities, not just with cognitive and executive function, but with the level of dependence on family and social resources.

Falls in patients with dementia are common. A study of 179 dementia participants over 65 years old demonstrated an eight-fold incidence of falls over 12 months. Dementia patients have a worse recovery than those without cognitive impairment [13]. In the general population, the prevalence of any bone fracture is higher when dementia is present. Dementia is a risk factor for hip fracture in the dialysis population for various reasons. Dialysis patients age more rapidly than the general population and have fragile bones.

Stroke

A stroke is an injury to the brain caused by a vascular event. It is a leading cause of death and disability. There is a 43% greater risk of stroke once the GFR falls below 60 mL.min.1.73m^2. Dialysis patients have a ten-fold higher incidence of stroke and a higher mortality rate once a stroke occurs. Atrial fibrillation is ten times more prevalent in the dialysis population and may result in an embolic stroke. Uncontrolled hypertension also increases the risk of stroke [14].

Although strokes are often associated with an acute, catastrophic neurologic deficit, the most common ischemic strokes are insidious in the beginning. The lacunar infarction results from chronic high blood pressure leading to hyaline changes that injure tiny penetrating arteries in the deep areas of the brain. These may result in residual 1–3 mm cavities known as lacunae. Early symptoms of lacunar infarctions are mild cognitive impairment and are apparent in brain imaging studies. Subsequent infarctions lead to progressive global brain atrophy. The size and number of lacunar infarctions are associated with the risk of falling ($p < 0.05$), particularly in older patients and those with significantly decreased eGFR values [15]. Risk factors for falls in stroke patients are fatigue ($p < 0.001$), the number of strokes ($p = 0.035$), depression ($p < 0.001$), gait disorders such as timed up and go and gait speed, and reduced stride length [16, 17]. The inability of a recovering stroke victim to perform activities of daily living is independently associated with the risk of falling [18].

Category 2: Patients Who Are Over-medicated

Multiple medication use is a modifiable risk factor for a fall injury. Sedatives, hypnotics, pain medications, neuroleptics and antipsychotics, antidepressants, benzodiazepines, and opioids are all associated with the risk of falling and are called fall risk-increasing drugs (FRIDS). Participants aged 70–79 followed for 8.0 ± 3.1 years. Of 1764 sampled, 36% took ≥6 prescription medications per day, defined as polypharmacy. The fall rate among these patients was 31%. The fall rate without polypharmacy was 38 per 1000 person-years, and with polypharmacy, the rate was 50 per 1000 person-years. When FRID was combined with persistent polypharmacy, the HR was 1.22(95% CI 0.93–1.60), and in FRID use without persistent polypharmacy, the HR was 1.08 (95% CI 0.77–1.51). Reviewing medication lists and using fewer FRIDs may help reduce falls [19]. Diuretics are also associated with falls. In another study, the use of ≥5 medications was associated with falls with an adjusted odds ratio (OR) of 2.513 (95% CI 1.339–4.718). The use of diuretics was associated with a fall risk with an adjusted OR of 2.803 (95% CI 1.418–5.544) [20].

In this sampling, antihypertensives were not associated with falls in patients (adjusted OR 0.473 95% CI 0.319–0.700) [20]. In a national cohort study of discharged elderly patients (mean age 77; $n = 4056$), intensifying blood pressure therapy resulted in an increased risk of readmissions within 30 days, with an HR of 1.23 (95% CI, 1.07–1.42). The HR for serious adverse events was 1.41 (95% CI, 1.06–1.88) [21]. The performance and mobility assessment for this population was not decreased. Yet the risk of falling increases when patients have multiple chronic conditions. The risk of falling worsens with excessive antihypertensive therapy because of an exacerbation of adverse events such as postural hypotension, balance and gait impairment, and dizziness. A Medicare claims review of 4961 patients demonstrated that antihypertensive medications were associated with a 11.6% fall incidence in patients on moderate-intensity antihypertensive therapy and a 10.9% fall incidence on high-intensity therapy. In patients who were not on antihypertensive medications, the fall risk was 9.0%. In a one-year subgroup analysis of patients who had a previous fall, antihypertensive therapy doubled the risk of another fall compared to patients who were not on antihypertensive therapy [22].

A systemic review and meta-analysis of falls demonstrated that falls are more common in people with diabetes (Risk ratio (RR) 1.64 95% CI 1.27–2.11). The RR of falling was 1.94 (95% CI 1.42–2.63) in those managed with insulin compared to an RR of 1.27 (95% CI 1.06–1.52) in those not treated with insulin [23]. Hypoglycemia as a consequence of diabetes can be worse in type 2 diabetes, where there may be a mismatch of insulin release and use. The kidney plays a role in clearing insulin and in increasing gluconeogenesis. Coupling this with the altered metabolism of antidiabetic agents or parenteral insulin can result in hypoglycemia. For these reasons, there is controversy over how strictly one should control diabetes in CKD. The KDIGO Guidelines recommend using HbA1C as often as four times a year to monitor glycemic control in diabetic patients with CKD. The targets range from <6.5% for patients with mild CKD and few comorbidities. This group is expected to have available resources for blood sugar control, a low likelihood of developing undiscovered hypoglycemia, and a long-life expectancy. In patients with advanced disease but not being treated with dialysis, who have multiple comorbidities, a short life expectancy, and fewer resources to monitor hypoglycemia, the HbAIC should be kept at <8.0% in CKD patients treated with dialysis therapy [24].

In patients with advanced CKD, including dialysis, the recommendation is to use glycated albumin (GA) instead of the HbA1C as a marker of glycemic control [25]. The GA is a predictor of mortality in the dialysis population (HR, 1.143 per 1% increase in GA, 955 CI 1.011–1.292; $P = 0.033$). It is recommended that the GA be kept ≤25%. All-cause mortality is significantly better in dialysis patients with adequate diabetes control ($p = 0.024$) [26]. A glucose-free dialysis bath has been associated with hypoglycemia in as high as 40% of patients. It is recommended that 5.5 mmol/L glucose is used in dialysis baths, making hypoglycemia during dialysis treatments less likely [27].

The benefits of medications versus their risks are readily apparent in the outpatient dialysis setting, especially in the elderly population. Polypharmacy may be complicated when patients have mildly decreased cognitive function. Deprescribing initiatives have successfully reduced excessive medication use [28].

Category 3: Patients with Systemic Diseases Who Have Trouble with Balance, Gait, Muscle Weakness, and Vision

Falls may also be the consequence of underlying diseases and conditions. Kidney disease is a fall risk. Age and living alone without social support increase the risk of falling. Impaired vision and gait, mobility, or balance disorders, may increase the susceptibility to falling. An acute inner ear disorder can also affect balance and lead to falls. Clinical fall conditions include hypertension, diabetes, cardiovascular disease, and arthritis. Primary or secondary neuropathies related to diabetes, medications, or amyloidosis can present a fall risk. Acute conditions that relate to volume depletion, such as dehydration secondary to poor fluid intake, over-diuresis, vomiting, or diarrhea, may result in postural hypotension. This list of disease states highlights conditions that can precede a fall but are not inclusive.

- Kidney disease
- Age
- Living alone

- Impaired vision
- Gait and mobility disorders
- Chronic illness (cardiovascular disease, hypertension, diabetes)
- Arthritis and neuropathy
- Volume-related disorders

Kidney Disease

While kidney disease alone is a fall risk, any of the factors below may increase the chance of a fall. Data abstracted from literature searches incorporated 2357 patients aged 58–75.6 years of age. Only 30% of patients over 75 years old remained free of falls. Falls were less common in those under 65; 89.1% of that age-group were free of falls. The incidence of falls in kidney disease patients varied between 1.18 and 1.60 falls per patient year, and the major risk factor was age. Medications, particularly antidepressants, the number of prescribed oral drugs, depression, failed walking test, frailty, diabetes, high school education, and a history of a previous fall comprised the major risk factors. Falls are widespread in patients receiving HD.

Falls result in a 2.13-fold increased risk of death and a two-fold risk of hospitalizations. 57% of falls occur when people are ambulating. 31% happen when standing from a seated position, and the remaining 12% when rising from a lying position [4].

In one study of dialysis patients ranging from 20 to 92 years old, 28.4% of the participants fell. 71% of patients were hospitalized after falling, and 11.2% of patients had fractures. Abrasions and lacerations also occurred. Fortunately, head injuries and hip fractures were relatively rare [29]. Patients with chronic kidney disease are more likely to experience an in-hospital fall. In a retrospective case-control study, the mean age of hospitalized CKD patients who fell was 65 ± 15 years of age. Comorbidities that increased the risk of a fall included dementia, pneumonia, gastrointestinal disease, diabetes, and depression [30].

One year after a fall, 25% of older patients will die, and 76% will have limited mobility. Fifty percent of patients will become incapacitated to the extent that their activities of daily living will be limited [4].

In a retrospective cohort study in Taiwan, hemodialysis (HD) and peritoneal dialysis (PD) were compared concerning the risk of falls. The study consisted of 127,823 ESRD patients, 101,304 on HD, and 7584 on PD. The HD population was older and had more comorbidities than the PD population, but when adjusted and matched, the risk of serious falls was higher in the HD population (HR 1.27, 95% CI 1.06–1.52) [31].

Age

The risk of falling increases with age, and one-third of people ≥65 years of age fall at least once per year [32]. Nursing home populations of 1,015 geriatric patients (median age 73 years) without dementia were studied. CKD was present in 205 and was an independent risk factor for falling. (OR 2.59, 95% CI 1.19–5.66) Stage 3 CKD comprised 90.2% of the patients, and 8.8% had Stage 4 CKD. Among the geriatric CKD patients at risk for falling, sarcopenia was present 57.6% of the time, significantly greater than those not at risk for a fall (27.6% $P < 0.001$). Other factors that significantly ($p < 0.001$) influenced falling in elderly CKD patients were malnutrition, frailty, mental status, and the level of activity [33]. Another study of 1,000 elderly patients (mean age 79.4 ± 6.6 years) analyzed 38% of whom had a GFR of at least 60 mL/min/1.73 m^2) and 17% who had a GFR < 45 mL/min/1.73 m^2. Although the odds ratio of falling was 1.75 (95% CI 1.21–2.53; $p \leq 0.01$) among those with the GFR < 45 mL/min/1.73 m^2, when adjusting for multiple potential confounders, the OR dropped to 1.08 (95% CI 0.72–1.62). This study suggested that it was not CKD but the associated factors of living situation, medical history, intoxications, history of falling, polypharmacy, comorbidities, postural hypotension, body mass index, physical function, cognition, depression, functional assessment, blood tests, and cardiovascular disease that influenced falling [34].

Living Alone

The English Longitudinal Study of Aging is a national study of people over the age of 50 living in private households in England. A review of fall incidences from self-reports and hospitalizations revealed that 52% of people self-reported having fallen. Fewer than 10% had a fall-related hospitalization. There was a 17% risk of falls among individuals who lived alone (HR 1.17, 95% CI 1.05–1.30). In the hospital group, the HR was 1.29, 95% CI 1.10–1.51) [35]. This study did not distinguish which patients had CKD.

Impaired Vision

A prospective analysis of 251 patients with a visual impairment aged 65–92 years of age assessed the outcomes and risks of accidental falls. The incidence of falls reported over 12 months was 565.975. The odds of falling were higher in women (OR 2.71, CI 1.40–5.27), in smokers (OR 3.57, 95% CI 1.34–9.48), awakening at night (OR 2.08, 95% CI 1.15–3.79), difficulty walking or balance (OR 2.60, 95% CI 1.29–5.24), glaucoma (OR 3.12, 95% CI 1.15–8.44), retinal degenerations (OR 3.31, 95% CI 1.16–9.43), and visual acuity (OR 1.79, 95% CI 1.10–2.91). Outdoor activities were also associated with a greater odds of falls in the visually impaired elderly population that was studied (OR 2.71, 95% CI 1.40–5.27) [36].

Gait and Mobility Disorders

Gait disorders stem from various clinical disorders and, in the aging population, are associated with higher fall risks. The assessment of gait is part of the standard neurological evaluation. Inspection of walking patterns may reveal a neurological disorder (stroke, Parkinson's disease, ataxia, spastic, and frontal) or a non-neurological disturbance related to arthritis or peripheral vascular disease. Ataxic gaits are generally wide-based and unsteady. They are associated with poor balance. Gait disorders may be associated with neuropathy and loss of sensation, foot drop, and decreased reflexes. Patients with a frontal gait have a wide base, take short strips, and have difficulty lifting their feet. The patient with a parkinsonian gait may take small, shuffling, jerky steps, and festinate with a quick, short stride. They may not swing their arms when walking. Spasticity may be associated with scissoring, crossing one leg in front of another when walking. A proximal myopathy may be associated with a waddling gait [37]. In a study of 632 elderly patients with gait disorders, the fall rate was 39% (244 subjects). The average age of participants was 80.6 years of age. Neurologic gait disorders were more frequently associated with a slower gait velocity. Falls were associated with moderately severe neurological gaits (risk ratio 1.92, 95% CI 1.20–3.06, $p < 0.001$) [38].

Studies of the gait of older adults who fall reveal that they have a more constrained, less adaptable trunk movement compared to younger people and that the walking pattern is different from those who do not fall [39]. Other studies have demonstrated that while a decreased walking speed was not associated with falls, a decreased stride length was associated with falls in men over 74 years of age (OR 1.34, 95% CI 1.05–1.70 per 10 cm decrease) [40].

Sarcopenia and Falls

Muscle breakdown and production should always be in balance. When breakdown exceeds production, the catabolism of muscle is known as sarcopenia. CKD is among the disorders that potentiate the proteasomal breakdown of muscle. These disorders include inactivity, space travel, inflammatory diseases such as cancer or HIV, severe infections, starvation, and metabolic acidosis. Sarcopenia is also associated with advancing age and diabetes [41, 42]. Angiotensin II, vitamin D deficiency, and insulin resistance also accelerate muscle turnover and catabolism. Sarcopenia has been demonstrated in a systemic review that included 52,838 persons with a mean/median age of ≥65 years. Nearly half of the studies reported a significantly higher risk of falls and fractures in persons with sarcopenia [43].

Volume-Related Disorders

A study of health records from the University of Wisconsin identified 11,622 dehydrated patients. Among these, the odds ratio of a fall was 1.12 ($P = 0.002$). Dehydration was defined as a blood urea nitrogen (BUN) to serum creatinine ratio of >20, a serum sodium of >145 mg/dL, and a serum osmolality of >295 mOsm/kg. Dehydration was also associated with antipsychotic medications and loop diuretics [44].

Dialysis is associated with increased cardiovascular stress and can be related to hypotension, hypovolemia, hypoxia, hypokalemia, and cardiac arrhythmias at the end of treatment [45]. In addition to the adverse consequences of stress related to treatments, patients can have orthostatic hypotension. This is particularly true in diabetic patients who often have autonomic insufficiency. Standing and then walking unassisted when orthostatic hypotension is present may result in a post-dialysis fall. It was reported that while 34.8% of patients have orthostatic hypotension predialysis, 69.6 have orthostatic hypotension after treatment. Ultrafiltration complicated by the underlying cardiac stress of dialysis, the use of antihypertensive medications, autonomic insufficiency, and all too often large weight gains in the interdialytic period, predispose patients to postural hypotension, and the risk of falling [3].

Arthritis and Neuropathy

The odds of falling increase with osteoarthritis, depending on the number of joints involved. A systemic review determined that the odds of falling when one joint is involved is 53%, 74 with two joints, and 855 with three to four joints. Arthritis involving the knee is associated with an adjusted odds ratio (aOR) of 1.39 (95% CI, 1.02–1.88). Hip-related osteoarthritis is worse and associated with an aOR for falling of 1.60 (95% CI, 1.14–2.24) [46].

Chronic Illness (Cardiovascular Disease, Hypertension, Diabetes)

Many patients have trouble with balance, gait, muscle weakness, or vision as a result of the comorbidities of their diseases. Thus, they are at high risk for a fall. It has been well established that falls among the elderly are associated with the disabilities associated with chronic illness. This was demonstrated in 1986. A study of 79 consecutive admissions to intermediate care facilities showed that 25 patients fell recurrently. Risk factors associated with an increased fall risk included mobility, morale, mental status, distant vision, hearing, orthostatic hypotension, back examination, medications, and the activities of daily living score. In patients with seven or more factors, the fall risk was 100%. Those with 4–6 risk factors had a 31% chance of falling. Those with less than three risk factors were not identified as fallers. The mobility test was the best predictor of recurrent falling [47].

Advanced diabetes presents a fall risk mainly due to neuropathy [48]. However, other factors, such as diabetic therapy that results in hypoglycemia, may also result in fall-related injury. Patients with diabetes tend to have systemic vascular disease, vision loss, and kidney disease, which compound the risk.

The World Health Organization has mapped fall causality in the elderly. After a review of 1,127 articles culled from the medical literature, 101 papers from 34 countries were retained for a comprehensive review. Among the most common determinants of risk were diseases, health conditions and physical characteristics, daily behavior and attitudes, preventative measures, environment, a history of falls, and age. Aggregating this data helps healthcare providers clinically assess which patients are likely to fall and institute preventive measures [49].

Prevention of Falls

The most important means of preventing a fall is to anticipate it. In encountering many persons who fall, the one fact they share in common is that the fall was never expected. In contrast is the American football running back, who is sure to be tackled, or the bull rider at the rodeo, who realizes he will be thrown and strives to stay on the animal's back for at least 8 s. The data presented in this chapter highlights how common falls are in the elderly, especially in the dialysis population.

Preventing Falls Related to Medications

The prevention of a fall depends upon its etiology. Each patient should be assessed for the risk of a fall. Non-mechanical falls related to medications present real-world challenges because there is a benefit-risk ratio. Diabetes and blood pressure control have been shown to have better outcomes. Patients often rely on sedation and pain medications and are loathe to give up these types of therapy. Medications should be routinely reviewed with a practitioner, and patients should be assessed for any side effects, drug interactions, and for postural hypotension. Education, awareness, and suitable alternative therapy are the best options for many patients on multiple medications. Patients undergoing dialysis who are on antihypertensive medications must be closely monitored for hypotensive changes during treatment. The volume status and medication regimen should be appropriate. Patients on blood pressure medication must be closely watched at the end of their treatment when postural hypotension is most likely to occur.

Falls and Cognitive Decline

Falls related to permanent cognitive decline require the use of assistive devices such as a cane, walker, or wheelchair. This population also requires careful vigilance and aid because they cannot perform otherwise routine activities of daily living. The patient with a previous stroke may have a gait or balance disorder. Strategies to fall-proof one's environment may prevent a mechanical fall in an impaired patient. Despite the best efforts of providers and family, the patient with cognitive impairment or frailty may still fall. To the extent possible, maneuvers to mitigate the consequences of a fall should be considered. These can include assurance of adequate nutrition—particularly in the dialysis patient. Exercise programs may offer some benefits. These should include resistance exercises, balance exercises, stretching, and ambulation with assistance within limitations.

Randomized controlled trials in subjects aged 60 years and older reveal moderate evidence that intervention through mechanisms to improve nutrition is associated with improvement in cognitive markers. Protein, fatty acids, and polyphenols may improve specific cognitive domains, but the evidence is conflicting [50]. Twenty-five hemodialysis patients with low Montreal Cognitive Assessment results were randomized to treatment with thiamin combined with folic acid vs. no treatment. The study lasted 96 weeks. The treatment group had lower serum homocysteine levels ($p < 0.05$) and improvement in the MoCA score ($p < 0.001$). The treatment group also observed a lower mortality rate [51].

Patients with Chronic Illnesses

The elderly patient with a secondary chronic illness presents a common, unanticipated fall risk. The clinician should identify gait, muscle strength, and ability to balance. Referral to physical therapy may be beneficial for some patients. Personal trainers specializing in senior fitness management are also knowledgeable and can help patients reduce the incidence of falls through resistance and balance training exercises. Tai Chi classes focus on fall prevention and may be an enjoyable and rewarding way to decrease the likelihood of a tumble.

Patients with peripheral neuropathy or arthritis have an increased risk of falling. While medications can alleviate pain and discomfort, the use of an assistive device may be helpful to enable the patient to maintain balance. Appropriate footwear can help some patients remain steady.

Visual and auditory disturbances can contribute to falls. Retinopathy is common in diabetic patients, and the elderly often have glaucoma, cataracts, or macular degeneration. Decreased hearing can impact awareness of surroundings and may be a risk for the elderly patient crossing a busy street. Routine visits to eye and ear specialists can help alleviate many potential problems.

Preserving Muscle and Bone Loss

The growth pathways that build muscle can be controlled. Eating essential amino acids and exercise training will promote protein muscle synthesis [52]. Thus, exercise and a sensible diet can combat the muscle protein breakdown that naturally accompanies aging and kidney disease. Furthermore, controlling metabolic acidosis helps decrease the proteasome breakdown of muscle. Immobility, whether sitting or reclining, decreased muscle mass.

A systemic review of 27 clinical studies adjusted for bias included 1,156 participants undergoing peritoneal or hemodialysis. The studies demonstrated that the 6-min walk test distance, sit-to-stand repetitions, grip strength, stair climbing, dynamic mobility, and physical performance improved with exercise [53].

Walking may be beneficial to improve exercise tolerance, reduce BMI, improve cardiovascular status, blood pressure control, and quality of life [54]. The use of wristwatches with built-in accelerometers documents daily activity. In a nonblinded study of 73 participants with a mean age of 66.5 years spent an average of one hour a day walking, engaged in moderate-intensity activity for 0.7 h per day, and were sedentary for 13.2 h per day. Dialysis patients were less active than healthy controls, 15.5 milligravity units vs. 24.5 milligravity units, respectively [55].

Exercising may offer an additional advantage; it improves cognitive function in CKD. A randomized but unblinded 24-week study of patients ≥65 years with CKD patients not on dialysis demonstrated that structured group exercise training programs combined with home exercise significantly improved memory (exercise effect: 2.82, 95% CI: 0.46–5.19, $p = 0.03$) and recall scores (exercise effect: 5.97, 95% CI: 1.13–10.81, $p = 0.02$) [56].

Fall-Proofing One's Environment

The best way for an otherwise healthy person to avoid a fall is to anticipate it and be prepared. However, there are ways to minimize fall hazards in the home environment.

1. Add grab bars to showers and bathtubs.
2. Assure doorways are wide enough for a wheelchair.
3. Make sure bathroom floors are not slippery—use nonslip bathmats.
4. Add night lights to walls.
5. Minimize surprise steps that can be easily tripped over.
6. Assure that carpets are anchored and do not slip easily.
7. Do not leave clutter (clothes, shoes, papers) in the pathway.
8. Use electronic wrist alarms that can alert a friend, relative, or neighbor when one falls.
9. Encourage the elderly to wear a hat with a stiff rim to help buffer a fall when walking outside.
10. Make sure stairs have handrails.

An occupational therapist may also offer suggestions for fall-proofing one's home.

A program developed by the CDC, Stopping Elderly Accidences, Deaths & Injuries (STEADI) (SOURCE: https://www.cdc.gov/steadi/index.html accessed October 31, 2022), was adapted to chronic kidney disease patients in Staying Healthy with Kidney Disease [57].

Conclusion

Although falls are common in the elderly and patients with chronic kidney disease, they are primarily unanticipated. Anticipating the risk of a fall, when possible correcting underlying medical conditions, and in others, increasing strength and balance may reduce the incidence and damage related to a fall. Many patients will need an assistive device and increased vigilance because they are either cognitively impaired, frail, or have had a previous stroke. Creating a safe environment by fall-proofing, the home may be a simple step to help reduce the incidence of a serious fall.

Elderly patients undergoing dialysis are at a very high risk of falling and require an assessment to minimize the chance of a severe injury. The risk of falling is highest at the end of the dialysis treatment and may be related to postural hypotension.

References

1. Britting S, Artzi-Medvedik R, Fabbietti P, Tap L, Mattace-Raso F, Corsonello A, et al. Kidney function and other factors and their association with falls : the screening for CKD among older people across Europe (SCOPE) study. BMC Geriatr. 2020;20(Suppl 1):320. https://doi.org/10.1186/s12877-020-01698-2.
2. Abdel-Rahman EM, Turgut F, Turkmen K, Balogun RA. Falls in elderly hemodialysis patients. QJM. 2011;104(10):829–38. https://doi.org/10.1093/qjmed/hcr108.
3. Roberts RG, Kenny RA, Brierley EJ. Are elderly haemodialysis patients at risk of falls and postural hypotension? Int Urol Nephrol. 2003;35(3):415–21. https://doi.org/10.1023/b:uro l.0000022866.07751.4a.
4. López-Soto PJ, De Giorgi A, Senno E, Tiseo R, Ferraresi A, Canella C, et al. Renal disease and accidental falls: a review of published evidence. BMC Nephrol. 2015;16:176. https://doi.org/10.1186/s12882-015-0173-7.
5. Morse JM, Black C, Oberle K, Donahue P. A prospective study to identify the fall-prone patient. Soc Sci Med. 1989;28(1):81–6. https://doi.org/10.1016/0277-9536(89)90309-2.
6. Kono K, Nishida Y, Yabe H, Moriyama Y, Mori T, Shiraki R, et al. Development and validation of a fall risk assessment index for dialysis patients. Clin Exp Nephrol. 2018;22(1):167–72. https://doi.org/10.1007/s10157-017-1431-8.
7. Leggett AN, Polenick CA, Maust DT, Kales HC. Falls and hospitalizations among persons with dementia and associated caregiver emotional difficulties. Gerontologist. 2018;58(2):e78–86. https://doi.org/10.1093/geront/gnx202.
8. Morley JE, Vellas B, van Kan GA, Anker SD, Bauer JM, Bernabei R, et al. Frailty consensus: a call to action. J Am Med Dir Assoc. 2013;14(6):392–7. https://doi.org/10.1016/j.jamda.2013.03.022.
9. Searle SD, Mitnitski A, Gahbauer EA, Gill TM, Rockwood K. A standard procedure for creating a frailty index. BMC Geriatr. 2008;8(1):24. https://doi.org/10.1186/1471-2318-8-24.
10. Lu Z, Er Y, Zhan Y, Deng X, Jin Y, Ye P, et al. Association of Frailty status with risk of fall among middle-aged and older adults in China: a nationally representative cohort study. J Nutr Health Aging. 2021;25(8):985–92. https://doi.org/10.1007/s12603-021-1655-x.
11. Bolla LR, Filley CM, Palmer RM. Dementia DDx. Office diagnosis of the four major types of dementia. Geriatrics. 2000;55(1):34–7, 41–2, 5–6.
12. Semrau M, Sartorius N. What is new within staging of care for people with dementia? The IDEAL schedule and other recent work. Curr Opin Psychiatry. 2019;32(4):366–71. https://doi.org/10.1097/yco.0000000000000508.
13. Allan LM, Ballard CG, Rowan EN, Kenny RA. Incidence and prediction of falls in dementia: a prospective study in older people. PLoS One. 2009;4(5):e5521. https://doi.org/10.1371/journal.pone.0005521.
14. Power A. Stroke in dialysis and chronic kidney disease. Blood Purif. 2013;36(3–4):179–83. https://doi.org/10.1159/000356086.
15. Jin J, Wen S, Li Y, Zhou M, Duan Q, Zhou L. Factors associated with higher falling risk in elderly diabetic patients with lacunar stroke. BMC Endocr Disord. 2022;22(1):198. https://doi.org/10.1186/s12902-022-01122-3.
16. Sibbritt D, Bayes J, Peng W, Maguire J, Ladanyi S, Adams J. The association between fatigue severity and risk of falls among middle-aged and older Australian stroke survivors. Aging Clin Exp Res. 2022;34:2457. https://doi.org/10.1007/s40520-022-02179-9.
17. Bower K, Thilarajah S, Pua Y-H, Williams G, Tan D, Mentiplay B, et al. Dynamic balance and instrumented gait variables are independent predictors of falls following stroke. J Neuroeng Rehabil. 2019;16(1):3. https://doi.org/10.1186/s12984-018-0478-4.
18. Pang MY, Eng JJ. Fall-related self-efficacy, not balance and mobility performance, is related to accidental falls in chronic stroke survivors with low bone mineral density. Osteoporos Int. 2008;19(7):919–27. https://doi.org/10.1007/s00198-007-0519-5.

19. Xue L, Boudreau RM, Donohue JM, Zgibor JC, Marcum ZA, Costacou T, et al. Persistent polypharmacy and fall injury risk: the health, aging and body composition study. BMC Geriatr. 2021;21(1):710. https://doi.org/10.1186/s12877-021-02695-9.
20. Abu Bakar AA, Abdul Kadir A, Idris NS, Mohd Nawi SN. Older adults with hypertension: prevalence of falls and their associated factors. Int J Environ Res Public Health. 2021;18(16):8257. https://doi.org/10.3390/ijerph18168257.
21. Anderson TS, Jing B, Auerbach A, Wray CM, Lee S, Boscardin WJ, et al. Clinical outcomes after intensifying antihypertensive medication regimens among older adults at hospital discharge. JAMA Intern Med. 2019;179(11):1528–36. https://doi.org/10.1001/jamainternmed.2019.3007.
22. Tinetti ME, Han L, Lee DSH, McAvay GJ, Peduzzi P, Gross CP, et al. Antihypertensive medications and serious fall injuries in a nationally representative sample of older adults. JAMA Intern Med. 2014;174(4):588–95. https://doi.org/10.1001/jamainternmed.2013.14764.
23. Yang Y, Hu X, Zhang Q, Zou R. Diabetes mellitus and risk of falls in older adults: a systematic review and meta-analysis. Age Ageing. 2016;45(6):761–7. https://doi.org/10.1093/ageing/afw140.
24. KDIGO. 2020 clinical practice guideline for diabetes management in chronic kidney disease. Kidney Int. 2020;98(4s):S1–S115. https://doi.org/10.1016/j.kint.2020.06.019.
25. Fonseca V, Kohzuma T, Galindo RJ, DeSouza C. KDIGO recommendations for the evaluation of glycemic control in advanced chronic kidney disease. Kidney Int. 2022;101(2):420. https://doi.org/10.1016/j.kint.2021.11.020.
26. Isshiki K, Nishio T, Isono M, Makiishi T, Shikano T, Tomita K, et al. Glycated albumin predicts the risk of mortality in type 2 diabetic patients on hemodialysis: evaluation of a target level for improving survival. Ther Apher Dial. 2014;18(5):434–42. https://doi.org/10.1111/1744-9987.12123.
27. Jackson MA, Holland MR, Nicholas J, Lodwick R, Forster D, Macdonald IA. Hemodialysis-induced hypoglycemia in diabetic patients. Clin Nephrol. 2000;54(1):30–4.
28. Battistella M, Ng P. Addressing polypharmacy in outpatient dialysis units. Clin J Am Soc Nephrol. 2021;16(1):144. https://doi.org/10.2215/CJN.05270420.
29. Kutner NG, Zhang R, Huang Y, Wasse H. Falls among hemodialysis patients: potential opportunities for prevention? Clin Kidney J. 2014;7(3):257–63. https://doi.org/10.1093/ckj/sfu034.
30. Angalakuditi MV, Gomes J, Coley KC. Impact of drug use and comorbidities on in-hospital falls in patients with chronic kidney disease. Ann Pharmacother. 2007;41(10):1638–43. https://doi.org/10.1345/aph.1H631.
31. Wang H-H, Wu J-L, Lee Y-C, Ho L-C, Chang M-Y, Liou H-H, et al. Risk of serious falls between hemodialysis and peritoneal dialysis patients: a nationwide population-based cohort study. Sci Rep. 2020;10(1):7799. https://doi.org/10.1038/s41598-020-64698-7.
32. Chang JT, Ganz DA. Quality indicators for falls and mobility problems in vulnerable elders. J Am Geriatr Soc. 2007;55(Suppl 2):S327–34. https://doi.org/10.1111/j.1532-5415.2007.01339.x.
33. Heybeli C, Kazancioglu R, Smith L, Veronese N, Soysal P. Risk factors for high fall risk in elderly patients with chronic kidney disease. Int Urol Nephrol. 2022;54(2):349–56. https://doi.org/10.1007/s11255-021-02884-w.
34. Goto NA, Hamaker ME, Willems HC, Verhaar MC, Emmelot-Vonk MH. Accidental falling in community-dwelling elderly with chronic kidney disease. Int Urol Nephrol. 2019;51(1):119–27. https://doi.org/10.1007/s11255-018-1992-9.
35. Bu F, Abell J, Zaninotto P, Fancourt D. A longitudinal analysis of loneliness, social isolation and falls amongst older people in England. Sci Rep. 2020;10(1):20064. https://doi.org/10.1038/s41598-020-77104-z.
36. Shuyi O, Zheng C, Lin Z, Zhang X, Li H, Fang Y, et al. Risk factors of falls in elderly patients with visual impairment. Front Public Health. 2022;10:984199. https://doi.org/10.3389/fpubh.2022.984199.

37. Verghese J, LeValley A, Hall CB, Katz MJ, Ambrose AF, Lipton RB. Epidemiology of gait disorders in community-residing older adults. J Am Geriatr Soc. 2006;54(2):255–61. https://doi.org/10.1111/j.1532-5415.2005.00580.x.
38. Verghese J, Ambrose AF, Lipton RB, Wang C. Neurological gait abnormalities and risk of falls in older adults. J Neurol. 2010;257(3):392–8. https://doi.org/10.1007/s00415-009-5332-y.
39. Craig JJ, Bruetsch AP, Huisinga JM. Coordination of trunk and foot acceleration during gait is affected by walking velocity and fall history in elderly adults. Aging Clin Exp Res. 2019;31(7):943–50. https://doi.org/10.1007/s40520-018-1036-4.
40. Thaler-Kall K, Peters A, Thorand B, Grill E, Autenrieth CS, Horsch A, et al. Description of spatio-temporal gait parameters in elderly people and their association with history of falls: results of the population-based cross-sectional KORA-age study. BMC Geriatr. 2015;15(1):32. https://doi.org/10.1186/s12877-015-0032-1.
41. Rajan V, Mitch WE. Ubiquitin, proteasomes and proteolytic mechanisms activated by kidney disease. Biochim Biophys Acta. 2008;1782(12):795–9. https://doi.org/10.1016/j.bbadis.2008.07.007.
42. Reid MB. Response of the ubiquitin-proteasome pathway to changes in muscle activity. Am J Physiol Regul Integr Comp Physiol. 2005;288(6):R1423–31. https://doi.org/10.1152/ajpregu.00545.2004.
43. Yeung SSY, Reijnierse EM, Pham VK, Trappenburg MC, Lim WK, Meskers CGM, et al. Sarcopenia and its association with falls and fractures in older adults: a systematic review and meta-analysis. J Cachexia Sarcopenia Muscle. 2019;10(3):485–500. https://doi.org/10.1002/jcsm.12411.
44. Hamrick I, Norton D, Birstler J, Chen G, Cruz L, Hanrahan L. Association between dehydration and falls. Mayo Clin Proc Innov Qual Outcomes. 2020;4(3):259–65. https://doi.org/10.1016/j.mayocpiqo.2020.01.003.
45. Canaud B, Kooman JP, Selby NM, Taal MW, Francis S, Maierhofer A, et al. Dialysis-induced cardiovascular and multiorgan morbidity. Kidney Int Rep. 2020;5(11):1856–69. https://doi.org/10.1016/j.ekir.2020.08.031.
46. Doré AL, Golightly YM, Mercer VS, Shi XA, Renner JB, Jordan JM, et al. Lower-extremity osteoarthritis and the risk of falls in a community-based longitudinal study of adults with and without osteoarthritis. Arthritis Care Res (Hoboken). 2015;67(5):633–9. https://doi.org/10.1002/acr.22499.
47. Tinetti ME, Williams TF, Mayewski R. Fall risk index for elderly patients based on number of chronic disabilities. Am J Med. 1986;80(3):429–34. https://doi.org/10.1016/0002-9343(86)90717-5.
48. Berlie HD, Garwood CL. Diabetes medications related to an increased risk of falls and fall-related morbidity in the elderly. Ann Pharmacother. 2010;44(4):712–7. https://doi.org/10.1345/aph.1M551.
49. Zhu H, Hu K, Liu S, Kim HC, Wang Y, Xue Q. Systematic causality mapping of factors leading to accidental falls of older adults. Public Health Pract (Oxf). 2020;1:100045. https://doi.org/10.1016/j.puhip.2020.100045.
50. Solfrizzi V, Agosti P, Lozupone M, Custodero C, Schilardi A, Valiani V, et al. Nutritional intervention as a preventive approach for cognitive-related outcomes in cognitively healthy older adults: a systematic review. J Alzheimers Dis. 2018;64(S1):S229–54. https://doi.org/10.3233/jad-179940.
51. Lu R, Fang Y, Zhou Y, Che M, Shen J, Liu Q, et al. A pilot study of thiamin and folic acid in hemodialysis patients with cognitive impairment. Ren Fail. 2021;43(1):766–73. https://doi.org/10.1080/0886022x.2021.1914656.
52. Semba RD, Trehan I, Gonzalez-Freire M, Kraemer K, Moaddel R, Ordiz MI, et al. Perspective: the potential role of essential amino acids and the mechanistic target of rapamycin complex 1 (mTORC1) pathway in the pathogenesis of child stunting. Adv Nutr. 2016;7(5):853–65. https://doi.org/10.3945/an.116.013276.
53. Clarkson MJ, Bennett PN, Fraser SF, Warmington SA. Exercise interventions for improving objective physical function in patients with end-stage kidney disease on dialysis: a system-

atic review and meta-analysis. Am J Physiol Renal Physiol. 2019;316(5):F856–72. https://doi.org/10.1152/ajprenal.00317.2018.
54. Kosmadakis GC, John SG, Clapp EL, Viana JL, Smith AC, Bishop NC, et al. Benefits of regular walking exercise in advanced pre-dialysis chronic kidney disease. Nephrol Dial Transplant. 2012;27(3):997–1004. https://doi.org/10.1093/ndt/gfr364.
55. Nawab KA, Storey BC, Staplin N, Walmsley R, Haynes R, Sutherland S, et al. Accelerometer-measured physical activity and functional behaviours among people on dialysis. Clin Kidney J. 2021;14(3):950–8. https://doi.org/10.1093/ckj/sfaa045.
56. Otobe Y, Yamada M, Hiraki K, Onari S, Taki Y, Sumi H, et al. Physical exercise improves cognitive function in older adults with stage 3-4 chronic kidney disease: a randomized controlled trial. Am J Nephrol. 2021;52(12):929–39. https://doi.org/10.1159/000520230.
57. Fadem SZ. Falls in CKD patients and seniors: causes and prevention. In: Fadem SZ, editor. Staying healthy with kidney disease: a complete guide for patients. Cham: Springer International Publishing; 2022. p. 103–12.

Muscle Wasting in Kidney Disease

20

Stephen Z. Fadem

Introduction

Muscle wasting, commonly seen in both aging and in patients with kidney disease, is associated with a worsened quality of life and poor prognosis. Muscle fibers can learn repetitive tasks, and thus intact muscles are essential for balance and movement. They are in a constant state of breakdown and regrowth and respond quickly to environmental stimuli. The major pathways of muscle protein breakdown include ubiquitin-proteasome (UPS) digestion, lysosome-related autophagy, and apoptosis. CKD and its attendant morbidities are associated with the breakdown of muscle through insulin resistance, metabolic acidosis, angiotensin II, malnutrition, immobility, an impaired microRNA response, and inflammation. Inflammation activates UPS through myostatin, a member of the TGF beta family that is produced by myocytes. Muscle protein synthesis can be improved through the consumption of essential amino acids, resistance exercise, and decreased inflammation. Early treatment of metabolic acidosis and kidney disease may reverse the fibrosis associated with muscle breakdown.

What Causes Muscle Protein Loss?

Malnutrition and Hypoalbuminemia

Albumin is a negatively charged, water-soluble molecule that is synthesized by the liver. In the setting of negligible protein intake, its production by the liver decreases,

S. Z. Fadem (✉)
Section of Nephrology, Department of Medicine, Baylor College of Medicine, Houston, TX, USA
e-mail: fadem@bcm.edu

S. Z. Fadem et al. (eds.), *Complications in Dialysis*,
https://doi.org/10.1007/978-3-031-44557-6_20

leading to hypoalbuminemia. Yet, albumin synthesis is synchronized to dietary protein intake. When protein intake is decreased, albumin degradation decreases. Amino acid feeding immediately increases protein and albumin synthesis. A low serum albumin accompanies poor nutrition and a poor prognosis, despite the fact that major observations dissociate nutrition and serum albumin. Persons with anorexia nervosa have a loss of body mass that is distanced from any disease state yet maintain their serum albumin levels unless their health status approaches death. The Modification of Diet in Renal Disease (MDRD) study restricted dietary protein intake to 0.56 g/kg/day, yet the serum albumin levels remained >4 mg/dL [1].

The optimal time for dialysis was increased from one to three times a week through clinical observation over a three-year period in Seattle and balanced well-being with cost restraint. Later on, a mathematical relationship between urea equilibrium and the removal of solutes was established as the single pool Kt/V (spKt/V). The use of this formula in the National Cooperative Dialysis Study led the renal community to think that only when the spKt/V fell to less than 0.8 was the clinical outcome worse, resulting in shorter dialysis times. Shorter dialysis was supported by the confluence of industrial advancement, regulatory and economic necessity, and patient convenience. It was noted by the end of the 1980s that the mortality rate in the USA was worse than that of other countries that had longer treatment times [2]. This was associated with increased malnutrition in dialysis patients, and it was suggested that intradialytic parenteral nutrition (IDPN) could improve the nutritional status of malnourished dialysis patients [3]. Uremic factors activate protein-calorie malnutrition that continues until the uremic process is reversed, and it was not surprising that IDPN studies in conjunction with oral supplements did not improve mortality rate, BMI, or nutritional status when compared with oral supplements alone [4]. By 2010, there was still insufficient evidence that IDPN fed to malnourished patients bestowed either benefit or harm [5]. The more likely explanation for the low serum albumin in CKD has to do with the consequence of protein breakdown—uremic toxins, metabolic acidosis, angiotensin II, inflammation, and insulin resistance, factors that also contribute to muscle breakdown.

The Ubiquitin-Proteasome System (UPS) (See Fig. 20.1)

Muscle protein half-lives are carefully regulated. During starvation, immobility, sepsis, or acidosis, there is a preferential breakdown of muscle proteins to amino acids that can be either consumed for energy (isoleucine, leucine, valine) or transported to the liver for gluconeogenesis. This is done through the process of ubiquitination.

Ubiquitin is a 76 amino acid protein that is preserved through the evolution of eukaryotic cells from yeast to humans. These small proteins require metabolic energy and are activated by an ATP-AMP exchange starting with a ubiquitin-activating enzyme (E1) which is then conjugated by the E2 enzyme. In the final step, E3 ubiquitin ligase binds the c-terminus glycine of ubiquitin to the lysine amino acid of the target molecule or to another ubiquitin. Once tagged with five or

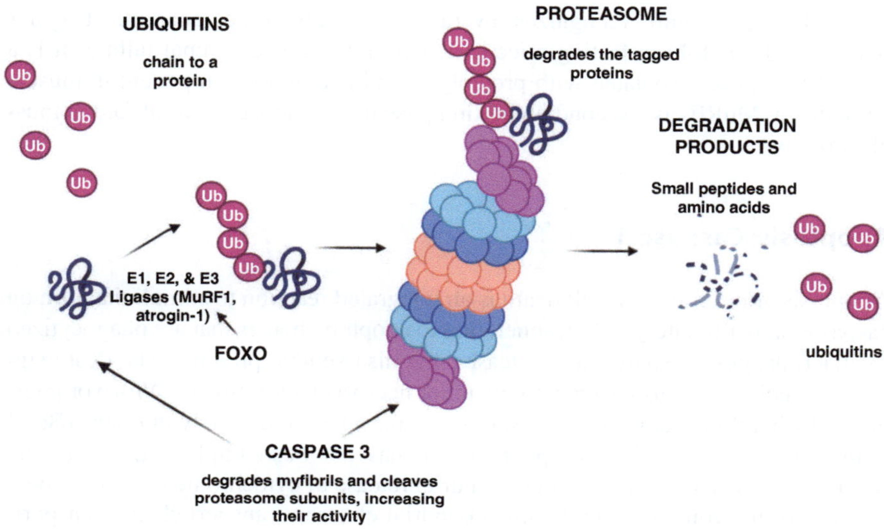

Fig. 20.1 Various stimuli activate ligases to tag ubiquitin to a targeted muscle breakdown product. The tagged complex is then degraded by the proteasome, and the small peptides are recycled. (Created with Biorender—(http://biorender.com))

more ubiquitin residues, the targeted chain is led to a 26S proteasome, a large barrel-shaped protease complex, where the protein is unfolded, degraded, and sent for recycling. For working out the multi-step ubiquitin-tagging hypothesis, isolating the three enzyme activities, and discovering the role of proteasomal degradation, Aaron Ciechanover, Avram Hershko, and Irwin Rose were awarded the Nobel Prize in 2004. The UPS is involved in DNA repair and transcription, protein quality control, the immune response, the hypoxia-inducible factor (HIF) activation leading to the erythropoietin synthesis, the degradation of damaged muscle fibers, and the cell cycle itself [6].

Uremia increases the mRNAs for ubiquitin, as does diabetes. Glucocorticoids are required for the mRNA encoding of ubiquitin and additionally promote muscle catabolism by inhibiting amino acid transport into muscle. Insulin opposes glucocorticoids, suppressing protein breakdown, but glucocorticoids in a non-fasting state can overcome the inhibition of insulin on muscle wasting.

Metabolic acidosis results in the conversion of amino acids from muscle protein to glutamine when glucocorticoids are present. Metabolic acidosis upregulates the mRNAs that encode the E2 conjugating enzyme, ubiquitin, and proteasomal subunits in the skeletal muscle [7].

Cytokines, along with glucocorticoids, also stimulate the UPS [8]. The suppression of E3 ligases associated with ubiquitination, atrogin-1, and MuRF1 prevents glucocorticoid-induced UPS activity [9]. Vitamin D deficiency, angiotensin II, inflammation, and insulin resistance also activate the UPS [10].

The E3 ligase family recognizes several of the targets of degradation. Atrogin-1 is increased ninefold in fasting mice and also in diabetes and renal failure. It is a critical E3 ligase associated with proteolysis and is a major component in muscle breakdown. MuRF1 is a second ubiquitin ligase that is induced several fold in muscle atrophy.

Apoptosis: Caspase 3

Apoptosis or programmed cell death is an integrated reaction to stimuli that turn on caspases and, ultimately, cell degeneration to apoptotic bodies that are phagocytized by macrophages. Caspases are proteases that disassemble proteins. The death signals can include extrinsic signaling by tumor necrosis factor-alpha *(TNF-a)* or internal mitochondrial pathways in response to the altered B-cell lymphoma (Bcl2) family proteins. Bcl2 is anti-apoptotic but has not been implicated in muscle. Intrinsic factors can signal the mitochondrial release of cytochrome C. Cytochrome C is one of the complexes in the mitochondrial electron-transport chain, transporting electrons between cytochrome III and IV. It is tightly anchored to the mitochondrion by cardiolipin. Reactive oxygen species (ROS) leads to the oxidation of cardiolipin, liberating cytochrome C from its anchored position and enabling its escape to the cytoplasm. Here it normally binds with apoptosis protease activating factor 1 (apaf1), caspase 9, and ATP. Caspase 9 activates caspase 7 and caspase 3. Cytochrome C can both be stimulated by increase in calcium and can potentiate the release of calcium from the endoplasmic reticulum.

In muscle cells, caspase 3 is involved in proteolytic enzyme processes that result in cell atrophy. It is involved in the cleavage of the subunits Rpt2 and Rpt6 from the 26S proteasome, amplifying its proteolytic activity. Caspase 3 has been shown to increase 14 kD actin fragments in rodent models by cleaving actin in the actomyosin complex. 14 kD actin fragments are biomarkers of muscle degradation and are elevated in CKD, in hemodialysis patients, and in post-operative hip surgery patients. In hemodialysis patients, 14kD actin fragments decrease with 18 weeks of endurance exercise. Caspase generally does not completely destroy muscle cells, but apoptosis is involved in the destruction of muscle nuclei in cases of disuse and aging [11].

Autophagy

Lysosomes are spherical organelles that enclose enzymes designed to digest worn-out cellular parts. This is an internal process that culminates in autophagy. Autophagy is appropriately named for the term literally means self-digestion. Aside from proteasomal degradation and to a far lesser extent, apoptosis, autophagy also plays a scripted role in the necessary breakdown of worn-out or defective organelles. It is regulated by the interplay between factors that stimulate the inhibition of the mammalian target of rapamycin (mTORC1) and those that stimulate it (FoxO). FoxO stands for Forkhead box, class O, and is a family of transcription factors that are targeted by the phosphoinositide-3-kinase (PI3K) and discussed below. When phosphorylated, they translocate to the nucleus and promote the transcription of genes associated with survival. They play key roles in autophagy. By inducing the E3 ligases, atrogin-1, and MuRF1, they also play a role in UPS. These pathways can control the cell recycling process, a conservation step that can be potentiated by starvation and is essential to survival. They are sensitive to external factors such as inflammation, diet, and fasting [12, 13].

Once a cellular target is identified, it is engulfed by an autophagophore that then elongates to become an autophagosome. The autophagosome then fuses with the lysosome forming the autophagolysosome. The autophagolysosome contains acidic proteases that degrade the targeted cellular components.

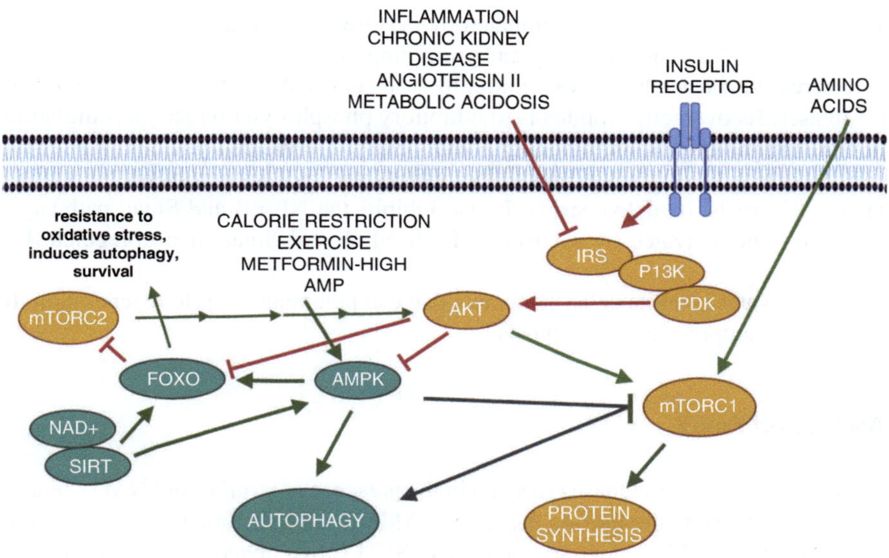

Fig. 20.2 Calorie restriction activates a system that either conserves energy through *AMPK* and turns on *FoxO*, a transcription enzyme that helps protect the cell from starvation and oxidative stress. Insulin, in the abundance of glucose, turns on an enzyme system that blocks *AMPK* and stimulates *mTORC1* to make proteins. The breakdown and synthesis of muscles are balanced, and both are necessary for healthy muscle function. *Akt* both stimulates *mTORC1* and is stimulated by mTORC2. (Mammalian/Mechanistic Target of Rapamycin Complex)—controls protein synthesis. FoxO (Forkhead Box Class O) proteins—stimulates (through transcription) resistance to oxidative stress and induces autophagy. *NAD* Nicotinamide adenine dinucleotide—is an essential cofactor that is involved in electron transfer and enzyme processes. *SIRT*—sirtuin (silent mating-type information regulation) moves acyl groups in enzyme reactions. It requires NAD+ and works along the sensing enzyme *AMPK* (AMP-activated protein kinase) senses low energy states—ATP/AMP ratios and switches on autophagy and lipid oxidation while switching off lipid, protein, and glucose synthesis—gluconeogenesis. Other abbreviations: *Akt* (Ak Strain Transforming—also Protein Kinase B), *IRS* insulin receptor substrate, *P13K* phosphoinositide 3-kinase, *PDK* 3′-phosphoinositide-dependent kinase-1. (Created with Biorender—(http://biorender.com))

The Metabolic Pathway (See Fig. 20.2)

Glucose entry into the cell is through glucose transporter-4 and is regulated through the binding of insulin to its receptor (IGF-1). Glucose entry is increased in the presence of insulin, while in fasting, insulin levels decrease. The insulin receptor substrate-1 (IRS-1) is not an enzyme but interacts directly with the insulin and IGF-1 receptor, and any hindrance affects downstream insulin signaling. It is implicated as a factor in insulin resistance. Proteasomal degradation of IRS-1 is increased by the inflammatory cytokine IL-6, delaying or inhibiting IRS-1 from complexing to phosphoinositide-3-kinase (PI3K), and activating the serine-threonine kinase, Akt1.

Akt1 is an enzyme that was derived from the studies of oncogenes. It is also referred to as protein kinase B. The deacetylation of Akt1 activates the glut 4 transporter, GLUT4, which leads to glucose entry. Akt1 can be blocked by several factors, including Nf-κB, angiotensin II, reactive oxygen species, and uremic toxins such as p-cresyl sulfate. It is stimulated by mTORC2 but results in the stimulation of mTORC1, blocking autophagy and promoting protein synthesis.

Decreased Akt leads to muscle atrophy, very likely through FoxO activation of E3 ligases. Its overactivation leads to inhibitory phosphorylation and accumulation of FoxO in the cytoplasm, blocking FoxO's entry into the cell nucleus. When Akt activity is low, FoxO translocates to the nucleus and induces autophagy, as well as factors that resist oxidative stress. It also inhibits the NF-κB and Smad pathways. Smad may be activated by myostatin. Both NFκb and Smad also upregulate E3 ligases.

Akt activates satellite cells, stem cells that can potentiate muscle regeneration. It induces the suppression of apoptosis.

AMPK and FoxO

AMP-activated protein kinase (AMPK) in the presence of sirtuins and NAD+ senses low energy states by monitoring the ratio of AMP to ATP. Its function is to conserve energy essential ATP. It does so, along with SIRT1, by enhancing FoxO transcription activity [14]. It promotes glucose metabolism to generate ATP and also conserves ATP by activating the inhibition of mTORC1-induced protein synthesis.

Inside the nucleus, FoxO has a high affinity for DNA, and a FoxO-recognized element (FRE) has been identified. It is involved in the control of a wide range of biochemical processes, including the promotion of the pro-apoptotic gene, Fas ligand, and promoting mitochondria-independent apoptosis. In combination with SIRT1, it forms a complex in response to oxidative stress and induces cell-cycle arrest and oxidative stress resistance. It also promotes the scavenger proteins manganese superoxide dismutase and catalase [15, 16].

Although FoxO induces ubiquitin proteasomal degradation of muscle, and its actions with respect to muscle may be ambivalent, it is also central to muscle energy homeostasis and mitochondrial metabolism [17]. It is tempting to think that this "ambivalence" may be controlled by external factors such as a judicious diet and both resistance and endurance exercises.

Myostatin

Myostatin, a member of the transforming growth factor-ß superfamily, is a negative regulator of muscle protein synthesis. Myostatin blocks Akt phosphorylation. It is mediated through the activin receptors and phosphorylates Smad protein which potentiates E3 ligase activity and increases UPS breakdown. Myostatin is increased in chronic debilitating conditions such as HIV, cancer, and heart disease. It is also elevated in aging and CKD, but gene expression is lower in hemodialysis patients. It may be related to uremic toxins such as indoxyl sulfate.

Indoxyl sulfate is associated with increased reactive oxygen species, inflammatory cytokines, and the enhanced production of atrogin-1 and myostatin. It is suppressed in the presence of antioxidants [18]. Endurance exercise for 12 months in CKD patients not on dialysis increases myostatin levels regardless of whether randomized to balance or strength training. In a 12-month study of 151 non-dialysis CKD patients randomized to a combination of balance or strength training in combination with endurance, sarcopenia remained the same and did not worsen from baseline. The plasma myostatin levels increased from baseline. However after 12 months exercise training maintained muscle mass and prevented sarcopenia [19]. This was an unexpected finding since the skeletal muscle atrophy in dialysis patients has long been known to improve with exercise training [20].

Exercise and Muscle Growth

Using ultrasound to assess the cross-sectional area of muscle, it was shown that quadriceps muscle volume significantly increased from baseline ($p < 0.001$) following a 12-week exercise program in CKD patients [21]. While a sedentary lifestyle in dialysis patients contributes to morbidity, mortality, muscle atrophy, and functional capacity, clinical trials have demonstrated benefits from regular exercise. Twenty-one clinical trials were reviewed in a meta-analysis that included 667 participants. Aerobic capacity, walking capacity, and quality of life improved with over 8 weeks of combined and aerobic exercise [22]. Exercise training for 6 months increases cross-section fiber area by 46% and increases the muscle capillary networks [20].

Nutrition

Poor nutrition, to the extent associated with decreased circulating amino acids, can lead to stunted growth in children. The mTORC1 pathway requires amino acid availability to integrate protein synthesis. Starvation potentiates AMKP and FoxO and is associated with the inhibition of mTORC1 and the induction of autophagy as well as UPS breakdown of muscle [23]. The use of a low-protein diet along with ketoanalogues reduces the loss of glomerular function in patients with advanced CKD. Acidosis and hyperphosphatemia are also controlled [24]. The plant-based diet has become a popular and useful way to treat patients with advanced CKD, not on dialysis, providing adequate nutrition, and as well managing metabolic acidosis [25, 26]. Once the patient begins dialysis, either peritoneal or hemodialysis, protein calories are essential. In both modes, nitrogen balance is negative in diets providing less than 1.2 g protein/body weight per day. PD patients should receive at least 1.3 g protein/body weight per day. Dialysate losses of protein, as well as the catabolism that accompanies dialysis, may contribute to losses. Studies demonstrate that 1–2 g protein may be lost in the dialysate with conventional therapy. These may be much higher with high flux dialysis. Peritonitis may result in a 5 to 15-g protein loss [27]. Compromised protein intake in dialysis is associated with muscle atrophy.

Although the mechanisms that lead to muscle atrophy in CKD patients are highly complex, we can confirm that insulin resistance, metabolic acidosis, and inflammatory cytokines are joined by decreased nutrition as major factors [28].

Rescue with Dialysis

In a study of muscle fibrosis in patients with CKD, 14 patients with stages 3 and 4 underwent a muscle biopsy. Twenty patients with CKD stages 4 and 5 were biopsied. Muscle biopsies were also performed on 16 control subjects. Four of the previously biopsied CKD patients advanced to chronic kidney disease. Although patients with CKD demonstrated fibrotic transformation of muscle, downregulated angiogenesis, and altered pathways toward stem cell renewal, the initiation of dialysis was associated with decreased fibrosis, lessened muscle atrophy, and increased strength and endurance. The study demonstrated a relationship between worsening kidney function and progressive muscle fibrosis. Fibrosis was felt to result in a decrease in the density of capillaries that came into contact with muscle fibers, promoting intramuscular hypoxia. Angiogenesis also decreased. The associated fibrosis decreased satellite function and abundance, limiting muscle regeneration. Although this would be expected to increase HIF/Notch signaling, Notch signaling was downregulated in CKD. This pattern is similar to aging, where Notch signaling is also impaired in aging mice until exposed to the circulation of young mice. Although dialysis may not restore "youth serum" to the patient, it is likely that circulating uremic toxins present a circulating factor that impairs Notch signaling. The reduction in inflammation associated with rescue dialysis may also play a role in regenerating muscle fibers [29].

In another study, CKD patients were followed for 2 years. Changes in muscle mass and functional assessments vary, but changes in muscle mass occur as CKD advances and are most pronounced in the pre-dialysis population. These changes reversed in the second year in 39%. There were also decreases in muscle mass that occurred during dialysis. This also reversed the second year. The study concluded that loss in muscle mass could be reversed with dialysis. The study suggested that earlier starts of dialysis might prevent significant muscle losses [30]. The transcription factor, MyoD induces skeletal muscle differentiation and continues at low levels in adults. It is capable of activating satellite cells [31] and may be blunted in CKD [32].

While the mechanisms by which dialysis reversed muscle fibrosis have yet to be clarified, the results of this study are enticing and engendering hope. One must also anticipate that kidney transplantation would help reverse muscle fibrosis.

Test of Muscle Function

Physical activity is a risk factor for mortality in dialysis patients. It was shown that a 10-min-per-day increase in physical activity resulted in a 22% reduction in the risk of mortality. Other studies have confirmed a lower death risk with increased activity in patients with reduced kidney function. To encourage and support exercise in CKD, one must have valid means of measuring muscular fitness [33].

Locomotion and Balance

The National Institute on Aging has developed a royalty-free assessment tool known as the Short Physical Performance Battery (SPPB). The website http://sppbguide.com/ offers links to a smartphone app, training videos, and tips, as well as background articles. SPPB was evaluated in 1122 subjects over a four-year period. The subjects were not disabled at baseline, but those with the lowest performance scores were 4.2–4.9 fold as likely as those with the highest scores [34].

Lower limb function determines mobility limitation and is associated with sarcopenia. It is worse in aged patients. The time needed to stand ten times from a chair was assessed and found to change significantly ($p < 0.0001$) with age. It was initially described in 1985 [35]. An alternative version is to ask the patient to perform as many sit-to-stand repetitions as possible within a 60-s period. The modified sit-to-stand test correlates with the quadriceps thickness [36]. Another alternative is to have the patient stand from the sitting position five times as quickly as possible.

The sit-to-stand test is incorporated into the SPPB and is part of the scoring system. In addition to the sit-to-stand test, walking speed and standing balance were assessed. The methods for these tests were established in 1994 and administered to more than 5000 elderly individuals. Balance studies include the tandem, semi-tandem, and side-by-side stand for a minimum of 10 s each. In the semi-tandem stand, the heel of one foot is placed next to the side of the first toe of the other foot. This is a 10-s test and is followed by the full tandem test, where the patient places the heel of one foot (right or left) in front of the other and holds this position for 10 s. The side-to-side position is an alternate position. Walking speed is tested along an 8-foot course. Subjects are asked to walk 8 feet at their comfortable speed and can use an assistive device. The faster of two timed tests is used. The sit-to-stand test involves rising from a sitting position in a straight-backed chair five times as quickly as possible. Tests are scored between 0 and 4. In the 0 category, subjects are unable to complete the side-by-side stand. Category 1 subjects can complete the side-by-side test but cannot perform the semi-tandem stand for over 9 s. Category 2 subjects can complete the semi-tandem stand but are unable to successfully complete the full tandem stand for 2 s. Category 3 subjects can perform the full tandem stand for between 3 and 10 s, and the fourth category subjects can complete the full tandem stand for 10 s. For the sit-to-stand and the 8-foot walk, scores were determined between 0 and 4 depending on the ability to perform the tests and the speed needed to complete them. The tests correlated well with activities of daily living and with walking a half mile and climbing stairs [37].

The hand dynamometer is an affordable and reliable tool to measure isometric handgrip strength. The handgrip test is a means of assessing muscle strength in CKD and is a diagnostic tool for sarcopenia, measuring functional and physiological impairment. It is useful for assessing muscle mass and fitness in dialysis patients and can offer immediate feedback to patients and health professionals [38].

The SPPB and handgrip strength were used in a population of 35 dialysis patients with a mean age of 70.1 years old who completed the baseline assessment. Subjects were studied at baseline and 3 and 6 months. The baseline median SPPB score was 6, grip strength 55 kg, and gait speed 0.76 m/s. SPPB scores improved from the first to the third visit in 49% of the patients and declined in 28%. Grip strength also improved in 40% and declined in 24% at the third visit. Gait speed improved in 25% and declined in 21% by the third visit. Thirty-one percent were unable to perform the sit-to-stand study because of knee pain or the need to use their arms. The SPPB and hand grip assessment have been standardized and validated. They were found to be valuable in helping identify vulnerable patients in the elderly dialysis population.

Conclusions and Take-Home Messages

Muscle breakdown in hemodialysis patients leads to poor outcomes, decreased quality of life, falls, and frailty. The physiology of muscle is balanced by stimuli that induce breakdown as well as factors that rebuild muscle. Cellular processes tie into the energy-sparing pathways that involve glucose metabolism, Akt signaling, mTOR activation and inhibition, and FoxO and AMPK regulation. They can either lead to muscle protein synthesis or promote conservation-related breakdown and recycling. Both breakdown and regrowth need to be balanced for healthy muscle preservation. Uremic toxins, inflammation, metabolic acidosis, angiotensin II, immobility, and starvation promote muscle degradation. Judicious eating, the control of metabolic acidosis, endurance and resistance training, and the control of inflammation promote muscle building. Muscle breakdown can be rescued with adequate dialysis. Standardized tests can be used to assess muscle and gait function and help clinicians detect the most vulnerable members of the dialysis population.

References

1. Friedman AN, Fadem SZ. Reassessment of albumin as a nutritional marker in kidney disease. J Am Soc Nephrol. 2010;21(2):223–30. https://doi.org/10.1681/asn.2009020213.
2. Fadem S. Milestones in dialysis. Issues in dialysis. New York: Nova Science Publishers; 2012.
3. Chertow GM, Ling J, Lew NL, Lazarus JM, Lowrie EG. The association of intradialytic parenteral nutrition administration with survival in hemodialysis patients. Am J Kidney Dis. 1994;24(6):912–20. https://doi.org/10.1016/s0272-6386(12)81060-2.
4. Cano NJ, Fouque D, Roth H, Aparicio M, Azar R, Canaud B, et al. Intradialytic parenteral nutrition does not improve survival in malnourished hemodialysis patients: a 2-year multicenter, prospective, randomized study. J Am Soc Nephrol. 2007;18(9):2583–91. https://doi.org/10.1681/asn.2007020184.
5. Sigrist MK, Levin A, Tejani AM. Systematic review of evidence for the use of intradialytic parenteral nutrition in malnourished hemodialysis patients. J Ren Nutr. 2010;20(1):1–7. https://doi.org/10.1053/j.jrn.2009.08.003.
6. Nandi D, Tahiliani P, Kumar A, Chandu D. The ubiquitin-proteasome system. J Biosci. 2006;31(1):137–55. https://doi.org/10.1007/bf02705243.
7. Mutsvangwa T, Gilmore J, Squires JE, Lindinger MI, McBride BW. Chronic metabolic acidosis increases mRNA levels for components of the ubiquitin-mediated proteolytic pathway in skeletal muscle of dairy cows. J Nutr. 2004;134(3):558–61. https://doi.org/10.1093/jn/134.3.558.
8. Mitch WE, Goldberg AL. Mechanisms of muscle wasting—the role of the ubiquitin–proteasome pathway. N Engl J Med. 1996;335(25):1897–905. https://doi.org/10.1056/nejm199612193352507.
9. Castillero E, Alamdari N, Lecker SH, Hasselgren PO. Suppression of atrogin-1 and MuRF1 prevents dexamethasone-induced atrophy of cultured myotubes. Metabolism. 2013;62(10):1495–502. https://doi.org/10.1016/j.metabol.2013.05.018.
10. Rajan V, Mitch WE. Ubiquitin, proteasomes and proteolytic mechanisms activated by kidney disease. Biochim Biophys Acta. 2008;1782(12):795–9. https://doi.org/10.1016/j.bbadis.2008.07.007.
11. Dupont-Versteegden EE. Apoptosis in skeletal muscle and its relevance to atrophy. World J Gastroenterol. 2006;12(46):7463–6. https://doi.org/10.3748/wjg.v12.i46.7463.
12. Mammucari C, Milan G, Romanello V, Masiero E, Rudolf R, Del Piccolo P, et al. FoxO3 controls autophagy in skeletal muscle in vivo. Cell Metab. 2007;6(6):458–71. https://doi.org/10.1016/j.cmet.2007.11.001.
13. Masiero E, Agatea L, Mammucari C, Blaauw B, Loro E, Komatsu M, et al. Autophagy is required to maintain muscle mass. Cell Metab. 2009;10(6):507–15. https://doi.org/10.1016/j.cmet.2009.10.008.
14. Greer EL, Banko MR, Brunet A. AMP-activated protein kinase and FoxO transcription factors in dietary restriction-induced longevity. Ann N Y Acad Sci. 2009;1170:688–92. https://doi.org/10.1111/j.1749-6632.2009.04019.x.
15. Huang H, Tindall DJ. Dynamic FoxO transcription factors. J Cell Sci. 2007;120(15):2479–87. https://doi.org/10.1242/jcs.001222.
16. Yoshida T, Delafontaine P. Mechanisms of IGF-1-mediated regulation of skeletal muscle hypertrophy and atrophy. Cells. 2020;9(9):1970. https://doi.org/10.3390/cells9091970.
17. Sanchez AM, Candau RB, Bernardi H. FoxO transcription factors: their roles in the maintenance of skeletal muscle homeostasis. Cell Mol Life Sci. 2014;71(9):1657–71. https://doi.org/10.1007/s00018-013-1513-z.
18. Enoki Y, Watanabe H, Arake R, Sugimoto R, Imafuku T, Tominaga Y, et al. Indoxyl sulfate potentiates skeletal muscle atrophy by inducing the oxidative stress-mediated expression of myostatin and atrogin-1. Sci Rep. 2016;6:32084. https://doi.org/10.1038/srep32084.
19. Zhou Y, Hellberg M, Hellmark T, Höglund P, Clyne N. Muscle mass and plasma myostatin after exercise training: a substudy of Renal Exercise (RENEXC)-a randomized controlled trial. Nephrol Dial Transplant. 2021;36(1):95–103. https://doi.org/10.1093/ndt/gfz210. PMID: 31848626; PMCID: PMC7771980.

20. Kouidi E, Albani M, Natsis K, Megalopoulos A, Gigis P, Guiba-Tziampiri O, et al. The effects of exercise training on muscle atrophy in haemodialysis patients. Nephrol Dial Transplant. 1998;13(3):685–99. https://doi.org/10.1093/ndt/13.3.685.
21. Gould DW, Watson EL, Wilkinson TJ, Wormleighton J, Xenophontos S, Viana JL, et al. Ultrasound assessment of muscle mass in response to exercise training in chronic kidney disease: a comparison with MRI. J Cachexia Sarcopenia Muscle. 2019;10(4):748–55. https://doi.org/10.1002/jcsm.12429.
22. Huang M, Lv A, Wang J, Xu N, Ma G, Zhai Z, et al. Exercise training and outcomes in hemodialysis patients: systematic review and meta-analysis. Am J Nephrol. 2019;50(4):240–54. https://doi.org/10.1159/000502447.
23. Semba RD, Trehan I, Gonzalez-Freire M, Kraemer K, Moaddel R, Ordiz MI, et al. Perspective: the potential role of essential amino acids and the mechanistic target of rapamycin complex 1 (mTORC1) pathway in the pathogenesis of child stunting. Adv Nutr. 2016;7(5):853–65. https://doi.org/10.3945/an.116.013276.
24. Koppe L, Cassani de Oliveira M, Fouque D. Ketoacid analogues supplementation in chronic kidney disease and future perspectives. Nutrients. 2019;11(9):2071. https://doi.org/10.3390/nu11092071.
25. Joshi S, McMacken M, Kalantar-Zadeh K. Plant-based diets for kidney disease: a guide for clinicians. Am J Kidney Dis. 2021;77(2):287–96. https://doi.org/10.1053/j.ajkd.2020.10.003.
26. Kalantar-Zadeh K, Fouque D. Nutritional management of chronic kidney disease. N Engl J Med. 2017;377(18):1765–76. https://doi.org/10.1056/NEJMra1700312.
27. Wolfson M. Management of protein and energy intake in dialysis patients. J Am Soc Nephrol. 1999;10(10):2244–7. https://doi.org/10.1681/asn.V10102244.
28. Wang XH, Mitch WE, Price SR. Pathophysiological mechanisms leading to muscle loss in chronic kidney disease. Nat Rev Nephrol. 2022;18(3):138–52. https://doi.org/10.1038/s41581-021-00498-0.
29. Brightwell CR, Kulkarni AS, Paredes W, Zhang K, Perkins JB, Gatlin KJ, et al. Muscle fibrosis and maladaptation occur progressively in CKD and are rescued by dialysis. JCI Insight. 2021;6(24):e150112. https://doi.org/10.1172/jci.insight.150112.
30. John SG, Sigrist MK, Taal MW, McIntyre CW. Natural history of skeletal muscle mass changes in chronic kidney disease stage 4 and 5 patients: an observational study. PLoS One. 2013;8(5):e65372. https://doi.org/10.1371/journal.pone.0065372.
31. Wardle FC. Master control: transcriptional regulation of mammalian Myod. J Muscle Res Cell Motil. 2019;40(2):211–26. https://doi.org/10.1007/s10974-019-09538-6.
32. Zhang L, Wang XH, Wang H, Du J, Mitch WE. Satellite cell dysfunction and impaired IGF-1 signaling cause CKD-induced muscle atrophy. J Am Soc Nephrol. 2010;21(3):419–27. https://doi.org/10.1681/asn.2009060571.
33. Bakker EA, Zoccali C, Dekker FW, Eijsvogels TMH, Jager KJ. Assessing physical activity and function in patients with chronic kidney disease: a narrative review. Clin Kidney J. 2021;14(3):768–79. https://doi.org/10.1093/ckj/sfaa156.
34. Guralnik JM, Ferrucci L, Simonsick EM, Salive ME, Wallace RB. Lower-extremity function in persons over the age of 70 years as a predictor of subsequent disability. N Engl J Med. 1995;332(9):556–61. https://doi.org/10.1056/nejm199503023320902.
35. Csuka M, McCarty DJ. Simple method for measurement of lower extremity muscle strength. Am J Med. 1985;78(1):77–81. https://doi.org/10.1016/0002-9343(85)90465-6.
36. Costa MJC, Cavalcanti FCB, Bezerra SD, Araújo Filho JC, Fernandes J, Marinho PEM. Relationship between quadriceps thickness and 60-second sit-to-stand test in patients with chronic kidney disease. J Bras Nefrol. 2022;44(2):164–70. https://doi.org/10.1590/2175-8239-jbn-2021-0064.
37. Guralnik JM, Simonsick EM, Ferrucci L, Glynn RJ, Berkman LF, Blazer DG, et al. A short physical performance battery assessing lower extremity function: association with self-reported disability and prediction of mortality and nursing home admission. J Gerontol. 1994;49(2):M85–94. https://doi.org/10.1093/geronj/49.2.m85.
38. Leal VO, Mafra D, Fouque D, Anjos LA. Use of handgrip strength in the assessment of the muscle function of chronic kidney disease patients on dialysis: a systematic review. Nephrol Dial Transplant. 2011;26(4):1354–60. https://doi.org/10.1093/ndt/gfq487.

Disasters and Dialysis

21

Stephen Z. Fadem

Introduction

A disaster is a severe and sudden event that can cause loss of life, damage, and interruption of services. The size of the area involved depends upon the nature of the incident. Major natural disasters like wildfires, earthquakes, landslides, freezes, and hurricanes can affect geographical regions that extend over several miles. Other disasters include acts of terrorism, utility failures, and epidemics. The majority of disasters have features in common regarding dialysis care. Each can interrupt the ability to perform treatments through potential structural damage, lack of water, or lack of electricity. They may require disinfecting before reopening. Disasters may interfere with the accessibility of staff or patients to the facility. In worst-case examples, patients may have to temporarily relocate to a nearby facility. Thus care in a first responder facility may surge well above its natural capacity.

All disaster deployment efforts require incident command coordination, including facility operations departments, vendors, and state and federal authorities. While transportation and the availability of food, water, pharmaceuticals, and supplies are taken for granted as routine, a disastrous event can interfere with each. All disasters require ongoing support and open lines of communication with biomedical teams to ensure that dialysis machines and water systems remain operational during increased times of stressful use.

S. Z. Fadem (✉)
Section of Nephrology, Department of Medicine, Baylor College of Medicine,
Houston, TX, USA
e-mail: fadem@bcm.edu

S. Z. Fadem et al. (eds.), *Complications in Dialysis*,
https://doi.org/10.1007/978-3-031-44557-6_21

Hazard Preparation

Hazard assessment and disaster mitigation planning are essential preparatory steps. http://ready.gov has resources to help assess the potential for hazards to occur. A dialysis center must appreciate what types of disasters are likely, and design plans for each. The planning team should determine what local services are available and select a disaster planning committee. First responder units should be identified, and the committees should be aware of and collaborate with network, local, county, state, national, and dialysis company resources.

Next, the team should have maps of the general area, including where fire hydrants, water mains, storm drains, and electrical transformers are. They should be aware of the water, electrical, and gas feeds into the facility and have a working knowledge of how the emergency generator operates. They should know where fire extinguishers and emergency supply kits are located, know the exit routes, and how to emergently disconnect and evacuate a patient during treatment. They should review readily available topographical information and understand the surrounding areas most likely to flood.

While disasters have much in common, each category has specific mitigation strategies. As an illustrative example, this chapter will review the approach taken by DaVita Med Center (DMC) Dialysis Facility when Hurricane Harvey impacted the Houston community with torrential rains and floods in August 2017.

Illustrative Example: Hurricane Harvey—2017

DMC is a 72-station dialysis center, one of the largest in the nation, and the regular home center for 350 patients. It has a backup generator and a redundant water system. DMC has been through several previous crises and served as a reference center for patients transferred from New Orleans after Hurricane Katrina in August 2005 and as a first responder after Hurricane Ike pummeled Galveston, Texas, and then destroyed the Houston electrical grid in September 2008.

Houston is the nation's fourth largest city and has a sizeable end-stage kidney disease (ESKD) population. On August 23, 2017, a tropical depression in the Gulf of Mexico was charted as heading toward Corpus Christi, Texas. By Friday, August 25, 2017, Harvey made landfall near Rockport, Texas, as a Category 4 storm with 130 mph winds. Rockport is a small resort community southwest of Texas and along the Gulf of Mexico. Flooding in Rockport was not extensive, but wind forces were treacherous and highly destructive, completely damaging structures, blowing off roofs and, downing many trees and power poles, interrupting electrical services until power could be restored.

Hurricanes can be highly destructive through wind damage. (see Fig. 21.1). But a hurricane that stalls over water will accumulate precipitation that can be unloaded when landfall occurs. In anticipation, many dialysis facilities activated their disaster plans. The Monday-Wednesday-Friday (MWF) and Tuesday-Thursday-Friday (TTF) schedules were combined, and dialysis times were shortened. On Saturday,

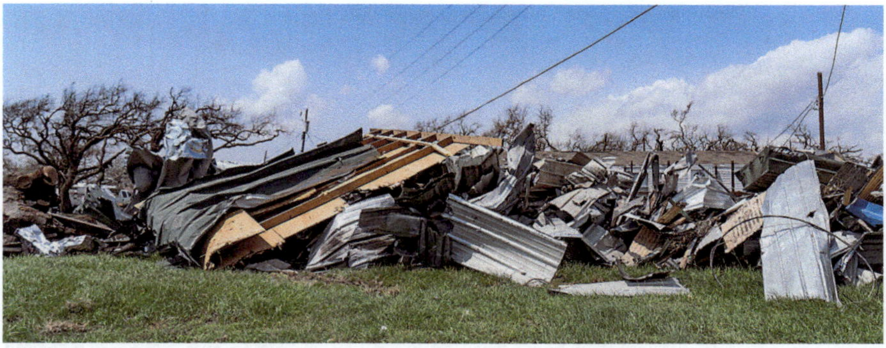

Fig. 21.1 Hurricane Harvey destroyed many sections of Rockport, Texas. (Photograph by Stephen Z. Fadem)

August 26, the rain was light, and DaVita Med Center continued truncated dialysis throughout the afternoon. Residents overwhelmed supermarkets, stocking up on bottled water, flashlight batteries, and nonperishable food. The facility governing body and core team held meetings to deploy emergency preparedness plans that had heretofore been training drills and exercises. Each patient was given instructions as to what to do regarding their personal safety, the safety and well-being of their families, diet and medication instructions, and phone contacts as to whom to contact regarding dialysis service availability. Patients were advised to stay home if their home was safe and start their fluid, salt, protein, and potassium-restricted diets. They were taught that perishable foods might become toxic without refrigeration. Excess salt intake will result in fluid gains. Patients were educated to keep portable radios, phones, smartphones, and other lines of communication open. If transported to an evacuation shelter, they were advised to let the relief worker know their status—whether they were dialysis patients, had diabetes, and what special medications they would require.

By Sunday, August 27, a solid 24 h of torrential rain arrived in Houston. Along the coast, storm surges were as high as 12 feet. Many of the areas in Houston received as much as 40 inches of rain. One Houston neighborhood, Cedar Bayou, received 51.88 inches of rain, setting the North American record. The consequence was a true paralysis of the city. Emergency services were interrupted despite many people trapped on their homes' rooftops, or second floors. Water levels rose as high as 20 feet in some areas, wiping out houses and vehicles. Many were rescued by neighbors using recreational boats. (See Fig. 21.2). Most streets in Houston had converted to rivers as the two large retention dams overflowed their boundaries. Bayous crested, making many roads impassable. (See Fig. 21.3). The loss of power and standing water further destroyed many homes because of mold and water damage. Thousands of people were suddenly homeless and were relocated to the George R Brown. Convention Center (GRB), which became an emergency shelter.

Fortunately, the flood waters on Almeda, the street adjacent to DMC, quickly receded, and no water entered or damaged the building. Several streets near the

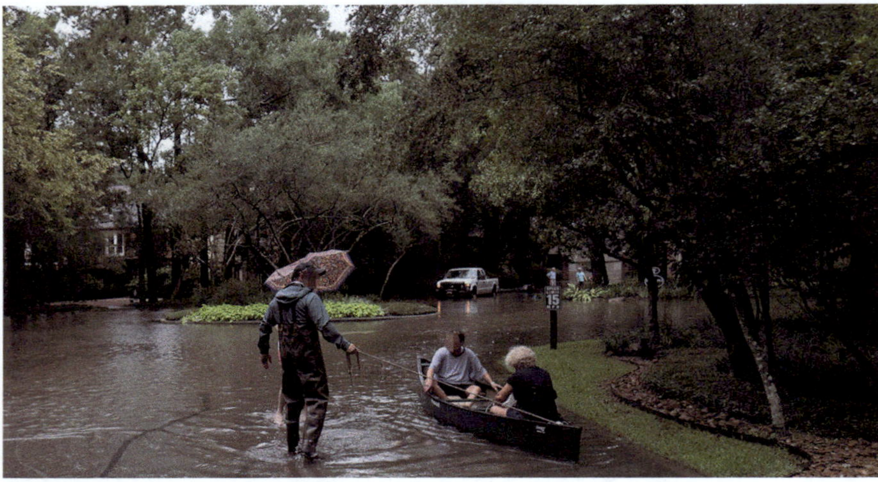

Fig. 21.2 Many Houston residents were rescued by neighbors in a small recreational craft. (Photograph by Stephen Z. Fadem)

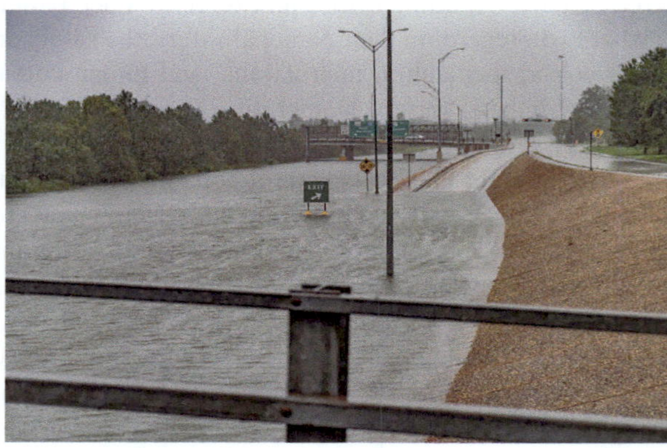

Fig. 21.3 Highway 288 in Houston remained a river after the storm. (Photograph by Stephen Z. Fadem)

facility were also passable. Thus, by Monday, August 29, DMC was quickly designated as a first responder unit. After the biomedical team ensured the structures were safe to support reopening and the emergency power system was deployed, the GRB started transporting busloads of under-dialyzed patients to DMC. Area hospitals and other facilities also redirected patients to DMC.

After the storm passed, the city was left with resultant logistics problems. The dialysis center immediately requested and received emergency pop-up pharmacy services, food, and supply resources. Gasoline at the pump was scarce. (see Fig. 21.4). Gasoline trucks were brought in to ensure that employees had ample fuel to go to and from the facility. Those who lived further away assured their families were safe and stayed in nearby hotels.

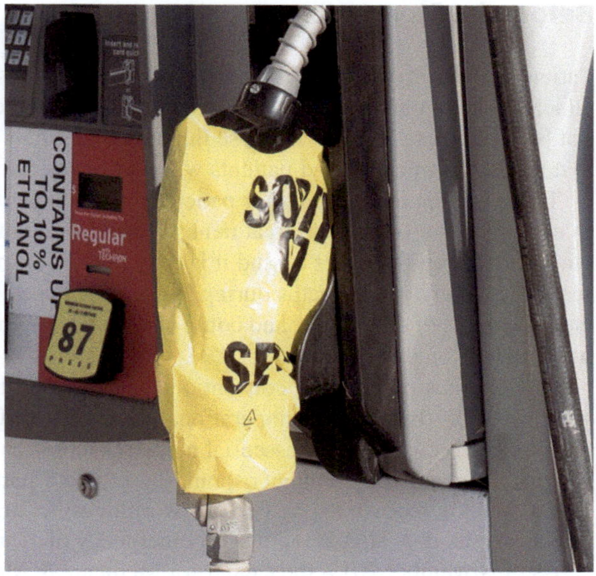

Fig. 21.4 Gasoline became a scarce commodity after the storm. (Photograph by Stephen Z. Fadem)

The medical director's job was to triage each of the 192 additional patients and help prioritize care depending upon need. Those patients who arrived short of breath were dialyzed first. Emergency stat labs were run off the generator to assess potassium levels. Some patients arrived from hospital emergency rooms and received priority treatment. The rest of the patients were managed for 2 h on a first-come, first-served basis. Contact with the primary nephrologist was attempted. Efforts to locate medical records led to suggestions for how electronic information could be handled. By the end of a hectic week, many area facilities had reopened and could resume their load of patients. Other facilities would not reopen for months.

Meanwhile, the governing body of DMC met to discuss continuous quality improvement processes that could improve their emergency preparedness routines. Storm-related disasters are recurrent events in Houston and many other areas. In February 2021, DMC dealt with another storm, this time with freezing weather but no electrical power, icy streets, with frozen pipes, and the loss of municipal water. Staff and patient access were again compromised. Lessons learned from Harvey enabled the team to again serve as a major first responder for our own patients, as well as for other dialysis centers, shelters, and hospitals. Top-level executives at DaVita ordered tanker trucks to fully supply our reserve tanks.

Before the Storm

Patient education is part of the emergency preparedness plan. Patients need to be educated on diet and fluid restrictions. Purchasing salted, nonperishable foods may not be wise because it will increase thirst and fluid gains. Disasters will necessitate that times be truncated, and patients with fluid overload present challenges to care.

There is a natural urgency for patients and dedicated staff to come to the center to either receive or provide treatment. In flood situations, it is often impossible to gauge how deep the water is, and it is easy to drive into roadside shoulders several feet deep. Many of the deaths during Harvey happened because people drove vehicles into areas of deep water and could not escape. Figure 21.3 shows a major highway in Houston during Harvey.

Communication through conventional means may be difficult as cell services will invariably be either nonoperational or overloaded. Patients should receive a hard (printed) copy of their essential medical records and keep them with them in a waterproof plastic bag. Patients should be issued a purple identification band that can be quickly recognized by persons working relief at shelters. This enables their easy triage to an available facility for emergency dialysis.

As of November 2017, the Center for Medicare & Medicaid Services (CMS) has required each dialysis facility which have an emergency preparedness plan. This plan needs to be developed and accepted by the facility's governing body. The governing body consists of the medical director, a regional operations representative, and the facility's administrator. The plan should also include a structured procedure for education, drills and rehearsals, and implementation. The drills are an ideal time to fine-tune and improve the procedures.

To aid in developing and implementing a disaster plan, CMS has prepared an extensive manual on emergency preparedness. https://www.cms.gov/medicare/end-stage-renal-disease/esrdnetworkorganizations/downloads/emergencypreparedness-forfacilities2.pdf.

Once the plan incorporates many potential contingencies and outlines how the deployment will be achieved, once this plan has been fully approved and accepted, it must be taught to the staff so that their roles will be understood. The plan needs to be rehearsed so care during the crisis will be as smooth as possible. These rehearsals and drills are essential and spell the difference between success and chaos. If the disaster is a flood, freeze, or impending hurricane, the team has the luxury of deploying the emergency preparedness plan in advance. This includes confirming that emergency systems for the local municipality have been notified to safeguard priority electrical and water services to the dialysis facility that will be a first responder. The staff leadership contacts local hotels to ensure that accommodation can be made so that patients who live far away have availability.

Large dialysis organizations fully cooperate in disaster management and have high-quality resources available. Patient checklists are available to distribute. They can be obtained through the National Kidney Foundation (http://kidney.org). Each state has a Network that has hotlines. A national emergency website has been established in Tampa, Florida—no stranger to hurricanes, and provides emergency resources. The Nephron Information Center also has resources that are published during hurricane season.

Prior to the storm, the facility reviews potential road closures, employee and patient accessibility, the possibility of power outages, and the potential for water supplies to become contaminated. Arrangements are made with the city or county in advance to ensure that dialysis facilities will receive the highest priority for required electrical power. Breaches in city water sources may require municipalities to add additional chlorine. Extra carbon tanks may be needed.

If the reverse osmosis system does not function, deionized tanks will need to be brought in regularly. If the city water pressure is too low, or if city water is not available, water trucks will be needed. Arrangements for backup water must also be secured in advance. The biomedical department reviews and makes sure inspections are as up-to-date as possible. The staff meets with patients and reviews the accuracy of their contact phone numbers and emergency contacts. The team also ensures that their phone numbers are up-to-date. Each person is advised to confirm that they have an ample supply of charged batteries so that access by smartphone can be continued.

In a city-wide emergency, there will likely be a gasoline shortage at the pump. This was true during the aftermath of Hurricane Harvey for several days. Therefore, the facility also assesses supply and fuel shortages and arranges contingency services for surges in care that will require additional supplies. Since teammates may be required to work long hours and nearby restaurants may be shuttered, food supplies and provisions should also be made. Each employee and patient must receive a curfew letter that can be shown to authorities if stopped after hours in the event of restricted travel.

Freezing weather can be an unexpected disaster, not just for dialysis facilities but for the homes of patients and staff. One essential is to "winterize" pipes by wrapping exterior pipes with pipe sleeves and keeping the water lines open by dripping water through the faucets.

Communication before the storm

- Verify the accuracy of emergency contact numbers for patients and teammates
- Curfew letters for patients and team
- Emergency management system communication—daily updates
- Contact with media for public service announcements on the radio for patients.
- Discuss the emergency plan with the team
- Set up a call to see who is available
- Call suppliers and stock up on anticipated equipment that will be needed during a surge

Each dialysis center should have a special designated "emergency box." This should contain vital patient information about patients, blank emergency forms, schematics of the water and electrical system, the patient census with shifts and critical information, mutual aid agreements, and lists of contacts for essential services—plumber, electrician, water system maintenance, deionization tank supplier, and water truck company. Understandably, dialysis providers will have this vital information available online, but a local disaster might make the internet and web services that are regularly relied on inoperable. Backup "nomad" internet services may be an option, however.

Prior to the storm, it is necessary to hold a governing body meeting to initiate the disaster plan, activate emergency orders, ensure emergency triage forms are ready, and that medical record packets have been distributed to all patients.

During the Storm

After implementing the disaster plan, the team players ensured the safety of their families and themselves. According to the Associated Press, Hurricane Harvey resulted in 122,300 official rescues. The Public Broadcasting System reported that there were 24,000 National Guard Deployed. There were also countless rescues by neighbors who had recreational boats. There were 660,200 claims made to the Federal Emergency Management Administration (FEMA) and 34,500 persons who occupied the major shelters. The American Broadcasting Company (ABC) reported that there were 56,000 emergency 911 calls attempted in the Houston area. From an economic perspective, three million barrels of oil output were lost daily. SOURCE: https://www.weather.gov/crp/hurricane_harvey

After the Storm (from CDC-CMS-FDA)

If the facility was not flooded but lost power, the team checks to determine that the facility is operational and has adequate water flow and pressure. A quick assessment should be made. In cooperation with the Food and Drug Administration (FDA) and CMS, the CDC has published disaster recovery technical considerations at https://www.cdc.gov/disasters/watersystems.html. These directions are for reopening a dialysis facility that has not flooded. The medical director should be familiar with these instructions and play an active role during this critical post-disaster period. The CDC-FDA-CMS technical considerations recommend flushing all pretreatment dialysis equipment to drain for a minimum of 30 min, as stagnant water from the system will need to be removed. The municipal water system will probably have higher than usual levels of chlorine and free chlorine levels of <0.5 ppm (or chloramine level of <0.1 ppm). If the water that is tested after the primary chlorine tank is out of range, the facility protocol for changing the primary carbon tank should be followed.

Once chlorine levels are in the accepted range, the reverse osmosis (RO) machine should be turned on. If possible, the distribution system should be flushed to drain, and the RO and distribution system should be disinfected and rinsed. The cartridge filters will need to be replaced. Note that if the trend of RO quality has worsened, it could indicate damage to the membranes. If total dissolved solids (TDS) are greater than 20% higher than previous readings, deionization (DI) tanks may be needed to polish the water. If municipal water TDS is higher, DI tanks may also be required. An ultrafilter should follow DI to minimize contamination by microbes.

Product water and chlorine testing will need to be performed each hour, and cultures and LAL testing begun immediately and be completed each week. The LAL is the limulus amebocyte lysate test that identifies whether endotoxin is present. LAL should ideally be tested each day during the crisis period.

Water pressure post-disaster may be erratic, and particulate matter in municipal water will probably increase. This calls for more frequent monitoring and backflushing if necessary. When possible, the RO membranes should be cleaned, a sample of product water sent for Association for the Advancement of Medical Instrumentation (AAMI) analysis, and the carbon tanks should be rebedded.

Dialysis machines will also need to be disinfected and rinsed and then tested for residual disinfectant levels to ensure that the rinsing effectively removed all disinfectant. Each machine that does not pass conductivity and self-testing should be taken offline and repaired.

If the dialysis facility is safe to open, appropriate authorities should communicate the role it will play as an emergency dialysis responder.

Boil Water Alert

Safe drinking water availability may be disrupted during a major disaster that affects a large geographic region. If the municipality has issued a "boil water" alert, patients and staff should be notified to avoid drinking any city water and use only bottled water for internal consumption. If water is reprocessed for human consumption, it must meet AAMI standards. Refer to the CDC fact sheet https://www.cdc.gov/healthywater/emergency/drinking/drinking-water-advisories/boil-water-advisory.html.

Infection Control After a Disaster

A severe disaster will displace patients who cannot bathe or carry out ideal hygiene. Many will be in shelters. The opportunity to spread communicable diseases is great. Respiratory infections were present during Katrina and Rita. The use of standard precautions—masking and social distancing—are highly familiar due to the COVID-19 pandemic and should be implemented. Refer to the CDC resource on respiratory hygiene and cough etiquette. https://www.cdc.gov/flu/professionals/infectioncontrol/resphygiene.htm.

The Evacuation Shelter

All persons who arrive in an evacuation shelter should make the relief workers aware of any chronic diseases like heart disease that might require blood thinners, diabetes that might require glucose testing and control, and chronic kidney disease that might require hypertension control and dialysis. Many shelters will have pop-up pharmacies that supply these medications on an as-needed basis to new arrivals, as there is a high probability that home medications will be lost.

Patients arriving in a shelter should immediately sanitize their hands. Many shelters have welcome kits that include small bottles of ethanol sanitizer. Sanitization is necessary before any contact or exchange with another individual. The shelter is an ideal area for norovirus to spread rapidly. Persons arriving at the dialysis center for emergency treatment will need to sanitize their hands and wear a surgical mask immediately.

Persons returning to their homes should be strongly discouraged from wading in flood waters. There were several cases of Vibrio vulnificus reported after Katrina.

If the Dialysis Unit Is Unsafe

If the facility is unsafe, patients will need to be rerouted to a first responder facility where emergency dialysis can be performed. Until the facility is considered safe, only emergency workers and rescuers should be allowed to enter the site until it has been checked by a structural engineer. Broken glass, water on the floor, active power lines, gas leaks, uneven concrete floors, damaged walls, "x" shaped cracks at the base of walls, and fallen roof sections are potential safety hazards that must be cleared. Entry into an unsafe area in a hotel was a cause of a fatal event during Hurricane Harvey (https://www.hotel-online.com/press_releases/release/missing-omni-spa-managers-body-found-at-hotel-after-flood/). Mold can also be a hazard; it takes 48 h for it to grow (https://www.cdc.gov/mmwr/volumes/68/wr/mm6821a1.htm).

If the Dialysis Unit Is Safe

Patients arriving at the facility are checked in and evaluated. This is ideally done in a quiet and private space adjacent to the lobby. If the patients bring their medical records, these are reviewed, and when possible, the primary nephrologist is notified. It is crucial to know what special needs must be met, the hepatitis status, the last date of dialysis, estimated dry weight, and dialysis prescription. Dialysis will need to be rationed, so patients must be reminded to remain on a survival diet. The facility medical director will review and approve all orders unless the primary nephrologist also has privileges at the first responder facility.

Arriving patients will be stressed, and some handle stress poorly. Staff should be trained to handle upset and frustrated patients and diffuse situations that could potentially become disruptive. The facility should have security on the premises. Staff should never transport patients, and emergency transportation services should be established in advance, taking into consideration road closures and flood conditions. Transportation must not be overlooked in planning. FEMA, city, and county cooperation are essential. One should not rely on emergency medical services to transport patients to or from the dialysis facility.

Emergency dialysis orders must be approved by the medical director or designate. It is ideal for a physician to be located on the premises and personally be involved with the triage of patients. Each dialysis machine must be set up with the same safety standards practiced routinely, and universal precautions must be maintained. The minimum dialysis time is 2 h at a maximum blood flow. Heparin dosing may vary. The specifics of the bath will vary but should be established by the medical director. They also resupplied the facility. During Harvey, DaVita established a pop-up pharmacy for essential pharmaceuticals as many patients lost all their possessions, including their medications.

Working long hours as first responders and providing care during stressful conditions is taxing to staff. The break room and lounge should be stocked with food and refreshments and offer an environment where staff can take a stretch break, rest, and take a nap. Stressful environments may be charged with excitement that wears off within a short time. Complacency and mistakes can occur during this let-down period, and the team needs to be re-engaged. Job rotation is often helpful.

The team needs to be aware of family issues. Education on emergency preparedness must be extended so that staff can ensure their families are safe and provided for. If there are concerns about the home situation, it will be difficult to secure adequate staffing. Several employees must care for children, pets, persons with special needs, and elderly relatives. Their personal obligations need to be considered. Ample backup staff is necessary. The dialysis providers can assist in providing relief nurses and technicians from units that have been damaged so that the first responder facility can remain operational until the others can reopen.

During a patient surge, housekeeping services will be required more frequently. It is essential that the area always appear clean and not chaotic.

Conclusion

Although this chapter highlighted experiences with a specific disaster, most natural disasters have much in common. They may interrupt services, interfere with the physical plant operations, and block access of patients and employees to the facility. Many facilities will be damaged during a disaster, and nearby facilities must be prepared to respond. This scenario is not dialysis facility or company-specific.

Preparation is key to successfully managing a catastrophe. The team must be organized and play out scenarios that can happen in advance. It is essential to pay attention to little details. A small factor can create havoc when a heavy load of ill patients depending on services are at the doorstep, and power and transportation are challenged.

After a crisis has passed, the team should meet and appraise how each specific event was managed. Hurricanes and other unforeseen weather events tend to recur. Appraising the situation and improving the facility's response are part of the dynamic that makes for a successful outcome [1–9].

References

1. Vora NM, Grober A, Goodwin BP, Davis MS, McGee C, Luckhaupt SE, et al. Challenges of service coordination for evacuees of Hurricane Maria through the National Disaster Medical System. J Emerg Manag. 2018;16(3):203–6. https://doi.org/10.5055/jem.2018.0369.
2. Sugisawa H, Shimizu Y, Kumagai T, Sugisaki H, Ohira S, Shinoda T. Earthquake preparedness among Japanese hemodialysis patients in prefectures heavily damaged by the 2011 great East Japan earthquake. Ther Apher Dial. 2017;21(4):334–44. https://doi.org/10.1111/1744-9987.12542.
3. Nihonyanagi R, Tsukasaki K, Itatani T, Nakai H, Toda D. Factors related to preparedness for emergency hemodialysis in the event of a natural disaster. Medicine (Baltimore). 2022;101(24):e29288. https://doi.org/10.1097/md.0000000000029288.
4. Morsch G, Chacko S, Randolph R. Disaster medicine: disaster preparedness planning. FP Essent. 2019;487:23–6.
5. Malik S, Lee DC, Doran KM, Grudzen CR, Worthing J, Portelli I, et al. Vulnerability of older adults in disasters: emergency department utilization by geriatric patients after Hurricane Sandy. Disaster Med Public Health Prep. 2018;12(2):184–93. https://doi.org/10.1017/dmp.2017.44.
6. Lempert KD, Kopp JB. Renal failure patients in disasters. Disaster Med Public Health Prep. 2019;13(4):782–90. https://doi.org/10.1017/dmp.2018.142.
7. Lee DC, Gupta VK, Carr BG, Malik S, Ferguson B, Wall SP, et al. Acute post-disaster medical needs of patients with diabetes: emergency department use in New York City by diabetic adults after Hurricane Sandy. BMJ Open Diabetes Res Care. 2016;4(1):e000248. https://doi.org/10.1136/bmjdrc-2016-000248.
8. Lameire N, Sever MS, Van Biesen W, Vanholder R. Role of the International and National Renal Organizations in natural disasters: strategies for renal rescue. Semin Nephrol. 2020;40(4):393–407. https://doi.org/10.1016/j.semnephrol.2020.06.007.
9. Atef-Zafarmand A, Fadem S. Disaster nephrology: medical perspective. Adv Ren Replace Ther. 2003;10(2):104–16. https://doi.org/10.1053/jarr.2003.50015.

Dialysis Safety

22

Stephen Z. Fadem and Brendan Bowman

Introduction

Although dialysis was first described in the 1850s, it was not until 1944 that the first dialysis was effectively performed [1]. This followed a series of deaths and was a trial-and-error endeavor. Along the way, modifications to the procedure resulting in stronger safeguards have been further developed, paralleling technology improvements. Yet, preventable errors that may result in harm to patients persist [2].

In the Institute of Medicine's landmark report, To Err is Human, safety was defined as "freedom from accidental injury," and medical errors were defined as " the failure of a planned action to be completed as intended or the use of a wrong plan to achieve an aim" [3]. The World Health Organization (WHO) defines patient safety as the "prevention of errors and adverse effects to patients associated with health care" [4]. Simplified patient safety is the pursuit of eliminating preventable errors that result in patient harm.

In the dialysis context, errors can be functionally grouped and include the administration of medications, fidelity to the dialysis prescription, and lack of adherence to infection-control techniques. Errors in setting up and maintaining the dialysis water system, mixing solutions, and setting up the dialysis machine also occur. Lastly, errors can occur with respect to dealing with patient-specific issues related to a new onset infection, coagulation, arteriovenous or catheter access, or

S. Z. Fadem (✉)
Section of Nephrology, Department of Medicine, Baylor College of Medicine, Houston, TX, USA
e-mail: fadem@bcm.edu

B. Bowman
DaVita Kidney Care, Denver, CO, USA

Division of Nephrology, Department of Medicine, University of Virginia School of Medicine, Charlottesville, VA, USA

S. Z. Fadem et al. (eds.), *Complications in Dialysis*,
https://doi.org/10.1007/978-3-031-44557-6_22

identifying the potential for a patient fall. These and others have occurred frequently enough that dialysis companies, inspectors, and organizations such as the Association for the Advancement of Medical Instrumentation (AAMI) and the Centers for Disease Control and Prevention (CDC) have developed guidelines and conditions for preventing them [5].

In dealing with complications of care, one must consider the event in context. Dialysis treatments are performed on a population of patients that are often older, have numerous comorbidities, and have little functional reserve. To avoid many of the complications described throughout this book requires vigilance, the ability to adapt, and adherence to policies. Despite the best efforts of caregivers, errors will occur, and strategies are designed to limit them from becoming sentinel events (an error resulting in death, permanent harm, or severe temporary harm) [6]. Most of the time, an error itself does not result in harm; it is when there is a compilation of errors that we have what James Reason has referred to as the Swiss Cheese model [7]. In this model, multiple barriers of protection (staff vigilance, machine alarms, policies, and procedures) fail concurrently, leading to a safety event. To help prevent errors from resulting in such catastrophes, dialysis governance implements quality assurance and performance improvement efforts (QAPI) that require individual dialysis governing bodies, under the leadership of their medical directors, to identify their weaknesses and develop, implement, and review adaptive strategic plans to mitigate consequences [8].

What Patients Expect

Each patient arrives at the dialysis facility with the expectation that the facility will be clean, warm, and welcoming. They expect their facility to be adequately staffed with qualified personnel, to start and end their therapy on time, and most importantly, a safe and effective treatment free of complications delivered in an environment that fosters satisfaction and trust. Dialysis is labor-intensive, and employees are constantly being trained and onboarded. Their supervision should be based on meeting the three expectations of safety, effectiveness, and respect. Controlling labor costs are essential for delivering cost-effective care in an environment where healthcare expenses are burgeoning and reimbursement is fixed. Thus, there is always a challenge to deliver care that meets the expectation and needs of patients in a way that is efficient. Errors are not just dangerous and threatening to the well-being of patients but are also costly to providers and the healthcare system. In addition to financial costs, there are psychological costs to the care team involved in the error where patient harm results. The longitudinal nature of outpatient dialysis therapy often fosters close bonds between dialysis staff and patients making patient harm events a "double hit"—affecting both patient and clinical staff [9].

Conditions for Coverage

In 2009, the Centers for Medicare and Medicaid Service (CMS) developed a series of rules that dictated the requirements that would become known as the Conditions for Coverage (CfC) [8]. These were the results of several rounds of comments and meetings by multidisciplinary technical expert panels. These conditions covered patient's rights, infection control, the physical plant, training and education of new personnel, the dialysate delivery system and maintenance of dialysis machines, and how both safety and clinical outcomes would be maintained and encouraged. They put a great deal of responsibility and accountability on the medical director—required to be a qualified and experienced nephrologist familiar with the dialysis procedure. A companion document used by Medicare surveyors, the ESRD Interpretive Guidance, notes that the QAPI process must track and investigate safety errors and events related to both patients and staff members [10]. Sourced from the Renal Physicians Association and the Forum of ESRD Networks, the "top five" safety focus areas are listed as:

- Hand hygiene
- Patient falls
- Incorrect dialyzer or dialysate
- Medication errors
- Non-adherence to unit policies or procedures, such as missing weights, blood pressure, and shortened treatments

While these are important areas of concern, they represent a limited view of potential sources of patient harm. Modern medical directors require a holistic view of safety that contemplates errors not just within the dialysis facility but in the interaction of the facility with the external environment.

How Decisions for Care Are Made

Returning to the IOM's report on patient safety, errors can be categorized as follows: errors of execution—the correct action does not proceed as intended; or, errors in planning—the original intended action is not correct. Errors in planning occur in the course of medical decision-making while errors of execution may occur within rule-based care or rote care if sufficient safeguards do not exist [3].

(a) Critical thinking—Decision-making that does not have a definite answer and care that must be achieved through accurate and complete information, reasoning skill, and experience.
(b) Rule-based care—Following procedures and adhering to policies. This takes training and understanding. Misapplying a rule can result in a hazard.
(c) Rote care—The setting up of a machine, passing out medications, wearing gloves during treatment, and then sanitizing hands are all automatic functions.

These safety breaches occur because the employee forgot or had a lapse in memory, slipped up and intended to do the right task, but either delivered it to the wrong person, or used the wrong technique, or intended errors that resulted from the employee feeling rushed and hurrying through the task.

Typical Hemodialysis Treatment

The delivery of the dialysis procedure, from when patients arrive in the facility to when they are picked up to go home, is the coordinated and multidisciplinary efforts of several individuals. Directly involved in the patient's care and management is the nephrologist and perhaps a nurse practitioner or physician assistant. The patient is visited on a regular basis, and the prescription is reviewed in the context of how the patient is responding to care. Patients new to the facility are assessed and evaluated at onset, at 30 days, and yearly [8]. An integrated team conference held monthly involves a social worker, registered nurse, dietitian, and nephrologist. Decisions regarding the patient require critical thinking and the combined experiences and observations of the entire team. The prescription that is developed or modified is then ready for implementation.

Rule-based care considers that dialysis is routine and entails several connected tasks. This care generally involves technicians who review water log records under the supervision of the nurse to ensure that the dialysate is free of chlorine. Biomedical teams assure the water system is operating appropriately, that conductivity will be within range, and that water pressure and flow are adequate. Potable water that is fed in from the city undergoes softening with brine to remove calcium and other minerals. Chlorine is removed when the water is passed over carbon in large tanks. Next, the water is sent to the reverse osmosis system that, through a series of interactions, forces out minerals and other toxins. At the chairside, the machine is set up by the technician, who then must guarantee that several steps have been implemented to ensure that conductivity is in range, that filters to prevent infection are placed, and that air is not present in the lines. They must set the flow rates and the pressure variables. They also assess the arteriovenous (AV) access for bruits and thrills that could indicate stenosis or any signs of infection or wall weakness that could represent a potential for rupture. If the patient has a catheter, the nurse must look for any sign of infection at the exit site. The AV site is cannulated following a strict set of procedures that ensure an infection will be prevented, that good needle flow is established, and that the needles are taped securely in place. The patient is generally anticoagulated during dialysis treatment.

Much of the care that occurs during this phase is routine. Personnel must follow care guidelines that they have learned and practiced repeatedly. These procedures are so routine that it is possible to forget a step or perform a step incorrectly. A common mistake is to not properly wear gloves or sanitize the hands when removing them. While skipping steps such as this may save time, they facilitate infection. The flow rate, arterial and venous pressure, air detection, and conductivity are constantly monitored during the procedure.

During the procedure, the dialysis prescription is followed to remove an adequate amount of fluid so that the patient achieves a dry weight, maintains blood pressure, and avoids cramps or hypotension. The blood flow, time on treatment and dialyzer size, and permeability coefficient determine how adequate dialysis will be. The staff must ensure that the access and the patient's head are never covered. This is because any change in the patient's clinical status or vascular state must be handled immediately to prevent a catastrophe. The patient is reassessed every 30 min; the blood pressure is taken and the machine settings are reviewed.

When the dialysis procedure ends, the patient is safely disconnected from the machine. The dialysis needles are removed, and the site is held until any sign of bleeding has stopped. After the treatment, the patient may be weak and unsteady, and the team must use judgment in how much assistance to offer when transporting to the scales and back to ensure a fall does not occur. When ready to return home, the patient may need assistance while waiting for transportation. How much assistance to provide is based on whether the patient is a fall risk. If there is a risk that the patient is going to fall, then assistance is necessary.

Error Prevention and Facility Safety Infrastructure

As the prior section illustrates, a safe dialysis treatment requires close coordination and cooperation of a large number of healthcare team members and the patient. Error prevention begins well in advance of the occurrence of any actual error. Ideally, a clinic possesses processes to allow for error intake, evaluation, and dissemination of any safety lessons learned. In addition, standing policies and procedures should be written with error reduction in mind and be periodically updated to benefit from safety lessons acquired in the course of patient care. The landmark Institute of Medicine report "To Err is Human" [3] noted the necessity of dedicated safety systems and the importance of providing legal protection and privilege to facilitate honest discussions of errors and address necessary improvements. The Conditions for Coverage (CfC) 8 -required the Quality Assurance and Performance Improvement (QAPI process) may serve a dual purpose as a home for safety-related work and traditional quality improvement (QI), or a facility may find that a separate safety forum is necessary. Regardless, safety information must be tracked and reported within the QAPI process, even if the analysis occurs outside.

At a minimum, the safety infrastructure at a dialysis clinic should include:

- A dedicated safety event/medical error reporting system optimized to capture dialysis care events
- A culture of safety, ideally led by the medical director, that encourages and allows safety concerns to be raised by any member of the dialysis team and addressed by leadership
- A standard methodology for the investigation of safety events/medical errors leading to the identification of root causes and mitigation actions
- A dedicated process for disseminating and implementing safety learnings

In addition to the above, error prevention is greatly facilitated by the use of standardized protocols and tools. These can be especially important in preventing errors due to communication—for example, during handoffs of care between unit personnel or when a patient is moving between different venues of care—whether from a dialysis unit to a skilled nursing facility or a back to the facility following an inpatient stay. Some examples of error prevention tools include:

- **S**ituation-**B**ackground-**A**ssessment-**R**ecommendation (SBAR)
- **C**oncern-**U**ncomfortable-un**S**afe-**S**top (CUSS)
- Safety Huddles
- **S**top-**T**hink-**A**ct-**R**eview (STAR)

Situation-Background-Assessment-Recommendation (SBAR)

The SBAR tool was originally devised to facilitate structured information exchange between personnel operating in high-risk environments in the U.S. Navy [11]. In the early 2000s, it was adapted to formalize information sharing with a focus on nurse-to-physician communication [12]. Since then, SBAR has been widely adopted in a range of clinical environments, often as part of QI and safety initiatives. The Institute for Healthcare Improvement (IHI) and many other healthcare quality organizations provide templates and examples of implementations in various clinical scenarios. The tool requires the initiating clinician (physician, nurse, technician, etc.) to provide a concise summary of a clinical issue, relevant background, a clinical assessment, and a recommended action. While initially used for urgent clinical communication, SBAR can be adapted for non-urgent issues and even administrative communication. For example, a clinic administrator can easily utilize the SBAR format to inform executives of supply or staffing shortages. While the SBAR technique is likely the best-known standardized communication protocol in health care, evidence of effect remains limited [13].

Concern-Uncomfortable-unSafe (CUS)

Errors may arise when communication is restricted within teams composed of individuals of varying levels of perceived authority or rank. In some organizational cultures, individuals may find it challenging to question those of a higher perceived rank within the group. This idea is akin to the "Power-distance" concept from Hofstede that describes differences in hierarchy behavior between countries [14]. Many examples exist in healthcare: a nurse that does not question a physician's inappropriate order; a medical trainee that does not share misgivings around a supervising attending's diagnosis. The CUS method has been developed to provide a framework for assertive communication. As shared by the Agency for Healthcare Research & Quality, each letter in CUSS represents a keyword used to escalate patient safety issues [15]:

- I am **concerned**
- I am **uncomfortable**
- This is a **safety** issue

Some use the phrase "I am **scared"** for the first S; Others have added a second S to CUSS—"We need to **stop**" to the original CUS concept as a further escalation phrase. Regardless, empowering frontline staff to share safety concerns with a communication framework like CUS can be a useful tool to overcome perceived barriers and improve a facility's culture of safety.

Safety Huddles

While no standardized definition of safety huddles exists, in general, safety huddles are brief (10—15 min) meetings of healthcare team members designed to enhance communication and collaboration around patient care [16]. Huddles have been implemented in a number of different clinical environments, though are part of safety and process improvement efforts [17]. The VA's Center for Healthcare Organization and Implementation Research reviewed 158 healthcare huddle studies and found nearly a quarter reported improvements in patient safety—most notably medication errors [18]. Huddles allow for two-way communication from the huddle leader, often a charge nurse, and the healthcare team members. For example, the dissemination of topical and important safety issues—think of unexpected supply chain shortages or updates to a critical facility policy, can be shared at the huddle. Staff members may, in turn, share concerns about a specific piece of equipment or changes in the medical status of a patient. Due to the fast-paced nature of a dialysis clinic, safety huddles must be efficient and focused while still encouraging participation. Structured communication protocols or agendas can help improve the effectiveness of huddles. Facilities may choose a daily huddle model following a first shift put on or multiple brief huddles on the treatment floor with each patient shift.

Stop Think Act Review (STAR)

Medical decision-making during procedures may be adversely affected by frequent interruptions and high levels of stress on staff members [19]. This scenario frequently plays out in the dialysis unit where a nurse or patient care technician may be attempting to multitask due to time pressures. Medication administration, addressing machine alarms, and addressing a change in patient status may all occur concurrently. To reduce the likelihood of errors occurring in high-stress situations, tools like STAR—Stop-Think-Act-Review—encourage a brief pause to reflect on a procedure or order about to be performed. Other tools besides STAR exist but operate similarly. Other checklist-based measures ensure medications are administered properly—the right drug at the right dose to the right patient at the right time.

Employing methods such as STAR provide a check on the urge to multitask and resulting attention loss to the task at hand.

Error Intake, Analysis, and Change

With approximately 480,000 patients on in-center hemodialysis in the U.S., nearly 70,000,000 treatments will take place in the course of a year [20]. Unsurprisingly, errors will occur. Most of these errors will not result in a patient or staff harm event, but a small percentage will, with some becoming serious adverse events or sentinel events. A medical director of a single facility rarely encounters serious harmful events, but when they occur, a framework for analyzing and implementing change is important. Not all events are suitable for a systems-based error approach and adverse events that are due to a healthcare member exercising extraordinarily poor judgment or flagrant negligence should be dealt with via existing human resources channels. Most errors are systems-based in nature and candidates for a systems-based analytic approach.

Immediate Actions

At the time a serious safety event occurs or is identified, a rapid assessment and action plan may be necessary to ensure no additional events occur in the short term and the facility is safe to continue to operate. For example, a patient fall precipitated by unnoticed moisture on the treatment floor must be assessed and remedied to prevent any additional injury. A similar assessment must be made in the case of improperly mixed dialysate. A medication administration error may require a different immediate assessment. Ad hoc safety huddles can be useful to clarify roles and assign tasks in such scenarios and medical directors must be informed and participate in initial error finding. In addition, perishable data from the event—data that is not captured by other systems and will be critical to future error analysis, should be recorded. Once a facility is deemed safe to continue operating, the particulars of the event should be recorded in the organization's safety event reporting system mentioned earlier. Depending on the severity of the event and plans for immediate changes, a governing body may be necessary.

Error Analysis

There are any number of methods, systems, and associated tools to identify contributory causes for medical errors. Optimal error analysis starts with the premise that errors have multiple causes and rarely a single point of failure. As such, an error analysis must contemplate multiple contributory factors. The Root Cause Analysis and Action (RCAA or RCA^2) framework is a method of analyzing patient errors followed by implementing and sustaining change [21]. While the name suggests a single "root" cause for an error, it is a misnomer in that contributory factors from many categories are analyzed: staff, policies and procedures, physical environment, patient factors, communication, etc. The RCA^2 approach specifically avoids blaming individuals and reviews errors from a systemic approach. Root cause analysis has been criticized in the past for challenges in leading to sustained systemic change [22]. The "action" component of the RCA^2 seeks to avoid the lack of follow-through in improvements that can plague the traditional RCA process and places emphasis on system improvement. Nonetheless, root cause analysis is specifically noted in Medicare's ESRD Interpretive Guidance as an expected component of error analysis [10].

A variety of tools from various safety methodologies may be used in the analysis phase of the RCA^2. A detailed listing of such tools is beyond the scope of this chapter, but frequently used components include Cause and Effect (Ishikawa/Fishbone) diagrams and Toyota's A3 analysis (so named because identified problems and solutions should fit on a single A3-sized page, 11.7 × 16.5 inches)—components of IHI's Model for Improvement and Learn, respectively. [23, 24]. While such activities are occurring, with much work done outside the formal QAPI process, medical directors should keep a facility's governing body apprised of status and findings. Additional analysis activities may involve staff interviews and a review of relevant policies and procedures. A strong safety culture in a facility will improve the likelihood of frank responses from all healthcare team members.

Implementing and Sustaining Change

Once the analysis phase is complete, developing recommendations for change to prevent future safety errors should follow. The VA's National Center for Patient Safety developed the Action Hierarchy to grade the relative strength of an intervention and the likelihood of preventing a future patient safety event [25]. The system grades interventions from Stronger to Intermediate to Weakest. Often, weaker interventions, like re-training, are the easiest to implement, while strong interventions requiring engineering or physical plant changes may be the most difficult. Strong interventions may also implement "forcing functions," which remove the ability to make the same error by ensuring a process follows the intended path. Removal of high-concentration heparin from a facility is one example. Interventions should also emphasize the standardization of processes or tools to eliminate variability a staff member encounters in the clinical environment. For example, multiple different types of dialysis machines in a single facility lead to confusion and increased cognitive load on cross-trained staff. Each RCA^2 should recommend an action plan that balances the ability to implement with a high likelihood of success.

Once specific action plans are settled, these should be presented to the Governing Body for adoption and subsequent monitoring. Ongoing monitoring can be challenging when assessing for rare safety events. For example, a dislodged fistula needle leading to hemorrhage and patient death is a rare event requiring an RCA^2. However, an action plan that calls for the reduction of deaths due to venous dislodgement does not represent a realistic plan as this scenario is rare and unlikely to be assessed at regular intervals. However, a plan that monitors for improvement in contributing factors like poor needle-taping techniques after access cannulation is likely more effective. Facility audits may expand from monthly hand hygiene to also include AVF taping policy adherence. A stronger action plan would be an engineering solution that shuts down a blood pump when dislodgement is detected (See Chap. 17). The RCA^2 team will be responsible for balancing efficacy and pragmatism in the final action plan.

Advocating for System Wide Change

In the modern era, dialysis facilities are not typically stand-alone entities but are often part of a larger dialysis entity where clinics may number <10 or over 2000. Regardless, the RCA^2 process of one facility is likely to benefit other clinics. A high-performing dialysis organization should seek to collate learnings from facility-level analyses and disseminate these learnings for the benefit of other clinics which may be faced with similar circumstances. As action plans are identified, these learnings must inform the development of new policies which incorporate lessons learned so that they may be disseminated across an entire organization. In this way, a facility's experience may contribute to an organization-wide safety collaboration.

Conclusion

Despite decades of advancement, providing dialysis care is a complex process that requires well-trained staff focused on the task at hand, strong policies and procedures, reliable equipment, and correct dialysis prescriptions. The sheer complexity of such an environment offers multiple pathways for errors to occur—some of which will result in patient harm. The CfCs require facilities to track, trend, and study safety errors as part of the overall QAPI process. As a complement to trend analysis, root cause analysis and action can be used to study the multifactorial nature of errors occurring in the dialysis unit. This avoids traditional, ineffective person-based blame and, when properly implemented, leads to stronger error prevention in the facility in the future. By sharing safety learnings between facilities, lessons can be disseminated and safety culture reinforced across an entire organization.

References

1. Kolff WJ, Berk HT, ter Welle M, van der Ley AJ, van Dijk EC, van Noordwijk J. The artificial kidney: a dialyser with a great area. 1944. J Am Soc Nephrol. 1997;8(12):1959–65. https://doi.org/10.1681/ASN.V8121959. PMID: 9402100.

2. Kliger AS. Maintaining safety in the dialysis facility. Clin J Am Soc Nephrol. 2015;10(4):688–95. https://doi.org/10.2215/CJN.08960914. Epub 2014 Nov 6. PMID: 25376767; PMCID: PMC4386259.
3. Institute of Medicine (US) Committee on Quality of Health Care in America. To Err is Human: Building a Safer Health System. Kohn LT, Corrigan JM, Donaldson MS, editors. Washington (DC): National Academies Press (US); 2000. PMID: 25077248.
4. World Health Organization Europe. Patient safety. https://www.who.int/europe/health-topics/patient-safety#.
5. Lindberg C, Downham G, Buscell P, Jones E, Peterson P, Krebs V. Embracing collaboration: a novel strategy for reducing bloodstream infections in outpatient hemodialysis centers. Am J Infect Control. 2013;41(6):513–9. https://doi.org/10.1016/j.ajic.2012.07.015. Epub 2012 Dec 7. PMID: 23219669.
6. The Joint Commission. Sentinel event (SE). https://www.jointcommission.org/-/media/tjc/documents/resources/patient-safety-topics/sentinel-event/camncc_20_se_all_current.pdf.
7. Reason J. Human error: models and management. BMJ. 2000;320(7237):768–70. https://doi.org/10.1136/bmj.320.7237.768. PMID: 10720363; PMCID: PMC1117770.
8. Department of Health and Human Services, Centers for Medicare and Medicaid Services: 42 CFR Parts 405, 410, 413 et al. Medicare and Medicaid Programs. Conditions for coverage for end-stage renal disease facilities; final rule. Fed Regis. 200873:20370–2-484. https://www.cms.gov/regulations-and-guidance/legislation/cfcsandcops/downloads/esrdfinalrule0415.pdf.
9. Edrees H, Connors C, Paine L, Norvell M, Taylor H, Wu AW. Implementing the RISE second victim support programme at the Johns Hopkins Hospital: a case study. BMJ Open. 2016;6(9):e011708. https://doi.org/10.1136/bmjopen-2016-011708. PMID: 27694486; PMCID: PMC5051469.
10. Center for Medicaid and State Operations/Survey and Certification Group: ESRD interpretive guidance update, Ref: S&C-09-01. Baltimore: Department of Health and Human Services, Centers for Medicare and Medicaid Services, 2008.
11. SBAR (SITUATION, BACKGROUND, ASSESSMENT, RECOMMENDATION). American Society for Quality. https://asq.org/quality-resources/sbar#:~:text=SBAR%20was%20introduced%20by%20the,improve%20safety%20is%20well%20documented.
12. SBAR tool: situation-background-assessment-recommendation. Institute for Healthcare Improvement. Cambridge. https://www.ihi.org/resources/Pages/Tools/SBARToolkit.aspx.
13. Müller M, Jürgens J, Redaèlli M, Klingberg K, Hautz WE, Stock S. Impact of the communication and patient hand-off tool SBAR on patient safety: a systematic review. BMJ Open. 2018;8(8):e022202. https://doi.org/10.1136/bmjopen-2018-022202. PMID: 30139905; PMCID: PMC6112409.
14. Hofstede G. Culture's consequences: comparing values, behaviors, institutions, and organizations across nations. Thousand Oaks: Sage Publications; 2001.
15. CUS tool—Improving communication and teamwork in the surgical environment module. https://www.ahrq.gov/hai/tools/ambulatory-surgery/sections/implementation/training-tools/cus-tool.html.
16. Huddles. Institute for Healthcare Improvement. Boston. https://www.ihi.org/resources/Pages/Tools/Huddles.aspx.
17. Scoville R, Little K, Rakover J, Luther K, Mate K. Sustaining improvement. IHI white paper. Cambridge: Institute for Healthcare Improvement; 2016. ihi.org.
18. Pimentel CB, Snow AL, Carnes SL, Shah NR, Loup JR, Vallejo-Luces TM, Madrigal C, Hartmann CW. Huddles and their effectiveness at the frontlines of clinical care: a scoping review. J Gen Intern Med. 2021;36(9):2772–83.
19. Bower R, Jackson C, Manning JC. Interruptions and medication administration in critical care. Nurs Crit Care. 2015;20(4):183–95. https://doi.org/10.1111/nicc.12185. PMID: 26084432.
20. United States Renal Data System. 2022 USRDS annual data report: epidemiology of kidney disease in the United States. Bethesda: National Institutes of Health, National Institute of Diabetes and Digestive and Kidney Diseases; 2022.

21. National Patient Safety Foundation. RCA2: improving root cause analyses and actions to prevent harm. Boston: National Patient Safety Foundation; 2015.
22. Peerally MF, Carr S, Waring J, Dixon-Woods M. The problem with root cause analysis. BMJ Qual Saf. 2017;26(5):417–22. https://doi.org/10.1136/bmjqs-2016-005511. Epub 2016 Jun 23. PMID: 27340202; PMCID: PMC5530340.
23. Cause and effect diagram. Institute for Healthcare Improvement. Boston. https://www.ihi.org/resources/Pages/Tools/CauseandEffectDiagram.aspx.
24. Myers JS, Kin JM, Billi JE, Burke KG, Harrison RV. Development and validation of an A3 problem-solving assessment tool and self-instructional package for teachers of quality improvement in healthcare. BMJ Qual Saf. 2022;31(4):287–96. https://doi.org/10.1136/bmjqs-2020-012105. Epub 2021 Mar 26. PMID: 33771908.
25. Guide to performing a root cause analysis (Revision 02/05/2021). Published by VHA National Center for Patient Safety (NCPS). https://www.patientsafety.va.gov/docs/RCA-Guidebook_02052021.pdf.

Index

S. Z. Fadem et al. (eds.), *Complications in Dialysis*,
https://doi.org/10.1007/978-3-031-44557-6

MIX
Papier aus verantwortungsvollen Quellen
Paper from responsible sources
FSC® C105338

If you have any concerns about our products,
you can contact us on
ProductSafety@springernature.com

In case Publisher is established outside the EU,
the EU authorized representative is:
Springer Nature Customer Service Center GmbH
Europaplatz 3, 69115 Heidelberg, Germany

Printed by Libri Plureos GmbH
in Hamburg, Germany